Resounding Praise for

Weathering

The
EXTRAORDINARY STRESS
of ORDINARY LIFE *in an*
UNJUST SOCIETY

"Arline Geronimus brings together a lifetime of research, scholarship, and experience to explain how continually battling back oppression hurts the human body. Her book offers an eloquent, comprehensive, and compassionate framework for understanding the physiological effects of societal harm and a path to healing."
— Linda Villarosa, author of *Under the Skin*

"Impassioned and persuasive, this is an essential call for change."
— *Publishers Weekly*

"Arline T. Geronimus, PhD, draws on her research to shine a light on what it means to age as a Black person in the United States."
— Kenrya Rankin, *Essence*

"Dr. Geronimus has published more than 130 papers, expanding and bolstering the evidence for weathering well beyond Black mothers... That body of evidence has turned her into an 'icon' and provided a framework for understanding health inequities that goes deeper than blaming poor health on lifestyle choices or flawed genetics."
— Alisha Haridasani Gupta, *New York Times*

"Superbly insightful. If this unique volume did nothing else, I would recommend *Weathering* as *the* book on health care disparities. But it also distills and delivers its scholarship and insight in engaging narratives, including compelling personal histories so that you will glean your education in racial health disparities—and how to end them—quite painlessly. In fact, reading *Weathering*, with its clear-eyed mixture of reality and hope, is a delight."

—Harriet A. Washington, author of
A Terrible Thing to Waste and *Medical Apartheid*

"The power of Geronimus's project remains the attempt to provide a conceptual framework for patterns that medical institutions, in their convenient recourse to individual failings, have yet to fully recognize." —Lauren Michele Jackson, *The New Yorker*

"One of the most significant public health research discoveries of the last few decades is this: when it comes to health and aging, how society treats us has more of an impact than how we take care of ourselves. In this monumental book, Arline T. Geronimus meticulously demonstrates that systemic injustice isn't just oppressive—it's toxic on the body; it's deadly."

—Ibram X. Kendi, National Book Award–winning
author of *Stamped from the Beginning*

"Crisp, backed with evidence, and rather heroic in spirit."

—Farrah Jarral, *The Guardian*

"As I learn more about the complexity of chronic diseases, and the reasons Black people who grew up like I did endure them more often than others, it provides me a peace of mind I didn't know was possible. This book brings clarity where I've long had confusion. No doubt, it will influence the broader discussion about health and race in this country on a macro and policy level. But more than that, it will be invaluable to folks who've faced anything like I did since I was a child."   —Issac J. Bailey, author of *Why Didn't We Riot?*

"A compelling contribution to the literature on the important issue of health care inequity."   —*Kirkus Reviews*

"In trying to understand the causes of group disparities in health outcomes, analysts have focused on features of the disadvantaged groups themselves—their genes, culture, income level, etc.—at the expense of environmental factors. *Weathering* corrects this bias. Better than any writing I've seen, it shows how the environments of the disenfranchised have a weathering impact on their health and longevity. Well written and accessible, it is a powerful book; indispensable to developing policies capable of reducing these disparities. And, more generally, it is a must-read for anyone interested in the nature of identity in American life. In short, it deserves the very broadest of readerships."
                         —Claude M. Steele, author of *Whistling Vivaldi*

Weathering

The
EXTRAORDINARY STRESS
of **ORDINARY LIFE** *in an*
UNJUST SOCIETY

Arline T. Geronimus

BACK BAY BOOKS
Little, Brown and Company
New York Boston London

Little, Brown Spark
Hachette Book Group
1290 Avenue of the Americas, New York, NY 10104
littlebrownspark.com

Originally published in hardcover by Little, Brown Spark, March 2023
First trade paperback edition, January 2024

Little, Brown Spark is an imprint of Little, Brown and Company, a division of Hachette Book Group, Inc. The Little, Brown Spark name and logo are trademarks of Hachette Book Group, Inc.

The publisher is not responsible for websites (or their content) that are not owned by the publisher.

The Hachette Speakers Bureau provides a wide range of authors for speaking events. To find out more, go to hachettespeakersbureau.com or email hachettespeakers@hbgusa.com.

Little, Brown and Company books may be purchased in bulk for business, educational, or promotional use. For information, please contact your local bookseller or the Hachette Book Group Special Markets Department at special.markets@hbgusa.com.

ISBN 978-0-31625-797-8 (hc) / 978-0-316-25807-4 (pb)

LCCN is available at the Library of Congress

Printing 1, 2023

LSC-C

Printed in the United States of America

Some names and identifying information have been changed to protect confidentiality.

Dedicated to the Balabostas, Sojourners, Hill Women,
Mentshes, and John Henrys,
including my grandparents,
Joseph and Anna Palejev Geronimus; and
Isadore and Annie Zarkin Moldveen
and my parents,
Lippman H. Geronimus and Miriam Moldveen Geronimus
Along with their indomitable counterparts among racialized, oppressed,
exiled, marginalized and exploited peoples worldwide.

Contents

Part II

The Way Forward

Weathering

Introduction

In August 1985, the US Department of Health and Human Services (HHS) published an eight-volume report detailing the stunning consistency and magnitude of what they referred to as "racial disparities in health" across a long and varied list of health outcomes, including cardiovascular disease, cancer, diabetes, low birth weight, and infant mortality. In the foreword, the Secretary of HHS at the time, Margaret M. Heckler, stated that its findings should "mark the beginning of the end of the health disparity that has, for so long, cast a shadow on the otherwise splendid American track record of ever improving health."[1] The year the report came out, overall life expectancy was 69.3 for Black Americans, 75.3 for white.[2]

In an effort to improve this "track record," HHS made reducing and eliminating racial inequities in health a high-priority national public health objective, and it reiterated this priority in the decennial *Healthy People* reports it published in 1990, 2000, 2010, and 2020, each of which set public health objectives for the subsequent decade.[3] The objectives set for 2010 were bolder than those set for 2000, and those set for 2020 were bolder than those for 2010—though none of the 2000 or the 2010 goals had been met. Not even close. In fact, despite many efforts and good intentions, racial health inequities in the United States remain as entrenched and pernicious today as they were in previous decades, and some have grown even larger since the Heckler report appeared in 1985.

The report consisted of statistics about health disparities and suggestions for potential avenues of research into the causes. The statistics compared rates of morbidity and mortality for non-Hispanic white, non-Hispanic Black, Hispanic, American Indian or Alaska Native, and Asian or Pacific Islander people—these being the basic racial/ethnic groupings the Office of Management and Budget required federal agencies to keep statistics on. Much of the report and subsequent political and scientific discussion was focused on Black Americans, because the health disparities between Black and white Americans were particularly and consistently large. The recommendations offered, however, are revealing, as they reflected the dominant thinking about possible explanations for Black/white disparities: There may be a genetic basis. There may be cultural influences. There may be differences in socioeconomic status and access to quality medical care. The primary recommendation of the report concerned improving individual health behaviors by expanding health education to minoritized individuals. The introduction to the first recommendation read:

> The disparity in the death rate between nonminority and minority populations in the United States (Blacks, Hispanics, Asian/Pacific Islanders, and Native Americans) is a compelling reason to investigate how health education can contribute toward reducing this disparity. Because many of the identified behavioral and environmental risk factors associated with the causes of excess deaths among minorities can be controlled, more work is needed to educate minority populations about the risk factors.[4]

By the 1980s, as a country, we had become focused on the role of unhealthy behaviors like smoking, consuming a high-fat or high-cholesterol diet, and living increasingly sedentary lifestyles as the causes of the kinds of chronic diseases—like cancer and cardiovascular disease—that account for the largest share of excess deaths in Black Americans compared to white. So it may have seemed a no-brainer to attribute bad health to the same behavioral causes. This conclusion led to a profusion of educational behavioral change interventions designed to disseminate information about the causes of poor health, and a prodigious market for self-help groups and publications. Eventually it led to more structural understandings of the barriers many Black Americans face when they try to maintain a healthy lifestyle. Such barriers include low incomes, lack of locally available healthy foods or safe exercise spaces, and the influence of targeted marketing for unhealthy products, particularly cigarettes and alcohol, ubiquitous in disinvested racially segregated neighborhoods.[5]

And then there was the blame narrative, sometimes dignified as the "personal responsibility" narrative. Those most invested in the blame game opined that Black Americans simply chose not to eat or exercise properly; that they didn't make the effort to become healthy. In their eyes, the fact that Black Americans exhibited worse health than Hispanic Americans in many outcomes—another finding of the report—ruled out societal causes. After all, both groups are disproportionally poor and subject to racial discrimination.

As for what could be done? Those who believed that the shorter life expectancy of Black Americans had a genetic basis suggested that perhaps there wasn't anything that could change that outcome. And for those who embraced the blame narrative, if Black Americans' shorter life expectancy was due to their eating fast food, drinking sugary sodas, and not exercising, well, there might be a role for health information campaigns, but not for anything more systematic or regulatory. In the eyes of those who took this view, it was hard to claim injustice if white Americans *earned* their health through personal restraint while Black Americans were dying from the effects of their own choices. This narrative weakened the political will necessary to support spending tax dollars to promote Black American health. Many thought to do *that* would be the injustice.

Many experts and public health professionals rightly rejected these blameworthy speculations as unscientific, even racist. But questions about why these health inequities occurred and what to do about them persisted, even if they were largely neglected by the mainstream. It was hard to make people in power care deeply about a difference of six years in life expectancy when both Black and white Americans were living well into their sixties and seventies. Moreover, large numbers of people weren't even aware of the Black/white health gap to begin with. Despite the Heckler report and a raft of subsequent literature on this health inequity, as recently as 2009 a national public-opinion survey found that fewer than half of American adults knew it existed.[6]

Fewer still grasped the full magnitude of these inequities, or their profound implications for the communities that suffer most from them, because average life expectancy, while certainly an important metric, is limited in what it can tell us about the health of the most marginalized communities. For example, while the difference in average life expectancy between Black and white Americans comes down to a relatively small number of years in old age, differences of decades separate the healthy life expectancies of Black youth in high-poverty neighborhoods like Central Harlem, the Watts area of Los Angeles, Chicago's South Side, or Eastside Detroit and their white counterparts in wealthier neighborhoods in the same metropolitan areas.

If, like many, you find yourself protesting that these decades-long differences are driven by homicides, AIDS, and drug overdose deaths—all of which can conveniently fall into the blame narrative—what if you found out that they were primarily accounted for by death from chronic diseases? What if you knew that these chronic diseases—including cardiovascular disease and cancer—were killing Black people starting at much younger ages than any amount of unhealthy behavior could account for? What if you knew that the excess deaths among Black residents of Central Harlem were largest not among the youth—too often viewed as irresponsible at best, predatory at worst—but instead among working-class adults in their thirties, forties, and fifties? Moreover, what if you knew that white Americans in high-poverty rural communities, such as in Appalachia, also face unconscionably high levels of early death and disability, also due largely to chronic disease? Yes, the much-publicized opioid epidemic plays a role in Appalachia, as do mining accidents. But chronic disease is the biggest killer by far. And these health inequities between Appalachia and the rest of the country predate the opioid epeidemic. So what's going on here?

My interest in this subject, and my early realization that the conventional theories and speculations had questionable basis in fact, stems from the research I began doing in college and graduate school. Just months before the release of the Heckler report, I received my doctorate in public health. My dissertation and first publications focused on differences in infant mortality rates, which were much higher for Black Americans than for white Americans—as they still are. I was interested in the impact of the mother's age on these mortality rates.

The conventional wisdom at the time—which is still widely believed—held that the Black/white infant mortality gap was importantly driven by Black women giving birth at too early an age, before they have achieved full reproductive or psychosocial maturity. The specter of the "teen mother" loomed over many social problems in the public mind in the 1980s through the mid-1990s. At that time, thirty to forty years ago, about 45 percent of Black first-time mothers gave birth in their teen years, a rate dramatically higher than the roughly 18 percent of white American mothers whose first births occurred in their teen years.[7] So, in the absence of a granular examination of the statistics, it was assumed that the prevalence of teen motherhood was a central explanation for the large Black/white infant mortality gap.

This idea dovetailed with the personal-responsibility narrative. If only young Black women would stop engaging in their (erroneously presumed) reckless and unseemly sexual behavior, and if only their parents would provide them with adequate supervision and moral education, they would avoid teen pregnancy, and infant mortality rates would plummet. From there, it followed that the government and nonprofit agencies should launch a public health education program that discouraged teen births. Several decades of such programming did indeed coincide with a great reduction in the incidence of teen motherhood. Now, only about 16 percent of first-time mothers in the Black community are teenagers, and rates among white teens have fallen too, to less than 7 percent.[8]

And how has that affected infant health? Not as hoped. There has been no commensurate reduction in infant mortality inequities. In fact, the absolute rates of babies born with very low birth weights have increased, while the infant mortality rate for Black mothers remains roughly twice that for white mothers.[9]

What I found in my own research completely contradicted the conventional thinking about the causes of infant mortality in Black women. For Black women, giving birth during the teen years, in particular during the late teen years (which was when most such births occurred), led to *healthier* infant outcomes than giving birth later. Black teens were at the lowest risk of having their babies die, while Black women in their twenties through early thirties incurred higher risks. This is certainly not an argument in favor of encouraging teen births. It is instead an argument for trying to get to the bottom of why the babies of older Black women are more at risk. And it's not just their babies that are at risk. It's the women themselves, for the maternal mortality rates of Black women rise with age and are far higher than those of white women, a phenomenon I will discuss in depth later in this book.

As I continued my research trying to understand why the risks of infant death went up, not down, as Black mothers aged through their twenties and early thirties, I started to assemble statistics about other Black/white health inequities that were much more alarming than those reflected in the Heckler report. And none of the common-sense speculations about what caused them were consistent with my growing findings.

In a study we published in the *New England Journal of Medicine*, my research team found that the number of Black youths living in disinvested high-poverty areas who could expect to live long enough to celebrate their forty-fifth birthday was smaller than the number of white youths nationwide who could expect to live to old age. This shocking disparity was attributable not to guns or needles but, much more importantly, to chronic disease. In subsequent research, we found the odds of a young Black person in a high-poverty area (or their white Appalachian counterpart) reaching age fifty alive and able-bodied was a mere 50 percent; the vast majority of US white youth can expect to both survive and be able-bodied at fifty, with decades of healthy life ahead of them. In the disinvested high-poverty Black and white locales we studied, we found that those who hadn't died by middle age spent as much as 30 percent of their lives disabled.[10]

These findings demand an explanation. Why are these young people so vulnerable to the depredations of chronic disease and disability? Research I've conducted over the past few decades, along with that of many others,[11] refutes or complicates the conventional speculations about the underlying causes. How can entrenched Black/white health inequities be largely due to genetics if there are pockets of impoverished white Americans in the country whose health is as bad as that of impoverished Black Americans? If Black people with college educations have worse health than white people who never completed high school, how can we attribute racial inequities in health to lower socioeconomic position or educational achievement? Can we really call it unequivocally irresponsible to bear your first baby before age twenty if your baby will be less likely to die in infancy than if you wait even just a few years?

How can unhealthy behaviors be the primary driver of inequity in deaths from chronic disease that become apparent as early as the twenties and thirties, if it takes decades for the effects of unhealthy diet, sedentary lifestyle, smoking, and alcohol and drug abuse to progress to end-stage disease? In fact, Black Americans start to smoke and drink at later ages than white Americans. Study after study has found that individual behavioral patterns play at best only a small part in accounting for excess deaths in marginalized populations.

This is not to suggest that it wouldn't be a good idea to improve the access of all populations to healthy lifestyle opportunities— parks and other green spaces where we can walk and exercise safely, food markets and farmers markets where we can buy healthy fruits and vegetables, etc., instead of the overpriced, low-quality offerings available in the food deserts where so many low-income Black people live. These are things that much of white America takes for granted. But making such environmental improvements in Black communities will not move the needle as far as one might hope if we continue to embed these improvements in a framework of blame and personal responsibility.

To understand what accounts for America's stark health inequities across racial and class lines, we must move beyond the conventional explanations. Our preoccupation with genetics, individual health behavior, and personal responsibility have blocked our view of other possibilities. So, unlike the drunk who looks for his keys under the lamppost because that's where the light is, we must ask ourselves if there are more promising places we should be looking for our answers.

I know there are.

After almost forty years of research in public health and a lifetime of wrestling with questions of racial and class injustice, I have concluded that a process I call *weathering*, a process that encompasses the physiological effects of living in marginalized communities that bear the brunt of racial, ethnic, religious, and class discrimination, is critical to understanding and eliminating population health inequity. Weathering afflicts human bodies—all the way down to the cellular level—as they grow, develop, and age in a racist, classist society. Weathering is not measured in number of steps walked, cigarettes smoked, opioids used, alcohol drunk, or calories eaten. It's not primarily measured by your years of education, the size of your paycheck, or your bank balance. It's not essentially about emotional despair, either. Weathering is about hopeful, hardworking, responsible, skilled, and resilient people dying from the physical toll of constant stress on their bodies, paying with their health because they live in a rigged, degrading, and exploitative system.

Weathering has dynamic physiological and psychosocial dimensions. The physiological dimensions are often activated by the psychosocial ones. As a shorthand, in the book I will often call the sum of these dimensions *biopsychosocial*. And I will explain that our colossal failure to achieve anything resembling health equity is the inevitable by-product of our general lack of understanding of this fact: Race is not rooted in any meaningful biological categories. Race is a biological fiction, an *invention* that keeps some people, those deemed by those in power to fall on the "wrong" side of an arbitrary color line (or a religious, class, ethnic, gender, sexual-orientation, or gender-identity line), in their place. If we limit our ideas to reigning folk notions about race, we will never truly get to the roots of the problem, and such discovery is a prerequisite to promoting health equity.

To understand weathering, we must first understand the power differentials and psychosocial dynamics between the *dominant culture* and *marginalized cultures* in our multicultural society. The practices, values, language, and common sense of a dominant group in a multicultural society are deemed to be the authoritative knowledge in a society—the knowledge that counts, irrespective of whether it is universally or empirically true.[12] The authoritative line in the US is to deny the existence of class and to be conflicted about diversity.

This imposition of values and practices is maintained systematically by power historically derived through might and hubris, and maintained by institutional control and greater economic resources of the dominant group.

Racialization is a powerful means by which the dominant culture sets groups apart as more or less deserving of, or entitled to, resources, esteem, or power; or, instead, as worthy of contempt, punishment, deprivation, stigma, oppression, and exploitation. The distinction between a *racialized group* and a *race* is fundamental to weathering. It is not what we call race, per se, that impacts health—being Black, for example, does not mean being inherently vulnerable to poor health. Rather, it is society's *racialization* of certain groups as being essentially "irresponsible," "inferior," "deficient," "naturally suited to harmful occupations," "insensitive to physical pain," and "threatening"—a classification scheme in which both dominant and marginal groups are fluent—that damages their health.

To racialize is to create a social identity based on a group's common superficial physical characteristics, ancestry, or national origin. Such groups are composed of people who may or may not primarily identify themselves with that classification, and who could just as easily have been sorted into different groups based on other characteristics. (Similar distinctions, such as those of gender or sexual identification, exist within racialized groups; and there are also intersectional differences in status, authority, and social-role expectations, such as differences in lived experience between white women and Black women.)[13] Once identified, a racialized group can be portrayed in terms that naturalize their oppression, exploitation, and exclusion. Through this same classification system, members of more-powerful groups are viewed as superior, responsible, and deserving. This pervasive social dynamic of superiority and inferiority, power and oppression, sets differently racialized groups on diverging health trajectories, leading to shorter or longer life expectancies. Reorienting our understanding of, and approach to, health inequity, so as to include the weathering implications of active and sustained racialization, is essential if we are to realize Secretary Heckler's now widely shared ambition to end the health disparity.

In the United States, the concept of race most often brings to mind Blackness or whiteness; and racism is often synonymous with anti-Black bias, which is particularly persistent and pernicious in America. But racialization is fluid. Early adverse racialization of Native Americans and Mexicans facilitated land grabs, genocide, and the forceful separation of Native American children from their families when the children were sent to abusive boarding schools. The explicit intent of this kidnapping was to obliterate tribal culture and children's meaningful social connections with members of their families and tribes. This practice, euphemistically portrayed as "civilizing" native youth (whose tribes had been racialized as "savages" since Columbus arrived in the fifteenth century), began in the mid-seventeenth century and continued into the twentieth century. Many Native people subjected to these boarding schools are alive today and remain traumatized.

Adverse racialization of Japanese Americans was intensified during World War II to the point where the US government felt justified in ordering them to internment camps. Here, too, many Japanese Americans who spent their formative years in these camps are alive today.

Chinese immigrants who were mercilessly racialized, exploited, and excluded throughout the nineteenth century and into the early twentieth were heralded as a "model minority" by the dawn of the twenty-first century.[14] Despite this partial reprieve, once COVID-19 was venomously misnamed "the China Virus," all Asian-origin people in the United States were targeted for violent hate crimes by some non-Asian Americans.[15] The spike in hate and suspicion of Muslims after September 11, 2001, is another palpable example of nearly instant racialization.[16]

Even Blackness and whiteness are fluid. Historically, the demographic groups welcomed under the umbrella of whiteness have evolved over time, which tells us much about how arbitrary their boundaries are. For example, Irish, Italian, and Eastern European Jewish immigrants to the United States in the early to mid-twentieth century were classified toward, and sometimes *on*, the "Black" side of the binary. It is equally well known that these groups were effectively reclassified toward the "white" side of the binary starting around the 1950s.

And in a Northwestern European Protestant white supremacist culture, the adverse racialization and exploitation of some groups of Northwestern European Protestant origin as "white trash" or "hillbillies" is more proof that race is a fiction. This conflation of class distinctions with race distinctions couldn't happen if race were a biological truth, but it can and does happen. What has not been fluid, however, is the systemic anti-Black racism that has remained a reality throughout US history, although its manifestations and legality have changed, and in some ways substantially improved, over the last century.[17]

Many scholars, writers, and activists have addressed the material, educational, legal, political, and environmental injustices caused by systemic racism. In this book, I seek to add an important piece of the puzzle to this public conversation, a truth to which I have dedicated my career: that the ideologies that sustain racialization and other forms of cultural oppression—racism, classism, sexism, ageism, xenophobia, homophobia—have real, measurable consequences for health, above and beyond the economic and educational inequities they create that segregate people into well-resourced or disinvested and environmentally toxic neighborhoods.

My research shows that pervasive racist and classist ideologies activate biological processes that wear out the physical and mental health of people of color *across all economic classes*, if to different degrees. In a particularly perverse irony, Black people who have achieved a measure of socioeconomic security or upward mobility—those who most actively counter the concrete threats of racism to their well-being and live in sync with core American values of "working hard and playing by the rules"—face unique assaults on their health. Weathering explains how and why racial inequities in health persist across class lines. In my research, I have studied the health profiles of white, Black, and Latinx groups who have suffered, or are actively suffering, under various forms of racialization-related or class oppression. With a weathering framework we can see how the marginalization of, for example, impoverished Appalachian white Americans and urban Black Americans are simultaneously linked and distinct.

Each of us is the product of the time and place in which we grew up. For me, the neon lights of ethnic and racial discrimination—and questions about who belongs where and when and why—have been flashing in my eyes all my life. As the grandchildren of Eastern European immigrants who fled genocidal pogroms, my sisters and I were named for family members who had been slaughtered in Europe, either by Russian Cossacks or later by German Nazis. Growing up in the greater Boston area, I had first-generation Irish-American classmates whose parents still spoke of the "Irish need not apply" statements punctuating the help-wanted signs they saw in shop windows during their youth. I also had classmates who were proud Daughters of the American Revolution, and who departed our public school for elite private day or boarding schools by seventh grade.

The civil rights movement absorbed my youth. I was close in age to Ruby Bridges when she walked into the otherwise all-white William Frantz Elementary School. I watched her on TV as she did so, small and alone, yet quiet and dignified, flanked by several federal agents to protect her from the angry shouting mob who surrounded her. I watched Bull Connor sic large dogs and fire hoses on Black children. The specter of death always lingered—the deaths of my extended family in Europe, the loss and trauma my living relatives personified, the assassination of a president and of a presidential hopeful, the murder of civil rights leaders and peaceful protesters, state-orchestrated bombings of the homes of Black activists, the nightly death counts of American soldiers, the much higher ones of Vietnamese, and, in my own home, my mother's early death from cancer when I was still a child.

Because of my positioning in my family, neighborhood, and the country, and the historical moment in which I grew up, I have focused my research largely on the weathering consequences of the US Black/white binary, of class distinctions shaped by poverty, working-class employment, and affluence, and of the subjection of immigrants to xenophobia; and, of course, on the intersections among these and with gender. These are not the only social identity groups that experience weathering. And while the specific contours of the weathering I have studied are clearly American, biological weathering can and does happen in culturally unequal multicultural societies across the globe. I highlight these facts to explain why specific marginalized groups are emphasized in this book, and also to clarify that weathering is a human process that pertains to any oppressed, marginalized, or exploited group.

Given their varied personal origins, current students of weathering are extending its application to other marginalized groups. For example, in ongoing work with students and younger colleagues, we are finding evidence of the cumulative toll transgender Americans are paying with their health as they navigate a society and institutions that were neither made for nor are welcoming of the LGBTQ+ community—a toll that in the United States appears largest for Black trans feminine and nonbinary people assigned male at birth.[18] Whatever your community, if the idea of weathering resonates with you, please see this book as an open door to consider its application to other populations and settings.

I am neither a historian nor a cultural anthropologist. As

someone who was raised to take pride in coming from a family of working-class, Eastern European Jewish immigrants, I've made use of stories from my youth and from my parents' and my grandparents' time to demonstrate the ways that racialization can shift over time. When Eastern European Jews first migrated to this country, escaping persecution and pogroms, they were looked down upon not just by the Protestant mainstream but by the Jews from Western Europe who had preceded them in coming here. I remember well how this affected my forebears and even, ultimately, myself. My personal stories are written from lived experience.

I also write from decades of experience researching and teaching in public health. But science—in any area, but especially in subjects related to the fiction of biological race—is at least as fraught as it is illuminating. And science at the nexus of race, culture, and biology is arguably the most dangerous of all. I am keenly aware of the complications involved in casting a scientific eye on the fundamentally moral problems of social justice, compassion, and social change. Certainly, all interpretations remain my own. As a scientist, I welcome sincere critique, debate, and the testing of alternative hypotheses. But false facts about race and health have been culturally unfalsifiable for too long.

There is a popular truism: If you always do what you've always done, you'll always get what you always got. If we are committed to health equity, it's long past time to admit the inadequacy of conventional approaches and take our efforts in new, evidence-based directions. In our system, unearned benefits for some and undue burdens for others will be the rule until we all see and reject certain core American myths and racist ideology. I offer the fruits of my labor, as a constant gardener in the field of health equity research, in hopes that my perspective can help spark new narratives and new understandings that will pave the way to new paths toward achieving health equity.

Part I

The Erasure, the Erosion, and the Withstanding

We have always been told that we have to suffer as Christ suffered; but I think in terms of what David had to do. David was a shepherd boy, but there did come a time in his life where he had to slay Goliath.

—Fannie Lou Hamer[1]

Every day in America, a broad swath of people see their chances for a long, active life diminished in the crucible of racialized social identity. The accidents of birth that assign us to either a socially valued or a marginalized and looked-down-upon group can impact life expectancy, not just through the obvious economic determinants but through the slow drip of stealth ideas about race and personal responsibility. Some of our most cherished beliefs as a culture activate or intensify these harms.

There are inescapable consequences of marginalized social identity. Whether members of a socially identified group are valued, welcomed, affirmed, and able to live their lives in culturally meaningful ways or are, instead, "othered" or exploited by dominant groups, is critical for their physical well-being, their rate of aging, and their life expectancy.

In members of groups that are othered and demeaned, who must struggle for validation or success against strong headwinds, a set of physiological pathways are chronically activated that can lead to cardiovascular disease, cancer, accelerated aging, weakened immune systems, and other life-threatening vulnerabilities. The triggers of these physiological processes are social and dynamic, even while they occur in individual bodies.

Thus, weathering is a stress-related biological process that leaves identifiable groups of Americans vulnerable to dying or suffering chronic disease and disability long before they are chronologically old. Through weathering, members of marginalized populations age prematurely, no matter how well they follow the social contract, the American Creed, or the latest dispatches from the front lines of healthy behavioral science. Sometimes *because* they do.

I chose to name this process *weathering* because the word is a contronym, that is, a word with opposite meanings. Weathering can describe deterioration and erosion, as in "that rock has been weathered by geological processes over millions of years," but also signal strength and endurance, as in "the family weathered the recession very well." With regard to health and aging, it can and does signify both, because, against all odds and in defiance of all the stereotypes and allegations about their sinister motivations, deficient capabilities, and dysfunctional family life, marginalized groups create networks of caring people, encompassing both extended family and friends, who do everything they can to support one another. In the absence of any government safety net, these networks help them weather the storms created by the society they live in.

In Part One, I elaborate on the societal sources and biological mechanisms of the physiological erosion that is weathering. Racial classifications and hierarchy are initially imposed by the dominant culture, even as great heterogeneity among individuals exists within any marginalized group. Still, once branded as members of this or that "race" or "class," people within marginalized groups do, indeed, share linked fates. For better or worse, the impacts of this derogatory branding are harmful to everything from their health to their income, their schooling to their job opportunities, where they live to how the justice system treats them. And when marginalized groups are defined as essentially monolithic and lesser, their individual identities—not just their autonomous identification as part of a cohesive group—are erased or demeaned in dominant narratives. Toward affirmation and survival, their now materially linked fates require them to forge and invest in collective strategies for social and economic support and personal and cultural affirmation as they express an abiding hope and determination to withstand, survive, and overcome their oppression.

In a cruel, if mundane, twist of biological fate, those among the devalued who engage in sustained acts meant to cope with and withstand racism, classism, or other ideological vectors of group marginalization often find that the sheer exertion required for the (inequitable) rewards they receive for even heroic exertion, and the indignities they still face as they make these good faith efforts, also contribute to their weathering. Further, as dominant cultural narratives erase or distort and stigmatize their efforts, those well-meaning members of dominant groups who are moved to address injustice arrive all too often at ineffectual or even damaging policy approaches, which at best may have some mitigating effects on weathering, but can also exacerbate it. In this section of the book, I will describe examples of these cruel social structures, the human biological processes they activate, and the conditions under which they have long-term health-damaging—weathering—effects.

1.

Is Working Hard and Playing by the Rules the Cure for What Ails Us?

Anyone who survived the spring of 2020—and many didn't—came face-to-face with a reality too many Americans have been familiar with for centuries, but which the more powerful among us have been able to ignore. Death is unfair. It comes sooner than it should to some, and it is no accident that those who die early are disproportionately people of color, members of the working class, and other marginalized groups.

In the spring of 2020 we were first introduced to COVID-19, a new, deadly virus that caused the worst pandemic in a hundred years. In the US, one million lives were lost to COVID in its first two years, and many of the people hardest hit were those we call essential workers—not just those in the health-care and medical professions, who were, of course, on the front lines, but the public-facing workers who keep our world functioning. And they, in turn, are disproportionately working class and people of color—like Jason Hargrove, a Black bus driver from Detroit. On April 2, 2020, after Mr. Hargrove died from COVID-19, Detroit's mayor, Mike Duggan, gave him a hero's send-off, telling reporters, "He knew his life was being put in jeopardy—even though he was going to work for the citizens of Detroit every day; and now he's gone."[1]

Let's spare a moment to find out a little something about Jason

Hargrove. We can look at his Facebook profile, which shows a photograph of him on his bus, wearing a face mask, and a hat with the Detroit Public Transportation logo. He surrounded the photo with hashtags: #CoronaVirus, #ICannotStayHome, and #I'mOnTheRoad4U—clear indicators of his fear about the danger he was facing just by doing his job, of knowing that he had no other option but to go out on the road every day and put himself in harm's way, and finally of his sense that his job was a public service.[2] On March 21, 2020, less than two weeks before he would die of COVID-19, Mr. Hargrove posted a video of himself on Facebook in which he described an unmasked passenger on his bus who had coughed repeatedly without covering her mouth.[3]

> We out here as public workers, doing our job, trying to make an honest living to take care of our families. But for you to get on the bus, and stand on the bus, and cough several times without covering up your mouth, and you know that we in the middle of a pandemic, that lets me know that some folks don't care.... This is real. I'm out here. We out here. We moving the city around back and forth, trying to do our jobs and be professional about what we do.

Although he expresses both his anger and his fear in the video, he makes it clear that he voiced none of that until after the woman and the other passengers left the bus.

> There's folks dying from this. And I am trying to be the professional they want me to be and I kept my mouth closed.

Having let us know that he did not in any way threaten or even admonish this woman, he also addresses his wife to reassure her that when he comes home, he will take off his uniform, put it in the wash, and take a shower before interacting with her or their kids, so that he can protect them from the threats he himself faces every day.

Having established that he is an honest, hard-working, responsible family man doing his best while keeping his mouth closed in the face of a woman who put him and his passengers at risk, Mr. Hargrove pleads:

But some point in time we need to draw the line.

For Jason Hargrove, that time has passed. Four days after making his video, he was diagnosed with COVID-19. A week later he was dead. While there is little mystery to how he was exposed to the virus, we have to ask ourselves why a fifty-year-old man, who took every precaution he could, died so quickly from it. Or at all.

That he was turned away at the hospital when he became symptomatic on March 25 couldn't have helped (though it is all too typical of the way Black people who seek medical attention are treated), but it's probably not the only reason he died, because at that point in the pandemic we did not have effective treatments or cures for the disease, so admission to the hospital might not have saved him.

I believe the answer to the question of why he succumbed so rapidly lies in the reality of day-to-day life for a hardworking, working-class Black man with a family. And we can see evidence of the stressors he constantly faced. In the video clip, the burden he so evidently carried, of having to prove both his worthiness and his self-restraint before voicing a reasonable grievance about someone coughing on him, is painful to see. He appears accustomed to the necessity of ensuring that he wouldn't be perceived as threatening or impulsive, no doubt because he lived in a systemically racist society where Black men in cities like Detroit are often reduced to stereotypes that can get them killed by police officers and other "law-abiding" citizens. Think about George Floyd, who died less than two months after Jason Hargrove, murdered by a police officer who kept his knee on Floyd's neck for nine minutes and thirty seconds while Floyd, surrounded by three police officers and in no way a threat to them, repeated "I can't breathe" twenty-eight times and then called for his deceased mama.

In the context of a society where Black, working-class men can never expect to be given the benefit of the doubt by their fellow citizens, it is easy to imagine that Mr. Hargrove intended his video to be self-protective and, indeed, strategic. Like most Black Americans, he was likely primed to be in a continuous state of vigilance about how others perceived him, and he managed his social identity in public accordingly.

But there is a physical price to be paid for that kind of sustained vigilance, for always having to tamp down reasonable anger, and you might even see it on the video as he repeatedly wipes his brow and opens his sweater to cool off while talking about what happened on the bus that day. These signs of anxiety can indicate that his physiological stress response—a series of physical reactions to stress whose effects on the body I will describe in the next chapter—is in overdrive. This was probably far from the first time he experienced such stress arousal in the course of his job, or even just walking the streets of Detroit. Navigating negative racial and stereotypic presumptions is exhausting. And it is damaging. It is part of the phenomenon of weathering.

Like Jason Hargrove, each of us, through a broad range of social classifications, becomes a gendered, racially defined actor in a cultural narrative that shapes our socioeconomic class, life, and health in countless and consequential ways. This narrative frees some of us to work remotely during a pandemic, or to voice our grievance if we are coughed on without first having to prove ourselves worthy and unthreatening. It consigns others of us to the repeated and sustained psychological and physical pressures that undermine our health and contribute to weathering.

Weathering

No matter how hard Black Americans like Jason Hargrove work, or how carefully they play by the rules, their bodies, like those of other poor, working-class, or culturally sidelined people, are subjected to weathering.

Weathering results from repeated or sustained activation of the physiological stress response over years and eventually decades. This means that a person's health and life expectancy depend more on their experiences, their interactions with others, and the physical environment they live in than on their DNA signature or lifestyle. For the more affluent members of marginalized groups, the housing, education, healthy food, and health care their money can buy might reduce or mitigate the harmful impacts of weathering, but they cannot eliminate them. Some specific triggers of accelerated aging processes are more likely to be activated in oppressed people when they find themselves in relatively advantaged settings, like colleges, suburban neighborhoods, and professional workplaces that are predominantly white, often historically designed to exclude Black Americans, and rarely designed with their needs in mind.

Hearing the stories of working-class Black people like Jason Hargrove, and learning the stark fact that Black Americans are more than twice as likely to die of the virus as whites, a broad swath of the American public was forced to take notice of something they had ignored until then.

Of course racism's clearest assault on Black bodies was demonstrated by the drumbeat of killings of innocent young Black men and women, including the murder of George Floyd in May 2020. In response, Black Lives Matter protests surged across the country, attracting many who had previously dismissed the group's concerns. In June 2020, polling showed 76 percent of Americans—including 71 percent of white people—called racism and discrimination "a big problem" in the United States, a 26 percent increase from five years earlier. The majority polled also said that the anger of Black Lives Matters demonstrators across the country was fully justified.[4]

Black Anger. Fully Justified. For the first time in decades, many acknowledged the wretched reality of structural racism—the way historical practices, entrenched dominant cultural beliefs, conventional wisdom, and "common sense" have allowed social and economic privileges to be cumulatively awarded to groups categorized as white, while denying or undermining opportunities, resources, and human dignity to Black people. (Disturbingly, few of the forty-four murders of trans women in 2020, nor the close to sixty in 2021—a record high number, who themselves were mostly women of color—were publicized to solicit outrage or empathy, indicating another way death is unfair.)[5]

Still, by summer 2020 a broad consensus of Americans agreed that dismantling anti-Black racism was urgent. Can this broad-based "road to Damascus moment" be harnessed to realize a global community that advances the justice for which it calls? Or will people soon forget, or, perhaps worse, decide that the proliferation of inadequate, underfinanced, ill-thought-out policy recommendations that often follow such moments—and that don't challenge the political economy that rationalizes class inequity through race fiction—will suffice to remedy all the problems?

Age-Washing

There is reason to worry that even the most well-meaning among us may be primed for the latter outcome. This is because in matters of life, death, and health, we have been age-washed. Age-washing is a term I have developed to describe a way of thinking that ignores the role of structural racism or classism and cultural oppression in the weathering of marginalized people's bodies by locating its causes elsewhere. We in the West tend to believe that there is a universally uniform growth and aging process and that, barring premature death from an acute virulent infection, a genetically linked disease, or an accident, everyone will have a long healthy life—*provided* they make disciplined, doctor-sanctioned, health-promoting choices regarding diet, exercise, and lifestyle. This view of growth and aging assumes that if we take personal responsibility and play by the rules of good health and good citizenship, our age will be an accurate predictor of our susceptibility to disease and death.

Early deaths like Jason Hargrove's and George Floyd's pose no challenge to our age-washed beliefs, if we view them as exceptions. They simply become the story of an unfortunate infection with a heretofore unknown lethal virus, or the tragic encounter with one rogue cop. And we hold tight to these beliefs, even as we begin to recognize that systemic racism—at least its low-hanging, most visible fruits—also contributes to life-expectancy inequities.

For example, it is arithmetically obvious that so-called essential workers, who are much more likely to be exposed to COVID-19 because of the exigencies of their jobs, would be disproportionately infected by it. We find no reason to be surprised that bus drivers like Jason Hargrove—or the nursing assistants, orderlies, and cleaning crews who handle the body fluids, human waste, and dead bodies of COVID-19 victims, or the line workers in overcrowded, badly ventilated slaughterhouses and meat-packing plants in the rural South and Midwest—all have higher infection rates, and therefore higher death rates. Nor are we surprised that these people are disproportionately Black or, in the case of slaughterhouse workers and meatpackers, Latinx. The labor market segmentation that disproportionately exposes people of color to the virus is itself a manifestation of systemic racism, one we may lament but don't really think about doing anything to address.

It is certainly true that disproportionate exposure to the virus helps explain the population inequities in COVID-19 infection rates. Yet the greater likelihood of exposure and, thus, infection does not on its own adequately explain why working-class people and people of color, especially young adults and middle-aged people like fifty-year-old Jason Hargrove, are more than twice as likely to *die* from it. The clearest demographic risk factor for dying from COVID-19 is being elderly. Even before the advent of vaccinations and treatments, well over 90 percent of younger adults who got sick from COVID-19 had mild to moderate symptoms—if they had symptoms at all—and recovered at home.[6]

So, why is it that from the start of the pandemic the young and middle-aged in marginalized groups, not just Black and brown but Indigenous groups and people in poor white rural communities, have been more likely to suffer severe COVID-19 and die from it than their white, more affluent counterparts? The answer is part of a broader question: Why are the largest health inequities between these groups and nationwide averages—whether in infectious disease or the early onset of chronic conditions of aging such as cardiovascular disease, hypertension, and diabetes—seen among those aged twenty-five to sixty-five?[7] The COVID-19 pandemic has thrown these inequities into stark relief. It's not just that Black Americans are nearly twice as likely to die of COVID-19 as white Americans.[8] Consider these statistics (among the many, many more you will see in chapters to come): Black mothers die during childbirth at an overall rate that is nearly three times as high as the rate for white mothers.[9] For Black mothers in their mid-to-late thirties, the figures are even more dire: They die at a rate five times higher than white mothers of comparable age.[10] Yet, the working- and reproductive-age years are those we have been led to believe should be the healthiest, following the higher-risk periods of infancy, childhood, and adolescence, and before the most serious risks of aging set in.

These are shocking figures, and people express surprise and puzzlement when confronted with them. They just don't match up with the age-washing mantra that taking personal responsibility and making "healthy" choices will typically lead to a strong and vigorous life that could extend well into your eighties or nineties, or even past a hundred. We believe that given the state of our medical technology and scientific knowledge, anyone and everyone can live to grow old. As the late James Vaupel, a prominent demographer of aging, optimistically wrote in the late 1990s, "Very long lives are the probable destiny of most people alive today. [...] Every successive generation is becoming healthier at older ages. [Today's young people] will live to age ninety-five or a hundred because they will be so healthy and active at age eighty."[11]

To hear the media tell it, even Vaupel's prognostications may now seem conservative. In 2015, a blond, rose-lipped baby stared out from the cover of *Time* magazine with the caption "This baby could live to be 142 years old."[12]

We have been bombarded by these age-washing messages for years. This one-size-fits-all, colorblind approach completely ignores the reality that in a race- and class-conscious society like ours, health is not just a matter of luck, personal choice, or responsibility.

I remember that on the morning after Martin Luther King Day in 2015, during a season of renewed and compelling debate on whether Black lives matter, when my Facebook feed was filled with hard news stories about incidents of racism and prejudice afflicting many different minoritized and marginalized people all over the world, the post that caught my eye was the only one to include the word stereotype. But when I looked at it, it turned out to be a post about Vladimir Yakovlev's Age of Happiness photo project.[13] The photos—almost all of them of white people—depicted a sixty-one-year-old pole dancer, a seventy-eight-year-old nude vegan bodybuilder, a seventy-two-year-old DJ, an eighty-year-old stand-up comedian, a ninety-six-year-old downhill skier, etc., under the heading "These 60-and-Older Seniors Will Destroy Your Age Stereotypes." I recognized this post as part of a continuing media narrative that had been gaining momentum for two decades, as popular culture anticipated the baby boom generation turning fifty. Media outlets from *Newsweek* and *Time* to PBS and NPR began to extol the ways baby boomers would redefine growing old. Rather than go quietly into that good night, we would rage on in new directions, going off on new adventures and meeting new challenges to both body and soul.

Consider Kate, profiled in a 2000 *Newsweek* article:

> The fifty thing started hitting Kate at 49.5. "I don't want to be that old," says the San Francisco psychologist. "It's a half-century." But when the big day came in January, Donohue decided to see it as a chance to fix the things in her life she didn't like. She made three resolutions: to worry less, to "make more space" for herself by not being so busy and to be more adventurous—more like the woman she was in her twenties and thirties when she routinely set off on solo trekking and biking trips. In August, she will head off to Africa to learn more about West African dance, a longtime passion."[14]

The popularized depictions of San Francisco boomers "reborn" on skateboards and Midwesterners celebrating turning fifty with their first tattoos and Harleys send the message that there is no good reason not to be healthy and active at least into one's eighties. It is a matter of choice. Indeed, in a 2000 special report in *Newsweek*, "How to Get to Your Golden Years," boomers facing fifty were admonished that they "still have time to choose between decrepitude and a vigorous old age. But time is running out."[15] That admonition was reinforced by a 2015 *Time* magazine issue on aging in which a reporter summed up the latest "science" by telling readers: "You're only as old as you bloody well choose to be."[16] The underlying message is that if you are aging badly, you have only yourself to blame.

Such optimism is undergirded by our fascination with technology, our uncritical acceptance of the primacy of the developmental view of the connection between age and health, and the obliviousness of our elites to the lived experience and compromised health trajectories marginalized populations face. But our "don't let them eat cake" ideology assumes both that most of us have healthy options and that, for those of us who are able to choose, these healthy options are the fundamental reason for our good health. In reality, such choice is only the organically grown cherry on top of many health-promoting privileges. For those who don't have those options, disproportionately Black people, and also members of other marginalized groups including Native Americans, Mexican immigrants, so-called hillbillies, LGBTQ+ people, and the poor and working class, the lack of resources is presumed to be the problem. However, it is not the only or even the worst problem, as we see when accomplished and affluent members of these marginalized groups manage to make their way into elite spaces and have the opportunity to make all those healthy life choices—yet still incur disabilities and early deaths at surprising rates. If you are a member of a marginalized group, you cannot educate or buy yourself out of weathering completely.[17]

The age-washed narrative has only been strengthened by the developments of the past century. People born in 1900 in the United States were expected to live forty-eight years. By 1930, life expectancy had climbed to fifty-nine. But by 2010, thanks to public health measures like improved sanitation, biomedical and technological advances, and our increased understanding of the health impacts of smoking, diet, and exercise, it was seventy-eight.[18] Today, increasing numbers of Americans take their good health for granted and expect to live long and active lives. The fact that this is not true for everyone—not true, in fact, for millions of people in marginalized groups—is generally ignored. In a 2019 issue of *The New Yorker*, Adam Gopnik described the process of aging in America as if it were a reality shared by all: "Decades pass with little sense of internal change, middle age arrives with only a slight slowing down—a name lost, a lumbar ache, a sprinkling of white hairs and eye wrinkles."[19] While this description likely resonated with many of Gopnik's white, educated, middle-aged or older readers, it is not the lived reality for many others.

Reams of epidemiological and demographic research, including my own, have been revealing for decades that large numbers of Americans experience death or disability long before they are chronologically old. One's health and rate of aging vary dramatically by social group. And contrary to Vaupel's faith in the prospect of an ever-increasing life expectancy, things don't just keep getting better for everybody. (Indeed, since the advent of the pandemic, life expectancy has decreased in the US. Even before the pandemic, life expectancy had stagnated or decreased among working-class Americans.) The magnitude of socioeconomic inequity in healthy life expectancy is not decreasing, despite medical and healthy lifestyle advances. Quite the opposite: the gap has been growing in recent decades.[20] And the primary causes of this growing inequity overall are cardiovascular disease and cancer, which are primarily diseases of aging, and now COVID-19—not guns or needles, as we might assume to be the case in high-poverty urban populations, nor opioids, as we might assume to be the case in impoverished rural communities.

As for living to be a hundred, that remains rare, although how rare varies dramatically across race, class, and gender lines. In the year 2000, my colleagues and I estimated that if that year's death rates remained constant over their lifetimes—we now know from hindsight they got worse—only 10 percent of Black youth living in high-poverty urban areas could expect to live to age eighty-five; and 50 percent of white youth living in affluent suburbs—the longest-lived group—could expect to live that long.[21] Living to a hundred is still exceedingly unlikely, and living to 142 is a purely theoretical proposition. That said, it makes perfect sense that the editors of *Time* put a blond baby on the cover of the magazine, because if anyone is going to make it to 142, a white child is much more likely to do it than a Black or brown or Indigenous child.

The Reality of Weathering Compared to the Distortion of Age-Washing

In elite academic circles, the big scientific question is: what are the biological limits of that period when all keeps going well? Eighty-five, ninety-five, a hundred, 142? Not nearly enough attention is being paid to why, for certain marginalized groups, there is no such extended period of well-being. How do we reconcile the notion that modern Americans have the potential to be healthy and vigorous well through middle and even old age with the stark evidence that many young and middle-aged Black, brown, Native American, working-class and poor white urban and rural Americans are not? How can we explain the rapid health decline of Black Americans and Appalachian whites which, according to a large body of research, including mine, begins in their twenties?[22] Is there anything other than the age-washed answer?

We have been inoculated from wrestling with these facts by the easy—but incomplete and wrongheaded—jump we make to individual behavioral explanations. This is the dark side of age-washing. It tells us that if we are each biologically capable of living a long, healthy life, then it must be something we do or don't do that leads some of us to have shorter and less healthy life spans.

Through an age-washed filter, we have come to believe that population differences in health and longevity will disappear if we each become educated and affluent enough to be able to put into practice the steps one must take to sustain a healthy lifestyle. We assume (insofar as we are aware of the difference at all) that because members of marginalized groups are more likely to suffer chronic disease and cancers during their prime years, they must be eating too much sugar, salt, fat, and processed food, while exercising or sleeping too little. Full stop.

We also tend to cordon off each specific disease for which there is a health disparity—hypertension, diabetes, cancer—as separate from the others, although they are often trees that are part of the larger forest. We think these diseases stem from having an unfortunate genetic predisposition. Or they are the result of making behavioral missteps in the realm of diet, exercise, or alcohol and drug abuse. Some people frame those missteps as the avoidable product of ignorance, sloth, or gluttony. Others, of a less accusatory mind-set, see them as systemically imposed: the product of impoverishment, of overwork for inadequate pay, of being redlined into neighborhoods without access to healthy food, good schools, reliable transportation, and good jobs outside the drug economy. Applied to COVID-19 inequities, we can hermetically seal our age-washed bubble if we tie infectious-disease death disparities to the greater likelihood that Black and brown people suffer from the pre-existing chronic conditions found to be statistically associated with a poor COVID-19 prognosis—like obesity, diabetes, cardiovascular disease, or respiratory disease. Each of these conditions is associated with specific unhealthy behaviors. But all these individual or disease-specific explanations can go only so far, and they fail to take into account the physiological processes that contribute to weathering, which increase health vulnerability throughout the body. Weathering might manifest as obesity, hypertension, diabetes, respiratory disease, or other chronic diseases of aging, but people who are weathered suffer stress-mediated wear and tear across their body systems long before they can be diagnosed with specific diseases or conditions. Focusing on the individual, these explanations also fail to grasp the systemic social forces that set the damaging physiological processes in motion.

Health is not an immutable consequence of one's genetic code, nor a reflection of one's character. Living life according to the dominant social norms of personal responsibility and virtue is not universally health-promoting. On the contrary: if you're Black, working hard and playing by the rules can be part of what kills you. For the Black community, such virtue is a cause of death that dates back centuries, because the stress of navigating presumptions based on stereotypes, all while working hard and keeping a low profile, has been killing Black Americans since the time of slavery and continues to do so in the twenty-first century. At a church in Harlem in 1964, civil rights activist Fannie Lou Hamer famously said that she was "sick and tired of being sick and tired."[23] These words resonate with many Black Americans to this day, because they describe a very real phenomenon, physiologically as well as existentially. The repeated or chronic activation of stress processes over years and decades—the measurable physiological stress you feel in the body—has both immediate and long-lasting consequences for physical health and longevity. In short, it can make you sick or disabled or even kill you.

The cascade of physiological processes that lead to heart disease, cancer, and other diseases associated with aging can be triggered every day in any of us, no matter our DNA signature, no matter whether we eat sugary, fatty processed foods from plastic containers while we smoke and watch TV on the couch, no matter whether we suffer genetic mutations from chemicals at our workplaces or pathogens in our air, water, and soil. Yes, we would be better off if, as individuals, we won the 23andMe lottery, if we didn't face toxic exposures or engage in those unhealthy behaviors. But none of these are the be-all and end-all of health inequity, or even its primary driver.

In contrast to what the age-washing narrative tells us, it is not a forgone conclusion that we can avoid disability and postpone death by following socially approved health protocols, having a college degree, or enjoying a stable income well above the poverty level. Depending on their lived experiences, relatively young people can be biologically old. That's why some population groups disproportionately suffer early onset of the diseases of aging—and even early death. This will continue to be the case no matter what they eat, how much they exercise, the size of their paycheck, or where they live or work, unless something changes in the society around them.

To understand how these accelerated-aging processes work, and to counter the prevailing belief that living to an advanced old age is more or less accessible to each according to his lifestyle, I have been exploring the process of weathering ever since I first posited it, decades ago. The disproportionate death toll of the COVID-19 pandemic on the poor, the working class, and people of color across classes lays bare the fact that weathered bodies are more vulnerable to the worst ravages of infectious disease outbreaks. Weathering has left them with dysregulated or exhausted immune systems, which makes them unable to mount proper immune responses and predisposes them to the dreaded cytokine storms that are often the immediate cause of COVID-19 related death. In general, it has been individuals aged sixty-five and up who are at highest risk of dying from COVID-19, but we fail to acknowledge that the effects of weathering have rendered certain populations biologically older than their chronological age, putting them at higher risk of severe chronic or infectious disease and death than would be predicted by their chronological age alone.

Sick and Tired of Being Sick and Tired

Weathering damages the cardiovascular, neuroendocrine, and metabolic body systems in ways that leave people vulnerable to dying far too young. Take Erica Garner. She became a tireless advocate for racial justice after her father, Eric Garner, was killed by a New York City police officer who placed him in an illegal chokehold for the crime of selling untaxed cigarettes. Her father's dying words, "I can't breathe," became a rallying cry for the Black Lives Matter movement. Afterward, though she was initially apprehensive, Erica became a major force in the movement for police accountability. She died at age twenty-seven in 2017, only three and a half years after the death of her father, and four months after the birth of her second child. Her own difficulty breathing, due to severe asthma, precipitated a major heart attack that killed her. According to her doctors, the pregnancy had stressed Garner's already enlarged heart, so her death was classified as a maternal death. But why did she have an enlarged heart at her young age?

In the weeks before her death, Erica Garner described the stress, exhaustion, and frustration she suffered as a spokeswoman for the

Black Lives Matter movement for police accountability. "I'm struggling right now with the stress and everything," she said. "This thing, it beats you down. The system beats you down to where you can't win."[24] Or as her sister, Emerald Snipes Garner, described it a week after Erica's death, "It was like a Jenga"; they were "taking out pieces, taking out pieces, ripping her apart."[25]

Weathering is a life-or-death game of Jenga. The Jenga tower appears strong and upright as the first pieces are removed, one by one. To all appearances, it continues to stand strong as pieces keep being taken away until the removal of one last fateful block exposes the many weaknesses of its interior, and the tower collapses. In spring 2020, COVID-19 turned out to be that last fateful block for tens of thousands of people of color. Every day, towers collapsed, as they continue to do, before our eyes.

It's long past time to do something. But what? It's not clear how we address it, or even how we talk about it. Weathering offers a new recognition of how deeply insidious systemic racism and classism are, and a better, more scientific understanding of the damage it does to the body. Through my decades of research, I have seen how cultural oppression and exploitation move from society to cells in the bodies of tenacious and hopeful working-class people, poor people, and people of color across class who are working hard and playing by the rules.

"The only thing I can say is that she was a warrior," Erica Garner's mother, Esaw Snipes, said after Erica died. "She fought the good fight. This is just the first fight in twenty-seven years she lost."[26] After she had spent twenty-seven years of battling headwinds, fighting the same system that had killed her father for selling a few cigarettes, those headwinds took their toll and killed her too. She was weathered to death.

I think the same could be said of Fannie Lou Hamer, who was the target of a drive-by shooting during her struggle for voting rights. The bullets left her unscathed. Or did they? She died at age fifty-nine, of breast cancer and complications of hypertension, and I think she intuitively understood the price she paid for her years of activism. After failing the literacy test in her first attempt to register to vote, she told the registrar of voters, "You'll see me every thirty days till I pass."[27] In later years, as she reflected on her persistence, her words suggest she knew she was being weathered: "I guess if I'd had any sense, I'd have been a little scared—but what was the point of being scared? The only thing they could do was kill me, and it kind of seemed like they'd been trying to do that a little bit at a time since I could remember."[28]

"A little bit at a time," piece by Jenga piece, the assaults on the body continue to accumulate as weathering. However, as the Reverend William Barber, cochair of the Poor People's Campaign, asserted in June 2020, "Accepting death is not an option anymore."[29] In an interview on MSNBC's *Morning Joe*, Barber was speaking of the demands for justice for Black Americans, including George Floyd and Breonna Taylor, the twenty-six-year-old EMT who saved lives in the pandemic and was shot by the police at least eight times while sleeping in her own bed during a mistaken surprise raid. But he emphasized that the imperative extends far beyond the issue of police brutality. Echoing Fannie Lou Hamer, he said, "In everything racism and classism touch, they cause a form of death."[30]

Barber's words read as metaphor, but they are the literal truth. The country is waking up to what Black Americans have known for centuries and what public health statistics have shown us for many decades: systemic injustice—not just in the form of racist cops, but in the form of everyday life—takes a physical, too often deadly toll on Black, brown, and working-class or impoverished communities. Contrary to popular opinion and accepted wisdom, healthy aging is a measure not of how well we take care of ourselves but rather of how well society treats and takes care of us. When society treats us badly, it doesn't just "cause a form of death," it causes damage that can literally age and kill us.

2.

Stress and the Human Biological Canvas

Stress is a strangely diffuse concept that everybody thinks they understand. The word stress is used loosely to cover a broad array of feelings, perceptions, circumstances, and physiological reactions. What any one of us deems stressful is influenced by our individual personalities and life histories, and is also partially a matter of how the social groups we are part of define stress.

For example, the stress of juggling the demands and deadlines of one's professional job—whether an accountant or a zoologist—with the needs and expectations of one's children is qualitatively different from the stress of being a soldier on a battlefield. But upper-middle-class working parents who perform that juggling act every day identify their constellation of personal and professional responsibilities as stressful, and they understand one another when they call this "stress." The stress of being "crazy busy" like those parents, within the context of having many options and resources, is also different from the stress experienced by parents working multiple minimum-wage jobs while battling with their landlords to fix the heat in their apartments and sending their children off to underresourced, physically toxic school environments. And it is different from the stress a bereaved Erica Garner described experiencing as she felt compelled to take on the mantle of a leader in the struggle to end police brutality.

How much of a toll such experiences of stress take on the body, both in the short and long term, and how they cause weathering, is the focus of this chapter. But this chronic physiological stress is very different from stress in the age-washing perspective, which views it as something largely within our control, if only we learn how to handle it.

Age-Washed Advice: Stress Less, Smile More

Part of the age-washing narrative is about stress. We are told that the key to a long life is not just to make the right lifestyle choices—to eat well, move more, and get a good night's sleep—but to stress less, and have a positive attitude. In a 2013 article on a site called the *Guardian Liberty Voice*, a reporter presented the statistical findings that stress in a woman's thirties is associated with Alzheimer's disease in her later years. So the prescription for avoiding Alzheimer's, she writes, is to "place your demons in a box, embrace your midlife crisis with a smile and high heels, and try to make amends with stress, for the less he visits you, the better."[1] Challenges, setbacks, and tragedies may be nonnegotiable parts of life, we are told, but how we face them is within our control. "The toll stress takes, research has shown, depends on how it is viewed," says the issue of *Time* magazine with the potentially 142-year-old baby on the cover. "The 70-year-old will always be 10 years older than the 60-year-old. But if you're talking about how many years both of those people have remaining, put your money on a happy, active 70 over a cynical, sedentary 60."[2]

Based on this description, we would certainly put our money on Kate's longevity. Yet, how representative is she of the baby boom cohort? My research shows that many baby boomers died or became disabled by age fifty. They didn't get to experience old age, let alone redefine it. So how well would Kate's decision to "worry less," and the *Guardian Liberty Voice*'s advice to put your demons in a box, smile, and make amends with stress, serve Beverly, a Black woman living in a Yonkers, New York, housing project who has experienced lifelong poverty and long bouts of unemployment? A *New York Times Magazine* article that profiled her as she, too, was approaching fifty, paints quite a different picture of what middle age looks like. According to journalist Helen Epstein, Beverly had

> asthma, diabetes, high blood pressure, rheumatoid arthritis, gout and an enlarged heart, and her blood has a dangerous tendency to clot spontaneously. She is 48, and she had her first heart attack in her late 20s. One of her brothers died of heart failure at 50, and another died of kidney failure at 45, as did a sister who was 35. A young cousin recently died of cancer. In the past three years, at least 11 young people she knows have died, most of them not from gunshot wounds or drug overdoses, but from disease.[3]

Do we really believe a positive attitude or the decision to become more adventurous and learn West African dance would cure—or prevent—what ails Beverly?

Being sick with such a litany of ailments is not unusual for low-income Black women. In a nationwide analysis, my colleagues and I found that 60 percent of all working- and reproductive-age Black American women suffer four or more stress-mediated chronic diseases by age fifty.[4] In her ethnographic study on welfare, children, and poor families in three cities, the sociologist Linda Burton found that 60 percent of the primary caregivers in the study suffered multiple morbidities, despite the fact that the vast majority of them were younger than thirty-nine years old.[5] For example, Barbara, age thirty-seven, suffered from a range of chronic health conditions that included diabetes, back injuries, kidney problems, high cholesterol, migraines, hernias, depression, and anxiety. Thirty-two-year-old Amanda had Sjögren's syndrome (an autoimmune disease), severe dental and gum disease, arthritis, acid reflux, and hypertension. Francine, age thirty, had stomach cancer. Even twenty-three-year-old

Hazel had gastric ulcers, asthma, liver disease, emphysema, dental and gum disease, and diverticulitis, and was clinically depressed. The mothers of many of these women were sick enough to require care. Many of the grandmothers had already died by their early fifties of cardiovascular disease, strokes, or cancer. This was an additional source of distress for their adult daughters as well as a window into their own futures.

One nineteen-year-old who lived in the same Yonkers neighborhood as Beverly reportedly lost so many loved ones to disease and accidents that whenever she thought about it, she was stricken with panic. "My heart beats so fast, and I can't breathe, and there's just death going through my mind the whole time." And in the three-cities study, Burton and colleagues found that in the most distressing of circumstances, cycles began to appear between parent and child, in which the chronic conditions of one exacerbated the conditions of the other. Fiona, whose ten-year-old son was diagnosed with depression, said: "He's depressed and worried about my problems and I feel guilty that he has taken my problems to heart."

The idea of living to age ninety-five or a hundred must seem mythical to these women; and their male counterparts have even shorter life expectancies, on average. Not that there are no "old old" (over age eighty-five) people in the communities I've studied, whether in Central Harlem, Eastside Detroit, the South Side of Chicago, or the Watts area of Los Angeles—they're just comparatively rare.[6]

Life Expectancy and Healthy Life Expectancy

So which children in high-poverty urban or rural areas can expect to make it to age eighty-five, ninety-five, or even a hundred? My research shows that prior to the pandemic a sixteen-year-old Black girl in Eastside Detroit had a 29 percent chance of living to age eighty-five; for a boy in the same circumstances, the likelihood dropped to 9 percent. For whites in high-poverty areas of Detroit, the odds were nearly as bad, with 30 percent of girls and 12 percent of boys likely to make it to eighty-five. Poor whites in Appalachian Kentucky fared a bit better than their urban counterparts, with 36 percent of girls and 16 percent of boys expected to live to eighty-five, but these figures are still far below nationwide averages.[7] For kids in any of these areas, even reaching retirement age—sixty-five—is an achievement. In Watts at the dawn of the twenty-first century, fewer than one out of two sixteen-year-old Black boys and two out of three sixteen-year-old Black girls could expect to survive through middle age. To put this into perspective: The average national odds of reaching age sixty-five are four out of five for sixteen-year-old boys and eight out of nine for sixteen-year-old girls.

If these grim statistics conjure up tabloid images of homicide deaths or drug overdoses, think again. Almost 50 percent of all early deaths among Black residents of the South Side of Chicago could be attributed to circulatory disease or cancer. Only 6 percent of early deaths among women and 14 percent among men were lost to homicide. That said, homicide *is* a significant cause of death for Black males aged fifteen to twenty-four on Chicago's South Side. But, importantly, the largest disparities in mortality between white and Black people, and between the poor and nonpoor, occur not among youth, but among those ages twenty-five through sixty-five.

We also found that Black residents of disinvested high-poverty neighborhoods who did survive to middle or old age—poor and middle-class alike—were more likely to have health-induced disabilities than white individuals across the nation who survived to the same ages. In fact, the differences between these groups in terms of *healthy life expectancy*—defined as the number of years of life lived without any health-induced disabilities—were huge. In one study, we found that twenty-eight years of healthy life expectancy separated Black teenage boys living in high-poverty areas from white teenage girls living in more affluent areas.[8] Among Black people in high-poverty areas of Chicago, the proportion of people who were likely to survive to age fifty without a health-induced disability was only 50 percent. For whites in Appalachian Kentucky, the proportion was similarly small.

As some of these statistics show, weathering is not all Black versus white. While I focus on specific racialized populations in this book—Black Americans in particular—it is essential we remember that weathering is a universally human physiological process. It just occurs more to members of oppressed and exploited social identity groups, who are often subjected to severe conditions of material hardship, toxic environments, social and cultural disruption, misrecognition, or erasure, and need to engage in high-effort coping to survive day-to-day. Indeed, since the 1990s, life expectancy has stagnated among the least-educated white Americans while continuing to grow to varying degrees for other groups, including low-socioeconomic-status whites in other Western nations.[9]

The most widely publicized interpretation of excess deaths among less-educated US white people is an increase in opioid overdoses, a cause that allows the age-washed perspective to consider their deaths preventable exceptions. But, horrific as the scourge of opioids has been, it is not the main cause of premature death in less-educated white people—just as homicide and drug overdoses are not the main cause of premature death in the inner city, despite what the tabloids would have us believe. Excess deaths of poor and working-class whites occur, in the main, as a result of chronic circulatory disease and cancer—diseases that are mediated by our stress response.[10] And I don't mean the kind of response where we meet the stresses of our daily life with a smile and a deep breathing routine, but rather physiological stress responses that are activated automatically.

Chronic Physiological Stress Responses and Weathering

Stress in the context of weathering refers to underlying and automatic biological processes that respond to lived experience. In the right measure and circumstances, these processes are protective and health-promoting. But when such responses are excessive and prolonged, they can cause damage. And since these physiological stress responses are indeed automatic, set in motion spontaneously by our bodies in response to various stimuli, they are not under our conscious control.

The inner workings of our bodies are always active and adapting, physiologically responding as necessary to changes in our environment. The late Rockefeller University neurobiologist Bruce McEwen referred to these adaptive processes as allostasis; they help us to maintain stability, or homeostasis, the tendency of the body to seek and maintain balance within its internal environment, even when faced with an external challenge.[11] Some external challenges are quite mundane, such as retaining our balance when we move from a seated to a standing position. Another example: our bodies physiologically work to maintain a temperature of 98.6 degrees Fahrenheit (37 degrees Celsius) by sweating in hot environments and shivering in cold ones. We don't decide to sweat or shiver; our hypothalamus, which we can think of as the hormone control panel of the brain, automatically activates the processes that heat and cool the body. That our bodies have this automatic capacity to calibrate our biological processes to respond to our environmental contingencies is a wondrous fact.

For the most part, our ability to quickly react to stressors and maintain homeostasis is health-protective. Your muscles precisely contract and relax in order to keep you balanced as you rise to your feet, thanks to quick signals between the cerebellum and vestibular system in your brain. You shiver long enough to get to your well-heated home, where someone awaits you with a hot cup of cocoa. You sweat long enough to get yourself to an air-conditioned movie theater. Even a massive stress response to a life-or-death threat is designed to be short. Seeing a cheetah in the savanna or a Big Bad Wolf in the forest triggers a release of hormones from the sympathetic nervous system, which in turn stimulates the adrenal glands, which release adrenaline and other hormones that activate increases in heart rate, blood pressure, and breathing rate. The result of all these actions is that oxygenated blood circulates to your large muscles quickly, preparing you to fight or flee. After the threat is gone, the body quickly returns to its pre-arousal levels. As the Stanford neurobiologist Robert Sapolsky so graphically puts it: "If you are a normal mammal, what stress is about is three minutes of screaming terror on the savanna, after which either it's over with or you're over with."[12]

During those three minutes, your body mounts an automatic response without your having to decide consciously that it was necessary. If mammals had to make a conscious decision about how to react to every threat, we would have gone extinct long ago.

In the context of meeting a cheetah on the savanna, this reaction works well; much better, presumably, than stopping to dazzle it with your smile and high heels, or taking a moment to meditate, feel gratitude, or cognitively reframe the situation. There's no time for cognitive reframing. The cheetah is there and it wants to kill you. Your cognitive capacities have been turned down spontaneously in favor of your affective ones. If you've ever had a sudden brush with death—say, a car barreling toward you while you're crossing the street—you've had some experience with this automatic physiological response.

Stress: Acute or Chronic? Or Both?

What happens if the threat never recedes, or if you face down one cheetah, only to spot ten wildebeests with their sharp horns in the elephant grass minutes later? Or what if you replay the terror of seeing the cheetah over and over in your mind after you've successfully fled? Maybe you've squared off with so many big bad wolves in this neck of the forest that you remain perpetually vigilant, rarely sleeping deeply because you need to be sure you spot the next one in time. In this state of constant vigilance, you'll react repeatedly to many things that, in life-or-death terms, will turn out to be false alarms; yet, better to overreact to a false alarm than to miss a true one. If, as in these examples, the physiological stress process is not completely deactivated, the body experiences overexposure to stress hormones. When this overexposure is sustained over a prolonged period, it causes the wear and tear on the body that is known, technically, as allostatic load, affecting all the major systems of the body: neuroendocrine, cardiovascular, metabolic, and immune.

When early humans staved off deadly threats on the savanna with short, intense bouts of fleeing or fighting, their biological functions readily returned to their routine levels once the threat passed, usually in a matter of minutes.[13] In modern life, we do not often face these life-threatening moments, but we do face a broad range of other stressors, which activate the same physiological stress response. For our ancestors, the stress response was a lifesaver. For us, depending on how prolonged and intense the response is, it can be a killer at worst, and a contributor to all kinds of disease and disability at best.

Modern stressors are often chronic or repeated, rather than acute and finite. They are most often psychosocial—encompassing recurring fears and anxieties, an ongoing experience of social injustice and/or material hardship, and a constant vigilance to threat. They can be relived or ruminated upon, without a clear endpoint. Traumatic experiences, for example, can continue to be stressful far beyond their actual occurrence, the extreme case being PTSD. In all these circumstances, the elevated production of stress hormones does not recede, because the anticipation of threat never recedes. Sometimes, the toothpaste cannot be put back in the tube. Elevated heart rates activated by the continued production of stress hormones can persist for hours and even days, including while you sleep. All the while, your body systems endure erosion. In these circumstances, no one specific moment presents you with the opportunity to simply take a deep breath and be done with it, especially if you are asleep.

Prolonged uncertainty about the future and anxiety about the present—how will you pay next month's rent, hold on to your job without childcare for your three-year-old, or get your recalcitrant landlord to remove the lead paint in your apartment?—can also have this effect. In these cases, physiological stress processes become a daily part of life.

Beyond the damage these chronic stress processes cause to the neuroendocrine, cardiovascular, metabolic, and immune systems, they can also influence brain structure. In the short term, stress-adapted brain structure can sharpen perception in ways that enhance problem solving in a high-stress environment.[14] I think of Damon Young's 2019 op-ed in the *New York Times*, in which he describes how growing up Black in a high-crime Pittsburgh neighborhood gave him an acute sensitivity to anticipating, avoiding, and responding to threats:

> I can sense when the stillness of the street is a precursor to danger, like the moment before a storm hits and the air adopts a menacing tranquility. I know the shuffle of someone carrying them tools in baggy jeans. I can feel it when the clamor at a nightclub shifts from festive to menacing. I know how to run. I know how to sit in public spaces (with my back facing a wall, so that I can see everything). I know how to park in lots (with the back in first, to make a quick getaway if necessary).[15]

Such "street smarts" can't always protect a person from a stray bullet or other danger, but this fine-tuned cognitive vigilance increases a person's chances of survival in some high-stress conditions.

There are costs, however. When exposed to long-term and traumatic stress, the hippocampus shrinks, adversely affecting one's short-term memory and ability to learn.[16] People with stress-adapted brains have been found to be more susceptible to anxiety and mood disorders, including depression.[17]

As a society, we often code outlooks like Mr. Young's as "overreactions" and encourage people who are inclined to them to turn to remedies like psychotherapy and journaling to exorcise the stress or try to reframe the threat as an invigorating challenge. But members of marginalized groups who have been conditioned by real-life, high-stakes hardships to be chronically vigilant are not overreacting. Nor are they "snowflakes." Nor are their challenges invigorating— often quite the opposite. They are adaptive. And while we sometimes devalue these reactions as "perceived," as if they are a figment of a person's imagination, it would be more accurate to consider them as evidence- or experience-based calculations that may have been triggered by a false alarm. Stressors that weather go well beyond the stresses you can consciously perceive and, possibly, reframe.

Other behavioral prescriptions for quelling the feeling of threat, like exercise and getting a good night's sleep, can be fraught for those who are Black. Exercise can be beneficial, but a Black person considering taking a run will be unlikely to forget that Ahmaud Arbery was shot to death while jogging because he was Black. And how can a Black person relax into restorative sleep knowing Breonna Taylor was shot to death by police as she slept in her own apartment?

For some of us, taking a deep breath and a moment to reframe or refocus our thoughts after an upsetting event will be enough to halt our physiological stress response. However, members of populations subject to weathering are rarely—if ever—responding to a single acute stressor. Their bodies are in constant biopsychosocial motion fulfilling their many and compelling responsibilities, which also steals their chances of having "me time." A 2004 ethnography of low-income mothers in Chicago (Black, white, and Latina) described the complex puzzle that many face to meet the basic daily necessities for their families.[18] Mothers commuted up to five hours a day (and rarely less than two hours), facing severe weather conditions and patching together the meandering routes of their underfunded public transportation systems. Long wait times and limited hours of availability at public-aid offices meant missing meals in order to navigate their schedules successfully. Not only was their discretionary time scarce compared to their more affluent counterparts, but the consequences of missed obligations were dire. The investigators wrote, "Mothers who received TANF benefits [Temporary Assistance to Needy Families]," for example, "faced work requirements that often did not take into account changing circumstances. If they showed up late for work because of sudden illnesses or emergencies, they often were docked prime hours or even fired. Changing family circumstances had continuing repercussions because public benefits could be cut or terminated when employment was lost." All in all, these strangling time constraints meant drastically reduced sleep, less family time, and less time to unwind from the day—the cruel irony being that more-structured stress meant less time to decompress. Two-thirds of the study sample led such "highly challenging" lives. One participant averred she "could never get a break." Another observed, "With working, the kids, and cleaning, [...] you just 'do' until you can just sit in a chair and nod off."

Another study of low-income mothers (Black, white, and Latina), using data from the same ambitious three-cities ethnography, exemplifies the kind of extraordinary stresses and choices faced in the communities most subjected to weathering.[19] Francine, a thirty-year-old mother of three, had no time to attend to her own stomach cancer diagnosis because she had to attend to her asthmatic son, as well as her mother who recently suffered a stroke and heart attack at the age of fifty. Lourdes, a thirty-four-year-old mother with diabetes and glaucoma, was expected to comply with welfare work requirements because her doctor insisted she could still work despite partial paralysis and blindness. As noted, 80 percent of mothers studied suffered from chronic conditions (83 percent of whom were thirty-nine or younger) yet could not afford regular doctor's visits, owing to either lack of income or "more immediate concerns," such as the need to attend to their child's health problems or their need to hold on to jobs that did not give them personal time off. It is hard to imagine a "more immediate concern" than an early-onset cancer diagnosis. That addressing it might not be an immediate priority reflects the constant juggling required in high-effort coping.

Tenuous housing can also be a focal point of chronic stress and health inequities for weathered populations. In her 1996 investigative report for the *New York Times*, Deborah Sontag laid bare the inhumane and illegal conditions that tens (if not hundreds) of thousands of tenants faced in New York City alone, as the government ignored negligent landlords, and left some 336,000 on waiting lists for public housing projects as part of its "homelessness diversion" policy.[20] The scenes read like something from the nineteenth century. "All-but-homeless," she reported, these residents were packed into basements, attics, and "coffin-sized cubicles" lacking "rudimentary amenities, like fire escapes and hot running water, mandated by early-twentieth-century housing laws."

Carmen, a resident of one of these residences in the Bronx, pondered: "Some days, I wake up and wonder how exactly we'll all die. Will we fall to our deaths when the floor gives way, or be crushed when the ceiling falls, or die in a fire because we can't make it out a broken window?" A resident in East Harlem, Martinez, "keeps a rope under his bed, preparing for a day when he will have no way out but a window with no fire escape." Their hypervigilance was well warranted, as fires and collapsed buildings regularly kill handfuls of tenants in these conditions. While these two ponder and take precautions against untimely death, others deal with smaller stressors daily, like the rats that crawled over Jose's family in Harlem. And there was eighty-three-year-old Maria, who was forced to scoop water from her toilet in order to brush her teeth. Not only are these conditions inhumane and illegal, but, as Sontag reported, city officials largely disregarded the often life-threatening complaints. Absent landlords racked up hundreds of violations, while the tenants could not dare organize a rent strike for fear of homelessness.

If this sounds hyperbolic, or like a sad state of affairs we left behind us in the mid-1990s, I wish you were correct. Unfortunately, housing conditions for the working-class or poor residents of America's major metropolitan areas have worsened as housing prices continued to spike into the twenty-first century, homelessness mush-roomed, and evictions and foreclosures happened with unconscionable frequency.[21] *New York Times* investigative reporter Andrea Elliott opens her 2021 book, *Invisible Child*, by describing the Dickensian housing conditions in which she first found the book's protagonist, Dasani, in 2012.[22] Dasani had been living for several years in a city-run shelter in Brooklyn with her family while waiting—along with another quarter-million New York residents—for her name to reach the top of a years-long wait-list for public housing. The conditions Elliott reports observing in the one-room "apartment" shared by Dasani's ten-member family include: mice scurrying across the floor; cockroaches climbing the walls; a mop bucket for a toilet; a propped-up hairdryer to keep the baby warm in the absence of any heating in the room; sawdust spewing from a gouge in the wall, chronically activating the asthma of family members forced to sleep near it for lack of space; and water leaking from the rusted pipes of the single small sink, among other equally appalling, stressful, and certainly unhealthy conditions.

Dr. Alexa Eisenberg, who worked with me while pursuing her doctorate in my department, led a study in Detroit that found a direct relationship between predatory investor-landlords and the exacerbation of "severe and racialized burdens of excess lead toxicity in low-income communities," particularly among children.[23] After the 2008 recession, Detroit failed to reassess property taxes for years, overcharging Detroit residents by at least $600 million as their home values dropped by about 80 percent and driving low-income families into foreclosure.[24] Once the homes reached foreclosure, the government auctioned them off, sometimes for as little as $500.[25] Today, investor-landlords own the majority of single-family homes in Detroit, a city once known for its high level of Black homeownership.[26] Many investor-landlords, seeing each home as simply a cheaply acquired piece of their massive portfolio, are quick to abandon homes that aren't turning a profit, and don't hesitate to withhold maintenance or demolish houses altogether.[27] In 2017, the Detroit Health Department found that children were likely to have excessive lead toxicity if they simply lived within 400 feet of a demolition.[28] Lead contamination is less obvious than scurrying mice, but at least as insidious: the consequences from early-childhood exposure include damage to the brain and nervous system, impaired language development, neurobehavioral disorders, and other developmental delays.[29] Homeownership, generational wealth, and children's futures are destroyed, while investors are handed the keys to the city.

The chronic stressors of everyday life for residents of high-poverty urban areas can be objective and environmental—for example, living through a very cold winter with no heat in your apartment and lead dust in the air you and your children breathe. They can be subjective, such as having sustained cognitive and emotional engagement with your landlord while trying to persuade him to turn on the heat. They can be massive and traumatic, such as when you experience a militarized drug raid of your apartment while your kids and elderly grandmother hide in the corners of the room, praying the police will realize they have the wrong address before shooting. Or they can be emotionally triggering, such as when you are exposed to the footage of your father being killed by the police, in looping news clips shown all over the city.

Whether your stress response is protective or damaging depends on whether the stressors you face are acute or chronic, whether you can achieve a satisfying outcome to them in a reasonable and predictable period of time, and whether you have sufficient health, support, resources, and power to do so. To the extent that you are marginalized racially, culturally, residentially, economically, or politically, you are more likely to face stressors that are constant, continuing, and long-lasting. This is what is known as structural violence, a major factor in weathering.

Structural Violence

Structural violence is the manifestation of systemic racism or classism through the complex web of overlapping and repeated harms faced by members of marginalized groups. It takes many forms, but in the context of weathering, structural violence refers to the chronic physical, environmental, material, and biopsychosocial stressors that members of a socially stigmatized and discriminated-against group face in their daily rounds. Structural violence can be perpetrated by an individual, as in the case of a police officer shooting an unarmed Black man or choking him to death over a minor civil infraction. Structural violence can be enacted by laws, such as the 100-to-1 crack-versus-powder-cocaine sentencing disparity that drove the mass incarceration of Black men and women in the 1990s.[30] Structural violence can also be enacted by institutions, such as by a municipal water department or a power company shutting off access to services for families who fall behind on their monthly bill in a recession (or a pandemic).

To illustrate, take the example of a building fire. Working-class and poor residents living in predominantly Black neighborhoods are more likely to suffer the loss of their homes and even their lives in building fires. Why? Consider this: you're living in an apartment building that is not up to code. The electrical system is archaic and prone to failure. So is the heating system. The fire doors don't automatically shut. The building is located in a neighborhood where there is limited low-income housing, and rents are rising in step with gentrification. The landlord has no incentive to make repairs or insulate or properly heat your building, because he can easily find a new occupant who will pay a higher rent. You don't dare complain too much, because there is a dearth of affordable housing in the area and you don't want to be evicted.

To keep your children warm in the winter, you turn to space heaters or opening oven doors. The result may be that a fire breaks out. Unfortunately, firetrucks don't or can't arrive quickly enough, because decades of municipal disinvestment have reduced the number of fire stations and firefighters in your neighborhood. The lack of funds may also mean that the garbage isn't collected regularly and the streets aren't plowed after snowstorms, which may impede access for the firetrucks. All these factors can be traced to racist policies of the last hundred years, but there is no one living person you can rightfully blame at the moment. You might point to the landlord, or to the mother who opened the oven door to keep her children or elderly parents warm. While their actions may have been the most immediate contributors to the fire, the resulting losses, injuries, homelessness, or deaths are fundamentally caused by the structural violence that placed these individuals in impossible situations and kept the damage from being minimized by any well-funded municipal infrastructure.[31] Structural violence is insidious, pervasive, and fateful. It is the fundamental cause of weathering, and it is entirely ignored in the age-washing narrative.

The stressors I've outlined in this example are primarily concrete—literal roadblocks, policy roadblocks, physical decay, cold temperatures. The biopsychosocial stressors are harder to see, but still damaging. How well would you sleep in an overcrowded apartment that is freezing in the winter and sweltering in the summer? Where your household has been invaded by rodents, while cockroaches regularly climb up your children's nostrils to lay their eggs? Where fears of eviction loom? Where you are constantly worried about house fires from your archaic, fraying, and overloaded electrical system or malfunctioning space heater?

Let's look back at Jason Hargrove. He worked in a closed bus during a pandemic in a hot-spot city. He may have been given a hero's sendoff in death, but in life his public-service job provided little support as he faced the incredible challenges of his job in pandemic conditions. Imagine the stress he felt when there was no one on board to ensure that everyone was masked, or to help him eject the woman who coughed on him—on top of all the stresses he routinely experienced as a Black man in a highly race-conscious and segregated city. Perhaps he should have tried to deal with his anger not by venting it on the video but by taking a deep breath and smiling. But that wouldn't undo having been coughed on during a pandemic, or protect him from having to get back on the bus the next day to take many more crammed busloads of often unmasked people to and from their destinations. He had restricted options and no power to create better ones. He could not simply walk away from his high-risk job, not if he wanted to feed his family, avoid eviction or foreclosure, and fulfill the American Creed.

Even though he literally sat in the driver's seat, he wasn't metaphorically in the driver's seat, and he was very aware of that. The sense of powerlessness he felt is itself a source of weathering, only one of many he endured.

The Inner Workings of the Stress Response System

What happens to the body over time from these various physical, psychological, and economic assaults? Many people are aware that too much fat and sugar in the bloodstream creates plaque in our arteries, which sets the stage for high blood pressure, diabetes, heart attack, and stroke. We think we can control these problems by eating a healthy diet. Perhaps some of us can. Fewer people are aware that, no matter your diet, chronic, repeated, unremitting stress sets you up for these same conditions. To get a bit technical: Recall that the physiological stress response increases breathing, heart rate, and blood pressure in order to quickly circulate oxygenated blood to large muscles. In order to accomplish this, the body activates the sympathetic nervous system (SNS) to release the stress hormones norepinephrine and epinephrine, and it triggers the hypothalamic–pituitary–adrenal (HPA) axis to release the stress hormone cortisol.[32] SNS activation causes the veins in our body to constrict, increasing blood pressure so the heart can pump with greater force. Meanwhile, the released stress hormones catalyze a breakdown of the triglycerides in fat cells, the proteins in nonexercising muscles, and the glycogen in other body cells.[33] Glycogen is a form of glucose—sugar—that is stored in reserve, mainly in the liver and the skeletal muscles. When energy is needed, glycogen can be quickly mobilized to deliver the fuel the body needs. Simultaneously, the cortisol prevents insulin in the bloodstream from storing these energy sources back into their cells.[34] The result of all these processes is that the bloodstream is flooded with glucose, fatty acids, and amino acids, which are used to fuel the muscles in the body and mount an immediate response to the stressor.

So, in the case of a person chronically subjected to stressors, the buildup of sugar and fat in their bloodstream does not rely on overconsumption of double-cheese pizza and beer or an exercise regimen limited to picking up the TV remote, but is at least, in part, due to physiological stress processes that unleash this complex cascade into our system over and over without letup. That the chronic cascade of stress hormones in the bloodstream may also physiologically propel us toward eating "comfort" foods high in fats and sugars, or to turn to alcohol or other drugs for relief, only makes this problem all the worse.[35]

The sustained activation of all these processes over a prolonged period of time takes a toll on the body in a multitude of ways, including the following: The increased blood pressure damages arteries and veins over time, while other biochemical processes create a buildup of atherosclerotic plaque in the damaged veins and arteries—this is known as hardening of the arteries—which further increases blood pressure and eventually leads to hypertensive disease. In the heart, high blood pressure can cause the muscles in the left ventricle to thicken, enlarging the heart and potentially triggering an irregular heartbeat. Disruptions in the rhythms of the heart can cause heart failure, while clogged circulatory systems or traveling plaque can obstruct blood flow, leading to pulmonary embolism, heart attack, or stroke. Elevated levels of cortisol in the bloodstream can eventually damage insulin-secreting cells in the pancreas or create insulin-resistance, leading to diabetes.

The Human Toll

Let's look back at Erica Garner's death at age twenty-seven, attributed to the stress of pregnancy overtaxing her enlarged heart. We could simply classify her enlarged heart as a preexisting condition; but we should ask why she had an enlarged heart at such a young age. Given her lifelong hardships and stressors, intensified by her father's very public, brutal death, and the difficult responsibilities she then assumed as an active spokeswoman against police brutality, it's easy to imagine the chain of weathering assaults that resulted in her enlarged heart. It starts with Erica's being chronically stressed, her arteries hardening, and hypertension developing. Her hypertension and narrowed arteries require her heart to pump more forcefully. With time, the effort needed to pump blood throughout her body enlarges her heart, just as intensely exercising any specific muscle will enlarge that muscle. Erica's enlarged heart then places her at greater risk of being unable to maintain a normal electrical heart rhythm and makes her vulnerable to irregular heartbeats (called arrhythmias), which can precipitate a heart attack and death.

Of course, her case could be idiosyncratic. Something specific about Erica Garner as an individual, or maybe something in her family's genetic heritage, might have predisposed her to her tragic fate. The age-washing narrative always tries to rationalize such a tragedy as an expression of bad luck or bad genes or bad behavior. After all, Erica Garner was overweight, grew up in Brooklyn with an often-unemployed dad who engaged in illegal activity, and was a single mom. This narrative would have us write off her death as exceptional—and preventable, if only she and her family had made better choices.

And yet, and yet...her early death is a scenario only too familiar in the Black community. The maternal death rates among women of Erica Garner's age are four times higher among Black mothers compared to white mothers. But what is particularly revealing, and relevant to the discussion of weathering, is that the maternal mortality rates for Black moms in their late twenties (Erica's age) are more than twice as high as the rates for Black teen mothers.[36] Why is that? A growing body of research, including my own, suggests that the longer a person is subjected to the kinds of stress we've been discussing, that is, the longer they weather, the more damaging the effects on the body. Through a weathering lens, we can see how chronic stressors over time could have contributed to Erica Garner's enlarged heart. Regardless of whether or not that's what happened in this specific case, there is reason to believe, on the population level, that the disproportionate rate at which Black women in the US start their pregnancies with life-threatening preexisting conditions is not due to chance, genes, poor attitude, or bad behavior alone—if at all.

For another example of premature death, not pregnancy-related but very clearly related to stress and "structural violence," let's look at the Browder family. Kalief Browder was jailed when he was sixteen years old after being accused by another teen of stealing a backpack (a charge that was later dropped). The Browder family did not have the $3,000 required for bail—an exorbitant sum, one might think, given the scope of the alleged crime. As a result, Kalief spent three years awaiting trial at the notorious Rikers Island jail, where he endured beatings by guards and 400 days in solitary confinement.

The Browders' story highlights the profound differences in lived experience that exist among Americans. Can those of us who have raised white teenage boys in affluent communities (I have raised two) imagine any of this happening to our sons? First, if one white teen accused another of stealing his backpack, it would almost certainly be worked out in school or between the parents—no police involved. In the unlikely case an arrest were made, however, one way or another we would find a way to pay the bail (which almost certainly would not be $3,000)—either with our own assets or with a loan from an affluent friend or relative or from the bank. Our sons would not be sent to Rikers Island to await trial for three years, let alone be beaten or placed in solitary confinement as minors for *allegedly* stealing another kid's backpack! Yet, what happened to Kalief and his mother, Venida Browder, was not an anomaly in their world.

After his release, Kalief took steps to educate himself and restore his life prospects. He enrolled in Bronx Community College, but he could not shake his suicidal depression, first induced by his incarceration at Rikers and the prolonged psychological and physical trauma he endured there. He attempted suicide several times at Rikers and even after he was released. In June 2015, he finally succeeded. The night before he hung himself, Kalief told his mother, "Ma, I can't take it anymore."[37]

We could point to Kalief's depression as a preexisting condition that explains his suicide, and it certainly was the immediate cause. By all accounts he did not suffer depression before he went to Rikers—his was a depression induced by structural violence. Consider that chronic exposure to physiological stress processes affects the brain as well as other parts of the body. It can enlarge the amygdala, which is the brain's integrative center for emotions, leaving people more susceptible to anxiety and mood disorders, including depression.[38] Stress and untreated depression can shrivel the hippocampus in a matter of months, impairing one's ability to engage in cognitive processes and to learn.[39] In a particularly young or sensitive person, and during critical periods of development including adolescence, prolonged toxic stress exposure can result in a propensity toward anxiety and vigilance and a low threshold for physiological stress arousal, which becomes biologically embedded.[40] This, in turn, can cause enduring changes in brain architecture and a low threshold for stress arousal, setting off negative recursive processes that weather mind and body.

For her part, Venida Browder fought for three years to get her son out of jail, visiting him every week at Rikers and bringing him books and magazines and fresh clothes. She showed up at each of his thirty-one court dates, until a judge finally dismissed the charges and ordered him released. She fought for more than a year until New York City's mayor prohibited the practice of solitary confinement at Rikers Island for sixteen- and seventeen-year-old inmates. After a protracted battle, Venida Browder also contributed to the passage of a new law named for her son, Kalief's Law, to ensure any future cases like his would go to a speedy trial. As did Erica Garner, Venida Browder took it upon herself to make a committed and public stand against the racial and class injustice that ultimately ended her son's life—and like Garner, she found such activism exhausting and stressful. It's easy to imagine how impossibly hard all of this must have been for her to endure—the three years of her son's imprisonment, the struggle to bring him back to civilian life after he was finally released, his suicide, and the battle to pass laws that would prevent what happened to her son from happening to anyone else. It's also easy to imagine what it cost her.

Venida Browder died from complications of a heart attack sixteen months after she lost Kalief. At age sixty-three, she died well before reaching the average life expectancy for Black American women in 2016, whether estimated as seventy-eight years (the life expectancy of Black women at birth) or eighty-three years (the life expectancy of Black women who have already reached age sixty). As her attorney, Paul Prestia, said, she died of a broken heart.

By all accounts, Venida had done her best to adopt a positive attitude. The city council member she worked with on reforming Rikers said at her funeral, "Despite the city failing her and Kalief, she firmly believed that we could work to create a more fair and just system. Venida was a woman of immense courage and boundless optimism. When you were with her, it was impossible to not feel hopeful about a better future."[41]

Even with her boundless optimism and resolve, Venida Browder was ripped apart by structural violence just as mercilessly as Erica Garner.

3.

Distressed Genes and Weathered Cells

When Emerald Snipes Garner said that the forces her sister Erica was fighting were "ripping her apart," she may have been speaking metaphorically. Indeed, when I first coined the term weathering, I was thinking metaphorically, too. In the decades since, scientific advances have provided insight into the concrete physiological mechanisms, down to the molecular level, that show us weathering is more than metaphor—it is a literal, physical process. And these advances challenge widespread beliefs about the role of genetics in health and life expectancy inequities across various populations.

Race and DNA, a Biological Fiction

Just as with the ill-defined and variable use of the term stress, we have certain vague and often unsupported ideas about the role of genetics in health. A common impression is that we have "disease" genes whose codes are fixed at conception, programming us for specific diseases at some point later in life. We also have a vague notion that families have "good" genes or "bad" genes that will determine how long members of those families are likely to live. And thanks to the eugenics movement, some may also think that whether your family's genes are "good" or "bad" is influenced by your race. Many believe that the inequities we observe in health and longevity derive from geographic ancestry (proxied by skin color) or "race" genes, which are bundled together in neat packages with disease genes. For example, diabetes, a disease that can be a manifestation of weathering, and is currently a disease found in disproportionate numbers among various marginalized groups, was once called a Jewish disease. During the first half of the twentieth century, its alleged higher prevalence among Jews was chalked up to a combination of bad genes and the bad behaviors and constitution seen as characteristic of Eastern European immigrant Jews, who at the time were racialized as Asiatic, Mongoloid or Negro, not white.[1] Now it's the currently vilified groups—Blacks, Latinx, and Native Americans—who suffer a disproportionate prevalence of diabetes. However, it is much more likely due to the weathering effects of cultural oppression than to "bad genes and bad behavior." These pervasive beliefs about the causes of diabetes, then and now, are simply incorrect. It's true that there are a few diseases that are determined by (or highly likely to develop due to) single genes, for example muscular dystrophy and Huntington's disease.[2] However, these diseases are not genetically linked to race.

Genetics and Epigenetics

Before attributing a disease to genes, we have to understand how genes actually work. The trillions of cells in each of our bodies contain the body's hereditary material: DNA. In the nucleus of each cell, the DNA molecule is packaged into threadlike structures called chromosomes. Genes are functioning subunits of DNA molecules. Each gene contains a particular set of instructions, or code. This code is the basic unit of heredity and is replicated as cells divide and proliferate. For the most part, your unique genetic code is fixed at conception and replicated in every cell in your body. (Mistakes can happen, but these are unusual.) This is your genotype. Personal genome sequencing would reveal it.

While our genetic signature is fixed, its expression is not. The basic code can be transcribed in numerous ways as different pieces of the code are either promoted (turned on) or suppressed (turned off) by biochemical processes, the result being widely varying expressions of the genes. The rapidly advancing field of epigenetics can help us to understand the mechanics of these gene variants. Epigenetics refers to events "above the genome" that regulate expression of genetic information without altering the DNA sequence.

As the mother of genetically identical twins (now young men), I see how the same initial genetic code written into their DNA gets interpreted in different ways every day. Genetic testing confirmed that my sons are monozygotic twins, meaning they began as a single fertilized egg (ovum) that split into two separate embryos in utero, probably within the first ten days of conception. Every cell across both of their bodies therefore has the same genetic signature.

In my eyes, they have always looked like brothers, but they have never looked or acted identically. Their health histories vary in important ways, too. Their dissimilarities occurred even though they grew up in the same family and neighborhood, attended the same schools through college, and shared an apartment right after college. Their environments, in a broad sense, have been remarkably similar.

Epigenetics explains on a molecular level how my DNA-identical sons can appear very different in some of their observable traits and health conditions. Twin research shows that as their environments diverge through adulthood, twins are likely to become less biologically identical, even though they will continue to have the same DNA signature.[3] My sons have the same genotype yet different phenotypes. Your phenotype is a description of your actual physical characteristics. Our health belongs in the category of phenotype.

Genotypes and Phenotypes

Gene-environment interactions can lead to different transcriptions of the same genetic code into varying phenotypes. Think about a straightforward characteristic of your phenotype, like your height. Your maximal potential height is certainly a product of your DNA, but how tall you end up being can vary with myriad aspects of your lived experience, such as your nutrition. Access to nutrients and other environmental influences begins in the womb and can vary even between twins. An extreme case is twin-twin transfusion syndrome, whereby one developing twin gets a greater amount of the blood supply from the mother, leading to increased growth relative to the other twin and the production of more amniotic fluid for the first twin.[4] This syndrome can result in substantial height differences between identical twins that can be lifelong. My twins did not experience this complication, but one was born with dangerously low blood sugar, while the other was not. The foods we eat, the chemicals in the air we breathe, the stressors we experience—all can result in epigenetic modifications. No two people are completely identical in the timing, nature, intensity, or full panoply of environmental exposures that can affect their phenotypes, not even identical twins developing in the womb!

As another indication, take the obesity epidemic of the last several decades. In the short time frame that US obesity rates have increased dramatically, genes related to obesity could not have changed. Instead, aspects of Americans' lived experience have altered our probability of becoming obese. There are a wide range of environmental suspects: greater exposure to endocrine disruptors in our air, water, soil, and cleaning products; increasingly sedentary lifestyles in the screen age; greater availability (and advertising) of fast and processed foods; the increasingly stressful rhythm of daily obligations; budget cuts suffered by public schools that have reduced opportunities for physical education or increased the reliance of school cafeterias on private contracts with fast-food distributors; or some combination of all of these and more that we have yet to discover.[5]

It's true that there is some genetic influence on weight.[6] But many gene variants (alleles) are involved, and which ones are expressed or suppressed is as subject to environmental conditions as height. So many gene variants are believed to have the potential to affect weight that you probably have some alleles that would statistically predispose you to a lower-than-average weight and some that predispose you to a higher weight. Outfits like 23andMe claim that they can calculate your "genetic weight," but all they can really tell you is that your weight-associated alleles might, on balance, predispose you to weigh X percent more or Y percent less than average.[7] While that percentage sounds quite precise, it is not dispositive. For example, my 23andMe report informed me that, on balance, my weight-associated alleles predispose me to weigh 9 percent less than average. Is this meaningful information? Not really. Even if my scale didn't beg to differ, as it does, what does it mean to have alleles, some of which are thought to predispose you to be heavy and some of which predispose you to be light, that balance out to 9 percent less than average? What is average? What is 9 percent? And if what matters to your phenotype is which genes are actually expressed, is this "balancing act" of alleles in your genotype relevant at all?

The report also advised me to keep in mind that lifestyle and environment have a big impact on weight. This is an artful understatement. The critical importance of the environment to obesity is clearly illustrated by the Akimel O'odham, of the Tohono O'odham Nation, a group of Native Americans in southern Arizona who are among the most obese populations worldwide, and who currently have among the highest prevalence of type 2 diabetes in the world.[8] That is only their current phenotype, however. This was not the case before the group's diet and culture shifted over the last century from agricultural crops to processed foods. Even today, O'odham living in

Mexico have substantially lower rates of obesity and diabetes than the genetically similar Akimel O'odham in Arizona. Despite our cultural fixation with genes, these examples illustrate that it is how environmental factors affect gene expression that matters most in the case of most complex diseases.

Environmental influences are so many and so diverse that they are impossible to enumerate or fully understand. As the phenotypic differences between my monozygotic twin sons suggest, our general concept of what constitutes the environment is too blunt an instrument to adequately describe all the environmental influences on health. My sons' phenotypic differences must have been shaped by factors we would loosely place under the umbrella of "environment." Yet these had to include factors or processes that are more subtle than those we usually put in the category of "environmental influences"—such as standard of living, toxins in the local environment, the environment in the womb, parenting style, school quality, diet— because my sons shared all of those and nonetheless turned out to be phenotypically different from each other.

A common misconception is that health differences between Black Americans and white Americans are due to essential genetic differences. By "essential," we mean that we take them as part of our genetic legacy, inherent to a bundle of genes responsible for both skin color and disease. Therefore, it may seem intuitive to speculate that, for example, since Black and white people vary in the distribution of gene variants influencing skin color (melanin production), the variations in their health outcomes must also be related to genes. But that speculation is false.

Gene variants for specific diseases do not come bundled with skin color genes.[9] Human genetic variation is the result of constant movements and migrations among people who mate with one another to produce continuous genetic variation across large geographic areas. Because of this history, each character or feature of human genetic variation varies nonconcordantly, that is, characters or features do not vary together in bundles for each individual. Indeed, the very concept of race is misleading. From a genetic standpoint, there are no subspecies or races; we are all human beings, each with our own independent assortment of genes.

When it comes to understanding social inequities in health, such as those between Black and white Americans, looking to genes is not much use.[10] The list of diseases that account for social inequities in health in the US is long and diverse; the diseases tend to be complex in their origins, and members of any racial/ethnic or socioeconomic group could be genetically susceptible to them under certain environmental conditions. For example, hypertension accounts for an important share of the overall poorer health and shorter life expectancy of Black Americans compared to white Americans. More than five hundred genetic variations have been associated with hypertension.[11] While these variations have been found more commonly in people with hypertension than in unaffected individuals, none are common causes of the condition. There is no hypertension gene.

The fact that there is no hypertension gene throws cold water on the idea that hypertension might come bundled with skin color genes. (And of course the spectrum of complexions between what we call white and Black is not based on a binary race gene, either.) If genes for skin color and hypertension were concordant, one would expect that in any and every context, darker-skinned populations would have higher rates of hypertension than lighter-skinned populations. Work by Richard Cooper and colleagues shows that this is not the case.[12] They studied African and European populations across several countries that would be likely to share genetic ancestry with their counterparts in the US. While hypertension rates were significantly higher in Black Americans compared to white Americans, findings about the other populations studied belied the belief that hypertension is genetically linked to Black people. The study found that the highest hypertension rates—higher than those of Black Americans—were among white people in Finland and Germany.

And Black Americans' hypertension rates were closer to the rates among white people in England and Spain than they were to Nigerians and Jamaicans, who had the lowest rates of hypertension among the populations in the study. That Black Jamaicans had such low rates of hypertension belies another popular but scientifically debunked theory,[13] namely that Black Americans were genetically selected for increased susceptibility to hypertension as a result of the abhorrent way they were treated by their captors during the Middle Passage. Yet, Black Jamaicans are descended from Africans who withstood the horrific trans-Atlantic voyage, too.

What about sickle-cell disease, which is a single-gene disease that occurs in disproportionately high numbers within the Black population of the US and is almost always thought to be a "Black disease"? Doesn't sickle-cell prove that a disease gene can be connected to genes for skin color? Not really. The trait for sickle-cell does not come bundled in a package with genes for Black skin. Its greater prevalence among African Americans is due to the fact that most African Americans are descendants of those who were brought here by the slave trade.[14] The sickle-cell trait helps confer resistance to malaria, and the slave trade drew from parts of Africa where malaria is endemic. The sickle-cell trait is also common in tropical Africa, southern India, and the Arabian Peninsula, other areas where malaria is widespread. But the sickle-cell trait is rare in South Africa, where there is very little malaria, and a mainly Black population.

As the geographer Jared Diamond has pointed out, if human races were based on the presence or absence of antimalarial genes, we would group Italians, Greeks, and Nigerians together as one race, while the Xhosas of South Africa would be grouped together with Swedes as another.[15] Each "race" group would include some European and some African populations and would exclude other white and Black populations. We would understand more about why African Americans are more likely than white Americans to have sickle-cell and other diseases by studying US history and geography, migration patterns, the slave trade, racial politics, and miscegenation and residential segregation laws than by studying genetics—or even malaria.

The links between racial identity and the environmental conditions to which an American is likely to be exposed underscore the perils of trying to understand population health inequities through the lens of genetic predisposition. Even if there were such predispositions—which there are not—single-gene diseases are not the ones that account for the lion's share of population differences in health and longevity. The reality is that your genetic heritage is only one influence on your ultimate health profile and life expectancy. Whatever contribution it makes to your individual chances of developing a disease, it is not particularly important on a population level. What populations do tend to have bundled together with skin color are lived experiences. In a racialized society, the likelihood of being exposed to particular chronic stressors—both ones that are objective and ones that are biopsychosocial—can indeed be linked to skin color; in fact, it's definitional.

Weathered Cells and Shortened Telomeres

If genes, per se, do not predispose some populations to weathering, what does cause them to weather at the molecular level? The cells that make up the body regularly divide. Cell division helps our bodies grow (by adding new cells) and helps maintain our health (by replacing damaged and worn-out cells with new cells). This process works well for repairing occasional cuts and bruises. It even enables us to heal from severe or life-threatening injuries, like those incurred in a car accident or a major surgical procedure. But if chronic stress responses damage our cells, they will stop dividing at an earlier age, endangering our health and longevity. Beginning in 2004 with the publication of a watershed paper by Professors Elissa Epel and Elizabeth Blackburn at UCSF, investigators are finding increasing evidence that chronic stress is associated with shorter telomeres and cellular aging.[16]

Whenever a cell divides, its DNA is copied and must remain safe and intact throughout the process. That's where telomeres come in. Telomeres are protective, stabilizing caps on the ends of chromosomes that serve as buffers to maintain the integrity of the coding DNA when the cell divides. One way to imagine telomeres is as though they are the plastic ends of shoelaces (the aglets) that keep the laces from fraying. Imagine that once an aglet is torn, the shoelace unravels from its ends onward, eventually affecting the integrity and functioning of the entire shoelace.

Each time a cell divides, its chromosomes' telomere buffers are shortened. Eventually the cell will die or enter "replicative senescence"—it will no longer divide and replenish. While the process of telomere shortening that leads to senescence, and ultimately to cell death, may take longer if we have been lucky enough to inherit telomeres that are longer to begin with, each of us will eventually reach a limit where cell division is no longer possible in vital tissues and organs, leading to frailty and death. As Elizabeth Blackburn, the winner of the 2009 Nobel Prize in Physiology or Medicine, discovered, some cells have a telomere-lengthening enzyme called telomerase that can restore shortened telomeres up to a point; however, eventually telomerase becomes inactive and the balance between telomere shortening and telomerase-mediated lengthening tips toward shortening.[17]

Telomeres help us understand how, on a cellular level, people who endure chronic stressors and other forms of structural violence can biologically age faster than their peers. People who are subjected to more threats to cell health will experience more-rapid cell division as the body attempts to repair damaged cells, leading to accelerated biological aging (shorter telomeres, more senescent cells) and the risk of premature death. Moreover, telomerase activity can be blunted by stress, accentuating the weathering-induced reduction of telomere length and undermining its chance of being restored.[18] In addition, as cells age, they respond to stressors increasingly weakly or maladaptively, whether the stressors are physical or psychological, literally adding insult to injury.

As telomeres shorten, chromosomes become more unstable. When telomeres can no longer protect the coding DNA during cell division, they signal the cell to cease dividing, to become senescent. You might imagine senescent cells as zombie cells. While dead cells are washed out of your body, senescent ones build up, sending toxic signals to other cells that can have adverse effects on health. As immune cells become senescent, you become more vulnerable to infections. Senescent cells in the walls of your blood vessels promote hardened arteries that can lead to heart attacks. Researchers suggest that cellular senescence may also be linked to increased cancer risk, as senescent cells secrete substances that trigger epigenetic modifications that "turn on" tumor-enhancing genes (oncogenes), while "turning off" tumor-suppressor genes.[19] This sets the stage for the activation and unregulated growth of cancerous cells.

When functioning well, telomeres emit protein molecules known as "anti-inflammatory cytokines" to help regulate the body's immune response to infections and trauma by suppressing or upregulating (increasing) the expression of pro-inflammatory cytokines as needed. This coordinated regulation of anti- and pro-inflammatory cytokines works well in cells with telomeres of healthy length in a person who is suffering from an occasional infection, acute injury, or physical trauma—like a C-section incision in an otherwise healthy woman. Immune cells respond to the signals and run to the rescue to help with wound healing. As the wound heals or infection clears, pro-inflammatory cytokines are suppressed. But in an aged cell with severely shortened telomeres, the telomeres can malfunction.[20] The cell signals for help (upregulating the emission of pro-inflammatory cytokines), but as a last gasp at protecting their prized DNA cargo, the telomeres keep even these helpers out when they come to the rescue! In that process, pro-inflammatory cytokines are continuously released and spread through the body, causing chronic, systemic inflammation. Chronic inflammation harms cells, tissues, and organs throughout the body.

Chronic inflammation plays a role in many of the diseases that members of marginalized populations are more likely to experience or die from at younger ages. For example, chronic inflammation leads to malfunctioning pancreatic cells, affecting insulin regulation and precipitating diabetes.[21] Chronic inflammation can trigger autoimmune diseases such as rheumatoid arthritis or lupus.[22] Chronic inflammation facilitates cancer growth in various organs and tissues.[23] The debris that builds up from the white blood cells of the immune system, thwarted in their attempt to repair damage, can trap cholesterol and form plaques that damage or block veins and arteries, inducing hypertension.[24] These plaques can rupture away from the blood-vessel walls to become blood clots, or embolisms, that travel to the lungs, heart, or brain, obstructing blood flow and resulting in dangerously low blood oxygen or blood pressure levels, heart attack, or stroke.[25] The buildup of white blood cells reaching bottlenecks as they futilely run to the rescue can also facilitate leukemia.[26] If bone tissue cannot be replenished due to a critical mass of senescent bone cells secreting pro-inflammatory cytokines, bone loss develops.[27] Asthma, COPD, and other diseases marked by poor lung functioning can be triggered or exacerbated by too many unstable or senescent cells in the blood vessels of the lungs.[28] Too many senescent brain cells can emit substances that kill your neurons.[29] Overall, and across body tissues and systems, persistent inflammation accumulates with age as telomeres are shortened and damaged over time by aging or, even faster, by chronically stressful lived experiences. This process is sometimes referred to as "inflamm-aging."[30]

As we have discussed, compared with more privileged groups, marginalized groups are prone to accelerated biological aging, early onset of chronic diseases of aging, weakened and dysregulated immune systems, and shortened life expectancy—all of which are the products of weathering at the cellular level. A critical reason for these health disparities is that marginalized groups face multifaceted, chronic, unremitting environmental insults that negatively impact gene expression and damage cells, thereby hastening telomere shortening and inflamm-aging.

While much remains to be discovered about the psychosocial, physical, environmental, and biological mechanisms of aging, particularly as they relate to health inequities, what we do know points us away from both the more common age-washing narratives and the genetic predisposition-to-disease explanations.

Weathering, which explains how cultural and economic oppression can manifest in a multitude of complex diseases, is a much more fruitful avenue of exploration. And, as we shall see, using a weathering lens rather than an age-washed or DNA-centric lens yields very different personal and policy approaches for how to promote health equity.

In summary, weathering is the accumulation and culmination of life experiences that are structured by historical and ongoing systemic racism and classism. To see how it erodes the health of oppressed working-class or poor populations, consider the lived experience of many Black residents of Eastside Detroit. Thanks to racialized residential segregation and disinvestment policies over the last century, the housing that is available and affordable to low-income Detroit residents is aged, deteriorating, and not up to code. The walls are often coated in lead-based paint. The insulation is asbestos, which in addition to being a toxic substance is also a lousy insulator, leaving your home too cold in the winter and too hot in the summer. Outside, the air is polluted, and decades of industrial activity have contaminated the soil and drinking water. Your community's diminished tax base leaves the roads with potholes and the schools chronically underfunded. Your commute to work is long and inefficient, and your work is difficult and sometimes dangerous. You have no control over how many hours you work, and the paychecks never seem big enough to pay the bills. Water and electricity shutoffs are imminent unless a family member can help you out—again. When a higher-paying job is posted, your application is rejected as soon as the employer sees your name and address. One emergency bill—a trip to the emergency room or a sewage leak in the base-ment—could jeopardize your monthly rent or mortgage payment; eviction, foreclosure, and homelessness are constant threats. As a Black, low-income resident of Eastside Detroit—as in many disin-vested and segregated high-poverty urban areas across the coun-try—you could lose your job for staying home with a sick child or to let the repairman in to fix the sewage leak in your basement. Your access to medical care is restricted and generally substandard even when you are able to get it. Shopping for healthy food means an hour-long trip on the bus, but fast food, as well as liquor, cigarettes, and street drugs, are all just down the block. On your walk or drive you may be subject to "stop-and-frisk" or traffic stops—and any mis-communication or false move could mean early death by police vio-lence. You have little political power to change all this.

Over time, these circumstances expose your body to physical, environmental, and psychosocial stressors that are chronic and unrelenting. This prolonged stress arousal exacts a physiological toll on your major bodily systems. Stress hormones, glucose, and fatty acids flood your bloodstream, your heart rate increases, and your large muscles oxygenate quickly, limiting blood flow to other parts of your body. At the molecular level, your cell environments are sub-ject to increased oxidative stress—an imbalance between the pro-duction of free radicals that are damaging to cells and antioxidant defenses—leading to maladaptive epigenetic modifications, muta-tions, and telomere shortening. Over the course of your life, these mechanisms increase your risk of developing cardiovascular disease, including hypertension, an enlarged heart, and hardened, clogged arteries that can rupture and send blood clots to the lungs, brain, or heart. They increase your risk of obesity, diabetes, and other metabolic disorders. Mood disorders become biologically embedded as your hippocampus shrinks, your amygdala enlarges, and your brain cells die off. Infections and infectious diseases become chronic, and autoimmune disorders develop as your immune system weakens or dysregulates.

The process and effects of weathering vary, not just from one social identity group to another but also among individuals within those groups. The extent of weathering will differ according to the range and diversity of chronic stressors people face in a given historical moment, and, as individuals, according to how these interact with the alleles and telomere lengths one was born with. In periods of xenophobia, immigrants will be subjected to weathering. When we are at war, those whom we construe as enemies in our midst will be subjected to weathering, as Japanese Americans were during World War II and as people perceived as Muslim or Arab Americans have been during our various wars in the Middle East and the war on terror. When we believe COVID-19 deaths are due to a "China virus," Asian Americans will be subjected to weathering stressors. When we hold tight to gender binaries and the preeminence of heterosexuality, transgender and other LGBTQ+ people will be subjected to weathering. Any individual or population can become weathered if subjected to oppressive conditions, whether in the form of economic pressures, the psychosocial pressures of negative stereotyping, or outright violence.

At a personal level, how weathering affects individuals varies a lot, and we cannot predict how well or badly a given person will be able to withstand weathering. But at a population level, we can say with confidence that those in oppressed groups will be subjected to greater weathering threats than others. As a result, they will suffer the consequences in both shortened life expectancy and greater incidence of disability and disease.

In a cruel irony, those in oppressed populations who face these challenges with tenacity every day over years and decades will be subjected to more of these threats than others. Those individuals continuously engage the bureaucracies, make the long commutes to work, experience the sleep deprivation of night shifts or double shifts or coordinating household labor with workplace responsibilities. They face competing obligations, perpetual indignities and microaggressions, and the need to keep their psychological armor on throughout the day. They are too often reminded how little they are valued, how little power they have to avoid these stressors, how unlikely they are to prevail in disagreements with those more powerful, and how underappreciated and undercompensated they are for the essential work they do. How persistently they are ignored and disrespected. How hard they must work to survive. They are weathered in both senses of the word—damaged by the physiological stress responses triggered by their stressful lives, and also by struggling against all the pressures they face. Their resilience is critical to facilitating their family's and community's ability to avoid or withstand the ceaseless barrage of weathering stressors, but their immense, unswerving effort to provide shelter also exposes them to the allostatic storm.

4.

Mothers and Babies in Jeopardy

"[A woman should stop having children] by age thirty-two, because if you get too old, it will be hard on you. Sometimes you can't take it," one sixteen-year-old told me. I was interviewing Black teenagers who were pregnant, some from a disinvested urban area in the North and others from an isolated disinvested area in the rural South. When I asked them at what age they thought a woman should complete her childbearing, they gave answers ranging from twenty-two to the late thirties, with most saying that, except for very special circumstances, thirty was the maximum age by which a woman should complete childbearing. The age range they saw as the tail end of childbearing fell well within the age range at which dominant cultural norms would have it *begin*.

When I asked them to explain their answers, many gave responses that spoke to weathering concerns and implied a very different understanding of how old one is at thirty, forty, or fifty from that held by the dominant culture. Concern for the health prospects of their elders was also on their minds.

"Well, the way I look at it, I think [a woman should stop at] thirty. [After that] I wouldn't recommend it. When the kid's ten and still needs a lot of attention, really hasn't grown up, then she's already forty-five. And then, here she is fifty, and the kid is like an adult, but she could be dying. So, I think thirty-five is too old," said one.

Note that the "kid" who is "like an adult" is fifteen years old, not an age that most Americans—Black or white—consider an adult. And her fifty-year-old mother is seen as facing a real chance of dying, also not the expectation of those in the dominant culture. The reality of weathering, and the young ages at which weathered people become sick or disabled, or die, are very present in this young woman's calculations about when one ought to bear a child. This perspective on age was repeated in others' responses:

"Some people wait until they are thirty-five. I don't think they should, 'cause you only got a few more years, you know," said another.

Another participant expressed concern for who would take care of the child in the face of the health problems she expected a woman might have by the time she turned fifty. She said a woman should stop having kids before her late thirties, "because she can raise the child until [the child] gets about my age [sixteen], you know, and if she get sick or something the child'll be almost grown at least. Be able to be on its own if something happened to the parent. [Otherwise] by the time you get fifty you'll have a ten-year-old and if something happen to you, somebody would have to take care of the child."

One participant was concerned about having children early enough that they would be ready and able to take care of their mother when her health falters—which she considered might happen in the mother's early thirties. She said a woman should stop having kids by about age thirty-three: "By that time [if you had your children younger] your children could be growing up. They can start taking care of you."

Another participant said: "Where I live at now, my grandmother got custody of three other little kids. [...] I let her go out to church because the kids be worryin' her, and she's so old, and she gets sick of that house, and she don't know nothin' else to do but yell and fuss. So, I keep the kids while she goes out."

I asked how old her grandmother was. I was imagining her as a doddering old lady of at least sixty-five, if not eighty-five. But the answer: forty-six! One might be tempted to think the interviewee's statement that her grandmother was "so old" was simply a measure of an adolescent's distorted idea of what constitutes being old. But health statistics back her experience up that a forty-six-year-old woman in her family could be showing signs of stress and aging.

A particularly pointed and poignant response revealed the conflict between the dominant cultural notion that a woman should get an education and become a fully mature person before she has a child, and the interviewee's experience that to postpone childbearing meant risking physical and mental incapacitation while her children were growing up and still needed her. She said a woman should stop having children " 'bout age thirty. They're too old. They have bad nerves and everything. She wouldn't be as fast as she was. She would know a lot but she wouldn't have the nerve to do it anymore."

One nineteen-year-old working-class Black mother spoke of what she learned from the experiences of her older sisters: "My thirty-four-year-old sister is dying of cancer. Good thing her youngest child is seventeen and she seen her grow up. My twenty-eight- and thirty-year-old sisters got the high blood and sugar. The thirty-year-old got shot in a store. She has a hole in her lung and her arm paralyzed. Good thing she had Consuela long ago. My twenty-eight-year-old sister wants a baby so bad. She had three miscarriages and two babies dead at birth. Doctors don't think she can have a baby no more. All my sisters weigh 250. I bet you wouldn't believe they looked [thin] just like me at my age. I'm sure I'll look like them when I'm old."

The lesson she drew from her sisters' experiences was that postponing childbearing, even to the mid-twenties, comes with increased risks, running the gamut from involuntary permanent childlessness to an inability to take care of your children to dying before they are grown.

In one of sociologist Linda Burton's ethnographic studies of poor Black families, one primary caretaker—a twenty-one-year-old mother of two—revealed a similar awareness of how her years for healthy childbearing might be cut short. "Me and my mom talk about how many problems I've had. I'm only twenty-one and I've had all these problems [asthma, gynecological tumors, and depression] and I worry about in coming years what's going to happen. There are women out there in their thirties having hysterectomies. Is that going to be me?"[1]

Through the interviews, I also saw how painfully aware the young mothers were of the compromised life prospects of their boyfriends. One particularly heartrending observation came from a sixteen-year-old describing her boyfriend's influence on her decision to carry her pregnancy to term.

> When I told him [I could be pregnant], he was in the hospital. [...] They didn't know if he was going to live or not, so I went to the hospital. [...] I told him that I was pregnant, that he couldn't die. [...] He said, "I can't die because I'm having a baby. Don't do anything to my baby." Before he had known that I could be [pregnant], but I guess I just needed him to know that I was. That he had to live for somethin'. [That influenced my decision to carry the pregnancy] because I felt as if somethin' happened to him, that he did leave somethin' behind. Even though I just wanted him to live so bad, I had to realize that he could die.

These young women are expressing views about pregnancy—the timing of it, what it means to them, the fears surrounding it—that may seem utterly foreign to affluent white Americans who abide by dominant cultural childbearing norms. Age-washing has taught us that the late twenties through early thirties are the universally ideal time for childbearing. Indeed, representative surveys of US white teens find they typically answer age forty as the end point for child-bearing, and many say there is no age limit at all. My privileged twenty-eight-year-old sons and thirty-four-year-old daughter—all of whom want to become parents someday—cavalierly dismiss me when I even ask if they've thought about when they might have kids. (I can't help but contrast my thirty-four year old daughter's outlook to that voiced by the research participant previously quoted, "My thirty-four-year-old sister is dying of cancer. Good thing her young-est child is seventeen and she seen her grow up"). The luxury my children have to be so nonchalant about how old they will be when they become parents is undergirded, in part, by their probably real-istic expectation that they have long lives ahead of them. They take for granted the likelihood of a future with good health, economic security, and a rich availability of life options. Weathering, however, robs young adults and even teens in culturally oppressed and eco-nomically exploited populations from experiencing that "whole life ahead of me, the world is my oyster" expectation.

Women in their childbearing years who find themselves at the intersection of racism, classism, and sexism must tread water per-haps harder and longer than just about anyone else to keep their families' collective heads above the surface. Like the woman who was trying to help her forty-six-year-old grandmother take care of the three children who'd been left in her custody, they feel responsi-ble for multigenerational kin networks, and they also need those networks for their child's survival ("if something happen to you, somebody would have to take care of the child"), and for their own ("[if you had your children younger,] they can start taking care of you"). The young women I've interviewed seem to have thought through their options very carefully.

These are the trade-offs and the high stakes they face—and they know how very little they can take for granted. Yet, the dominant American culture has branded teen mothers as incompetent, irresponsible, or worse. And US social policy has institutionalized this branding into its various programs and budget allocations.

Even the terminology we use here is problematic.

In the 1970s, the term teen childbearing (used interchangeably with adolescent childbearing and popularized as "babies having babies") was institutionalized as an explanation for all our pregnancy and childbearing woes and, starting around the mid-1980s, for a panoply of society-wide woes as well. Given the broad acceptance of this term, it may surprise you to know that it is flawed in every conceivable way. It's a misleading, imprecise, and incomplete description of a phenomenon that is much more complicated than is generally understood.

At the most obvious, the term teen birth is flawed because it fails to distinguish between mothers giving birth at thirteen and those giving birth at nineteen, ages that represent very different stages along a social and developmental continuum. Despite misleading and highly publicized phrases like "babies having babies," the lion's share of so-called teen mothers—about three-quarters—are eighteen or nineteen years old. Fewer than 2 percent of teen mothers are younger than sixteen, while thirteen-year-olds are an infinitesimally small percentage. A methodologically diverse scientific literature dating back to at least the mid-1980s finds that in marginalized groups, older teenagers consistently enjoy better pregnancy outcomes than mothers in their mid-to-late twenties and thirties. This was true when research on teen mothers was first done in the 1970s, and it remains true today.

I was first compelled to ask questions about the harsh branding of teen mothers as a new class of social deviant as it was being constructed, popularized, and scapegoated for many social ills. I watched as academic players and social policy makers first began to define these ills, hardening the vague concept of the deviant teen mother into an apparently factual analysis and driving it home to the public. Organizations exploited the term's chimeric flexibility to shift the definition and racialization of the alleged "problem" as changing political and organizational objectives warranted. As resonant—even if irrational—moral panics changed over time from concerns about the sexual revolution among baby boom adolescents, to fears of an alleged pathological Black underclass, or, more recently, xenophobia and replacement theories, the vague and imprecise term teen pregnancy could be applied as the cause of very different social problems—real, exaggerated, and imagined.

For example, as the sociologist Constance Nathanson elaborated, in the early stages (the late 1960s and early 1970s), cultural fears about teen motherhood were focused on middle-class and affluent white teenage girls who, at the dawn of the feminist movement and amidst growing tolerance of sex outside of marriage, might undercut their emerging educational and career opportunities by becoming mothers at too young an age, even though technology that could help prevent this outcome—the birth control pill— existed.[2] Highly educated white parents didn't want their teen daughters to hit a baby bump on the road to a very bright future, a bump that could be avoided by expanding their access to sex education and contraception.

Later, beginning in the late 1970s and continuing through the 1980s and much of the 1990s, the construct could be applied to a hyped Black urban "reproductive underclass" to stoke fear and political will to unravel the welfare safety net.[3] Now that teen childbearing among Black women has been dramatically reduced, Latina girls have become the latest target, and women as old as twenty-nine years of age are now sometimes the focus of the same contraceptive campaigns that were originally launched to prevent teen childbearing!

A lack of appreciation for health inequity and the implications of weathering was a silent partner in all three formulations. Highly educated white parents took for granted that their teenage daughters still had decades to become mothers after they had graduated college or even graduate school. Meanwhile, the fact that poor, working-class white teenagers and teenagers of color faced substantially shorter healthy life expectancies and substantially more constrained educational and work options has been consistently ignored.

Back in the mid-to-late 1970s, when I was taking advantage of new opportunities for advanced education for women as a senior at Princeton University and had a part-time job as a research assistant to the director of Princeton's Office of Population Research (OPR), I saw the transition in concept and representation of teen mothers from white to Black girls as it was being made—to serve changing political purposes.

During my time at OPR, I saw how many of its faculty members focused on and interpreted the problems associated with teen childbearing. No question there were—and still are—many severe problems statistically associated with teen childbearing, from poverty to infant mortality. However, association does not on its own imply causation. This basic tenet of quantitative research would be well-known to the Princeton University economics and sociology professors who constituted the OPR faculty. I am sure they applied it in other less value-charged or age-washed contexts. But perhaps by centering their own experience as affluent professionals who were most familiar with teenagers in their own affluent suburban families or as their students at Princeton, they may have taken it as a matter of common sense that all teen mothers must be upset by their pregnancies, would be harmed by them, and would have preferred to avoid them, just as most teens they knew well likely did. In terms of policy solutions, they understood these issues narrowly as questions of sex education and access to contraceptives. Their solutions might well have made the difference between their daughters or Princeton students facing a teen pregnancy or not, but they were woefully out of step with the lived realities of many young women they were ostensibly trying to help.

I probably would have held on to the same "common sense" assumptions if they were not at odds with what I was seeing through an internship I held simultaneously at a women's health clinic and alternative high school for teen mothers in the then high-poverty, predominantly Black city of Trenton, New Jersey. It was twenty minutes but worlds away from Princeton. There I saw women shouldering great responsibilities—both the pregnant young women and their mothers, some of whom I came to know as well. They faced substantial material hardships, psychological challenges, and unhealthy living conditions, yet they remained tenacious and hopeful as they worked to support their children and communities. Most of the young women expressed excitement about the new lives they were carrying. At the same time, as I accompanied them on their clinic visits and medical exams, I observed that they appeared physically worn and torn, in stark contrast to my peers at Princeton, who were roughly the same chronological age.

During these appointments, instead of speaking to the young women about their health, the physicians I observed often gave unsolicited lectures in medicalese to me, the white Princeton undergraduate, while directing my attention to various medical points of interest on the patients' bodies in ways that I suspect were a violation of privacy. I never observed a physician ask a young woman about any health concerns she might have had, or look her in the eye. The physicians I observed basically ignored each young woman as she lay exposed on the examination table, treating her as if she were not a conscious, intelligent, or even sentient human being. Chances are she was feeling many things in those demeaning circumstances, none of them good for her health or that of her developing fetus.

As for me, I wasn't even a premed or medical student. I was there to be the young woman's peer companion and to ensure against sexual assault. I never witnessed a physician commit sexual assault. But I had received no training in interrupting this other kind of assault, which was omnipresent: assault on the patient's dignity. Total erasure, replaced by projection.

For their part, the OPR faculty seemed unaware of and, despite my efforts to describe what I was seeing, uninterested in the pervasive health problems and social hardships facing these young women. They denied the possibility that any teenager could be excited about her pregnancy, assuming that she was pregnant because she didn't know any better. This was the "babies having babies" narrative, which prevented the women from being taken seriously and served as a powerful rationalization for such smug erasure.

To me, the idea that the broad range of entrenched problems these young women and their families lived with would disappear if they had just used contraception appeared wishful and uninformed. I was also quite aware that their contraceptive ignorance was overstated. They knew as much about contraception as I did, and had, in fact, used it in the past when according to their circumstances they thought they were too young to become mothers. Mansplaining contraception to them was unlikely to move the needle. Yet, the magical beliefs held by the OPR faculty, that the core problems among the young women were ignorance, lack of access to contraceptives, and sexual impulsiveness—hearkening to the racist Jezebel trope[4]—appeared impervious to questioning or, as I observed later when I began to compile evidence of weathering, even to facts.

The Influence of Weathering on Maternal and Infant Health Outcomes

Eliminating racial inequities in maternal and infant health has been a high-priority national public health objective for more than thirty years. Yet there is little evidence that much progress has been made. The US ranks 33 out of 38 high-income countries, and has almost 6 times the rate of Iceland, the country ranked #1.[5] But the rates are far worse for Black babies in the US, who die at more than twice the rate of white babies.[6] This inequity has only become entrenched over the most recent decades.[7]

The maternal mortality rate in the US is also disgracefully high — 23.8 maternal deaths per 100,000 births in 2020.[8] It ranks as the worst among all high-income countries.[9] It is also increasing, having more than doubled since 1990, and the greatest rates are seen among Black mothers.[10] In 2020, the overall non-Hispanic Black maternal mortality rate in the US was 55.3 per 100,000 births. The non-Hispanic white rate was much lower, at 19.1 per 100,000.[11] And for every US mother who dies for pregnancy-associated reasons, another 70 mothers come close to dying for such reasons.[12] They suffer what the medical profession calls severe maternal morbidity, which encompasses various life-threatening pregnancy, delivery, and post-delivery complications that can have enduring consequences for the mother's health.

The graph below illustrates both how dramatically the US maternal mortality rate increased between 1990 and 2015, a period when the maternal mortality rate was *decreasing in all other high-income nations*, and also how much higher our mortality rate is than that of other affluent Western countries.[13] This is true even as we spend more than $60 billion every year on maternity care, an amount that is dramatically higher per capita than that of other countries with much better maternal health outcomes. The WHO has gone so far as to call US maternal death rates a violation of human rights.

Trends in Maternal Mortality Rates in Wealthy Countries, 1990–2015

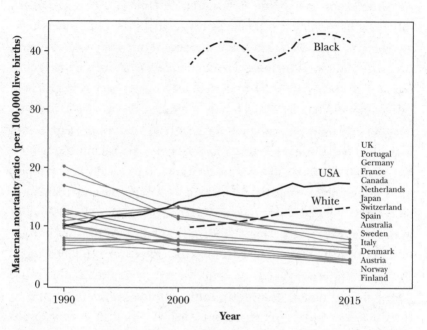

Note that the curves appear smoother for the other countries than for the US. This is because outside of the US, we only had data points for 1990, 2000, and 2015. For the US we had data points for every year from 1990 through 2015 for overall maternal death rates, and from 2000 through 2015 by race.

Teen Motherhood versus the Cost of Postponing Childbearing

When I present figures like these in talks, audience members are quick to venture that the primary explanation for this country's high maternal mortality rates must be the high rate of teen childbearing in the US relative to other countries, in general and among Black women in particular. The US does have a higher rate of teen births than other affluent countries.

The US also has greater income inequality and higher poverty rates, and it is the *only* high-income country without some form of universal health care and family- and maternity-friendly policies such as child allowances, postnatal home visits, and paid family leave. Interestingly, those highly pertinent differences between the US and other high-income countries go largely unmentioned in discussions of comparative maternal mortality rates. That audience members tend to ignore our lack of a safety net and turn first to teen birth rates as the probable explanation is emblematic of how automatically we resort to age-washing explanations to account for health and mortality inequities. If individual teens would just take the personal responsibility to not have babies at an age when, we assume, they are too physically undeveloped for healthy childbearing, the problem of high maternal and infant mortality rates might be solved. So goes the age-washed logic. But inequities in mortality are not that simple. Indeed, in many ways they are in complete contradiction to our beliefs about the risks of teen childbearing.

At the opposite end of the reproductive years, we, as a country, have come to believe that postponing childbearing, even well into the thirties or forties (or even, some believe, the fifties), is *not* problematic. In fact, certain segments of our society have been able to skirt the natural limits of biological reproductive aging by the extensive—and expensive—use of technologies now available to those who can afford them, whether through IVF, freezing your eggs when young for later use, using the eggs of a younger woman, or simply implanting a fertilized egg into the womb of a younger—and almost always lower-income—surrogate.

I am not trying to stir up a political hornet's nest (at least not until later in the book). I do want to ask you to be open to reconsidering what you think about the relationship between maternal age and adverse birth outcomes, without presuming you already know the (age-washed) answer.

Through age-washing, we have been taught to accept as true that there are universally "good" and "bad" ages to bear children, and that for all women, in every situation, "teenage childbearing" is the worst. But the facts tell a very different story. As illustrated in the graph below, over the thirty years that witnessed dramatic increases in maternal mortality, teen childbearing rates decreased, most dramatically among Black mothers.[14]

US Birth Rates of Mothers, Age Fifteen to Nineteen, by Race and Hispanic Origin, 1989–2019

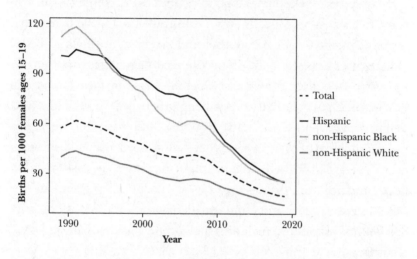

If teen childbearing were a driving force behind our statistically appalling maternal health outcomes, we would have expected that maternal death rates would have gone down as the teen birth rates went down. But they didn't. Instead, they went up.

In reality, in populations afflicted by weathering, teen childbearing does not contribute to these poor outcomes. It may even reduce them. Nancy, a midwife practicing in a high-poverty and predominantly Black clinic in Ohio, had this to say about her experience of delivering babies there: "What I found was that sixteen-year-olds did just fine at having babies. By twenty-five, we just automatically assumed we should be on the alert for trouble."[15]

I cannot count the number of comments to this effect I've heard from obstetric nurses, midwives, and obstetricians who work with a culturally oppressed, poor, or working-class clientele. And the empirical scientific literature supports their perceptions.

Maternal Age and Poor Infant Outcomes

Maternal death rates among oppressed populations do not go down with age. They increase. But what about the effects on the children they bear? Despite public and political opinion to the contrary, there is no universally applicable guideline for the best age, in terms of the health of the mother and the baby, at which to bear a child. For example, the graph on the next page illustrates the average risks, for Black mothers and white mothers who gave birth in the US between 2017 and 2019, of having a baby with a very low birth weight (VLBW; less than 3.31 pounds), according to the age of the mother.[16] VLBW reflects either being born preterm or being growth-retarded while in the womb; it increases the risk of infant death and, for those babies who survive, portends long stays in neonatal intensive care units and an increased risk of developmental delays and disabilities, including being blind or deaf, among other challenges.[17]

In addition to these human costs, the health-care costs in just the first six months of life for a single preterm and/or low-birth-weight baby are currently estimated to range from $76,143 to $603,778 per baby.[18] These financial costs are often paid by all of us—through the high cost of our health insurance premiums, our tax dollars, or the inflated costs of our own hospital stays to compensate the hospital for lost revenue.

Looking at this graph, we see that babies born to white teen mothers in the US do have a higher risk of VLBW than white mothers in their twenties. So do white babies whose mothers are in their thirties or older. However, the overall risk of a white baby being VLBW is small—no matter the age of the mother—when compared to the risk for a Black baby with a mother of the same age.

Very-Low-Birth-Weight First Births by Maternal Race and Age, 2017–2019

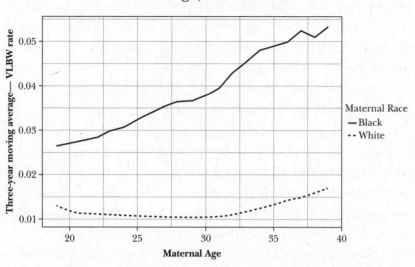

Rates of VLBW among Black babies are substantially higher than among white babies at all maternal ages. But what is most striking in the context of the condemnation heaped on teen mothers is that within the Black population, VLBW rates *increase steeply* with maternal age. For Black mothers, the lowest-risk ages are actually in the teen years! In the early twenties the rates begin to rise substantially. We and others have found similar divergence in risk by maternal age for a number of other poor birth outcomes among Black women, including for fetal, neonatal, or infant deaths,[19] and, as you will see in the next section, maternal deaths, too.

Furthermore, the Black/white inequity in any of these outcomes is much larger among older compared to younger mothers, especially for Black women in segregated, high-poverty areas. For example, among Black mothers residing in the Central Harlem Community District in 1990, we found infant mortality rates for Black teens—eleven deaths per thousand live births—were similar to those for white teens—ten deaths per thousand live births—nationwide.[20]

But in Central Harlem, the infant mortality rate for Black mothers in their twenties was twenty-two per thousand—twice that of Black teens—and more than three times that of white mothers nationwide who postponed childbearing beyond their teens—six per thousand. Of particular note, virtually all of the "older" Black mothers in Harlem were in their twenties, while the older, "non-teen" whites included many mothers giving birth in their thirties and forties. Neither Black mothers nor their babies escape the ultimate price of weathering.

I want to be clear that it would be a misunderstanding to interpret the policy implications of these findings to be that poor or Black teens should be encouraged or incentivized to bear children. That's no answer to the underlying problems revealed by these statistics. However, holding fast to the belief that early childbearing is always bad for mothers, children, and their families is not scientific or grounded in facts. Nor is it respectful of the lived reality of those in a culturally oppressed group.

If giving birth at a younger, less weathered age leads to better health outcomes for both mother and child, we must acknowledge that within society as it exists now, it is more important to remedy the causes of weathering than to focus on reducing teen births. As we will see in the following section, public health efforts aimed at encouraging weathered populations to conform to the dominant culture's imaginary optimal timeline for childbearing have had damaging, even fatal, consequences for mothers and their children.

The Cost of Delayed Childbearing in the Black Community

In 1990, 43 percent of the first births among Black Americans nationwide were among teenagers, with only 10 percent among those thirty-five or older. By 2019, the percentage of Black first births to teens had fallen by more than half—from 43 percent to 17 percent—while the percentage of Black births to women thirty-five years and older doubled—from 10 percent to 22 percent.[21] This shift to giving birth at older ages mirrors a larger trend within the United States. How positive was the result of that shift? Not what you might expect. In fact, this shift has had tragic implications for the health and survival of both mothers and their babies. The reason: Weathering intensifies with age.

Pregnant Facts

Pregnancy is a risky business, but it is far riskier for women in culturally oppressed groups whose health has been damaged by weathering. Weathering stressors are pervasive in the everyday lives of these women. They seep into any physiological cracks in a woman's body they can infiltrate, sometimes even crossing the placental barrier to affect fetal development. Lived experiences such as the ones we have been describing, prior to and during pregnancy, delivery, and the postpartum period, can impact the progress of a pregnancy and increase the risk of severe morbidity, delivery complications, and even death to mother or child. That is, weathering threatens the two most fundamental goals all parents have for themselves and their children: that babies be healthy at birth and that the mother's pregnancy and birthing experience leave her healthy enough to care for them.

Mothers who enter pregnancy with chronic diseases of weathering, in particular hypertension and other cardiovascular diseases, are at elevated risk of adverse outcomes. If a woman is hypertensive when she becomes pregnant, or develops hypertension during her pregnancy, she has an increased risk of developing life-threatening conditions including preeclampsia (high blood pressure with liver or kidney damage in mid-to-late pregnancy), eclampsia (when a pregnant woman with preeclampsia experiences seizures or lapses into a coma), stroke, and labor complications.[22] High blood pressure in the mother also compromises the fetus's access to oxygen and nutrients, retarding its growth. That, combined with the fact that the best hope of saving a mother with preeclampsia from developing eclampsia is to deliver the child, even if premature, increases a baby's risk of being a fetal death, stillbirth, or born preterm or low birth weight. Rates of preeclampsia in the US have been rising over the past three decades, and there appears to be a further jump in pre-eclampsia rates since the pandemic.[23]

As everyday weathering stressors continue or even increase during pregnancy, the activation of physiological stress responses that deliver blood to the large muscles will necessarily diminish blood flow to body functions that don't contribute to immediate survival— another way in which the developing fetus may be deprived of oxygen and nutrients it needs. Furthermore, the stress hormone cortisol, while buffered, especially in early pregnancy, can cross the placental barrier, exposing fetuses to impacts of the stress response in the womb.[24]

For mothers, blood vessels weakened by years of weathering increase the risk of hemorrhage during labor. Having a chronically weathered and dysregulated immune system increases a mother's chance of postpartum infection and lengthens the healing time of tears and incisions. Plaque buildup in her arteries due to weathering can cause blood clots that can be fatal if they travel to her lungs, heart, or brain.

Environmental racism encompasses all the ways in which people of color and the poor are disproportionately exposed to environmental hazards. Its effects can include living in neighborhoods where toxic waste sites and air-polluting industries are located, and in homes poisoned by toxic substances like asbestos, mold, and lead paint, lead pipes, or lead-contaminated soil. Rural populations are exposed to toxic pesticides in the fields, while coal dust looms in the air in Appalachian coal-mining towns. Tribal reservations near nuclear power plants, such as that of the Diné Tribe (also referred to as the Navajo Nation), across parts of northern Arizona, northeastern New Mexico, and southeastern Utah, find that babies have measurable toxic uranium in their bloodstreams and tissues at birth. A pregnant woman's exposure to the effects of environmental racism is a problem for both her and her baby.

Like uranium, other environmental pollutants such as black carbon and lead can cross the placental barrier, directly exposing the fetus to toxic levels of these poisons.[25] Maternal and fetal exposure to black carbon air pollution has been linked to miscarriages, premature births, and lower birth weights.[26] Long-term exposure to environmental lead (think, most infamously, of the lead in the drinking water in Flint, Michigan) can have similar results, increasing the risk of miscarriage, preterm birth, and low birth weight, as well as intellectual deficits, neurobehavioral disorders, developmental delays, and lower academic achievement in exposed children.[27] And while the Flint water crisis was finally being exposed, the deterioration and demolition of foreclosed houses in the aged housing markets of Detroit, about an hour and a half southeast of Flint, was introducing lead-containing dust into the nearby residential environment. As noted earlier, the Detroit Health Department found in 2017 that children were likely to have excessive lead toxicity if they simply lived within 400 feet of a demolition, implying that the lead burden on mothers was also increased by the cycle of predatory lending to poor households, subsequent foreclosure, and demolitions to the benefit of predatory landlords.[28]

When the lead circulating in a pregnant woman's blood crosses the placental barrier, the developing fetus will absorb it like a sponge. Breastfeeding is another route through which an infant can be exposed to lead stored in the mother's body.[29] Once absorbed, lead remains in the body for life, having only negative effects.[30] As women subjected to environmental racism age through their reproductive years, the store of lead in their bodies keeps increasing with every subsequent exposure, becoming ever more toxic. This may be one of the many reasons why older Black mothers have worse pregnancy and childbirth outcomes than younger Black mothers. We will return to this later in the book.

As Black women age from their teens through their twenties and thirties, becoming ever more vulnerable to the effects of weathering, they develop more conditions that are risk factors for pregnancy and childbirth. As noted earlier, women who enter pregnancy with chronic diseases of weathering, in particular hypertension and other cardiovascular diseases, are at risk for health- and life-threatening conditions such as preeclampsia, eclampsia, stroke, and labor complications. The baby is at risk, too, because the mother's high blood pressure can retard the growth of the fetus and increase its chances of being born prematurely.

Now consider the findings of one of my studies, which showed that the prevalence of hypertension among Black women increases from less than 20 percent at age twenty (which is actually just a shade higher than for white women of the same age) to 60 percent by age forty-five.[31] (White women do not reach that level of hypertension prevalence until they are in their sixties.) By age thirty, that probability has already increased to more than 35 percent for the Black mother.

And what about cardiovascular diseases in general? A study by Andrea Creanga and colleagues, which included a statistical analysis of pregnancy-related death rates across several populations in the US—including non-Hispanic white, non-Hispanic Black, Hispanic, and others—showed that the medical causes of maternal deaths shifted between 1987 and 2010.[32] Hemorrhage was by far the leading cause of maternal death in 1987, and remained a major cause of maternal death in 2010, yet the proportion of maternal deaths due to hemorrhage was cut by over half during this period as a new mix of causes took center stage. The proportion of maternal deaths attributed to cardiovascular conditions, cardiomyopathy, and infections each surpassed hemorrhage; cardiovascular deaths ranked first among the causes—accounting, in fact, for five times as many annual maternal deaths in 2006–2010 as they had in 1987. Given estimates that one in two Black women over age twenty have some form of cardiovascular disease, and cardiovascular disease is the number one killer of Black women, this further indicates that postponing childbirth until their twenties or beyond has put them at greater risk. And that's what we see when we look at the statistics. As illustrated in the chart below, pregnancy-associated death rates for Black women in their late twenties and thirties are higher than those among teen mothers (echoing what we saw when comparing infant mortality rates for Black teen mothers with that of older Black mothers).[33]

Maternal Mortality by Age

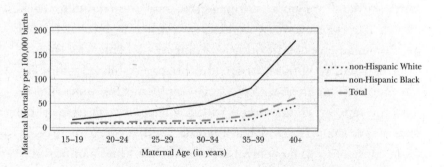

While for white mothers the aging-related risk of having a pregnancy-associated death rises very slowly and gradually until the thirty-five-and-over range, the risk for Black mothers increases substantially with every age increment beyond the teen years. By ages thirty-five to thirty-nine, a Black mother's risk of dying is approaching twice that of her early thirties; three times that of her mid-to-late twenties; four times that of her early twenties; and five times greater than that of her teens. Maternal death rates for Black women in their forties go through the roof (and are nearly seven times the rate for white women the same age). It's worth noting that these findings hold true despite the fact that mothers in their thirties, as a group, are more highly educated, have higher incomes, and are more likely to be married and have (private) health insurance than teen mothers. While the increase with age is steepest among Black women with no more than a high school education (not shown), regardless of socioeconomic position, Black women in the United States keep weathering over time as they are subjected to the stressors that afflict a marginalized, stereotyped, exploited, and looked-down-upon population.

Risks for Black Women — Rich and Poor, Famous and Not

Who are these Black mothers who are dying in their twenties and thirties? Many are poor, working-class, and less-educated Black women like twenty-seven-year-old Erica Garner, as one might suspect. But many are not. In 2016, according to the Centers for Disease Control and Prevention (CDC), the pregnancy-related mortality rates for Black mothers with a college degree was five times higher than the rate for white mothers with a college degree. In fact, the maternal mortality rate for Black mothers with a college degree or more education was 60 percent higher than for white mothers who did not graduate from high school!

Starting in 2017, the public began to get word of the maternal deaths of Black women we could not simply write off as "poor," "unhealthy" or "undeserving." A spate of highly successful Black mothers in their twenties or thirties who died or almost died in 2017 and 2018 gave a public face to weathering. Their cases seemed like inexplicable aberrations. But as the chart above makes clear, they weren't. Following are a few of those women:

Shalon Irving, PhD, was a member of the Epidemiology Intelligence Service at the CDC, the preeminent public health institution in the US. Among the tragic ironies of her death, Shalon was professionally dedicated to promoting health equity. "She wanted to expose how people's limited health options were leading to poor health outcomes," said Dr. Rashid Njai, her mentor at the CDC, "to kind of uncover and undo the victim-blaming that sometimes happens where it's like, 'Poor people don't care about their health.'" Yet, her own body may have suffered from the same structural violence she was working to name and undo. She died of complications of high blood pressure—a condition often seen in weathered bodies—just a few weeks after giving birth to her daughter. She was thirty-six years old.[34]

Sergeant Tahmesha Dickey was a dedicated, veteran police officer. She was described as "a true team player," who had been with the force since 2002, sixteen years to the day before her death, in January 2018. Those who interacted with her said she was always kind and helpful to the community. According to her spouse, "her work ethic was amazing" and she was "very generous, motivated, dedicated to her family. [...] She was just a caring loving person." Tahmesha Dickey's pregnancy had gone well; she was not classified as high risk and had regular prenatal visits. But during labor, Dickey began having trouble breathing. Within minutes, she went into cardiac arrest. She was thirty-eight years old—very young for a heart attack. But we know that heart attacks are among the cardiovascular results of weathering.[35]

Kira Dixon Johnson was a successful international businesswoman, a marathon runner, a licensed pilot, and avid skydiver who spoke five languages. She was the daughter-in-law of prominent lawyer and TV judge Glenda Hatchett and enjoyed a very affluent life. Yet, when giving birth by C-section to her second child, it all went horribly wrong. It is alleged that the planned (not emergency) C-section was rushed and performed recklessly. Apparently, her bladder was lacerated in the process. Despite showing clear signs that she was hemorrhaging internally—which may have been partially facilitated by having blood vessels weakened by weathering—doctors let her lie helplessly for ten hours before getting her into surgery, even while her family was pleading for assistance. She was thirty-nine years old.[36]

One woman who didn't die, but came very close, was Serena Williams, who, as a world-class tennis champion and superstar, needs no introduction. Whether you think she is the "greatest female athlete" or simply the "greatest athlete" of all time, her physical fitness and work ethic are unquestionable. To have become that champion requires incredible drive, discipline, resilience, and grit. Anyone who tuned into her reality show, *Being Serena*, saw a testament not just to her determination but to how strong and vigorous she was, even when she was fewer than six months postpartum. In that show, Serena was seen breastfeeding and pumping milk for her daughter, Olympia, while at the same time embarking on a grueling exercise and practice regimen to stage her elite tennis championship comeback. By nine months postpartum, she competed in the French Open, a Grand Slam tournament, and by ten months postpartum she won her way to the women's finals at Wimbledon. Yet, as her husband, Alexis Ohanian, ruminated after watching her recover at age thirty-six from a near-death experience shortly after giving birth to their daughter, her body, which had taken her to the greatest heights of athleticism, was also nearly her undoing. "Consider for a moment that your body is one of the greatest things on this planet, and you're trapped in it."[37]

Trapped in it? Serena was only in her mid-thirties, not even middle-aged. But he was right: Serena was trapped—trapped in the body of a Black woman in the US, and therefore likely to have been trapped in a body that had been weathered. Seen from this perspective, the life-threatening blood clots she experienced post-delivery were a manifestation of her weathering, which trumped all of her other advantages, including being extraordinarily fit and possessed of enough money to access the finest medical care available.

None of the Black women profiled here fit the conventional wisdom on health disparities. They were not stereotypes—none of them were poor, welfare-dependent, or teenage mothers. Yet, while we don't know how representative these specific mothers are, they are not anomalies. As we've seen, contrary to entrenched popular belief—and despite having more financial resources, higher educations, and better access to health care—Black mothers in their twenties and thirties are more likely to die within a year of childbirth than those in their teens. We've seen this is true for their babies as well.

Note also that these highly publicized cases cover a range of socioeconomic experiences. Sergeant Tahmesha Dickey had a solidly middle-class public service job; Shalon Irving and Kira Dixon Johnson had affluent backgrounds and graduate educations; Serena Williams ascended from a working-class childhood to superstardom and the wealth that typically accrues to such fame. Earning about $45 million in 2021, and with an estimated net worth well over $200 million, Serena Williams is a member of not simply the top 1 percent or even the top 0.1 percent, but roughly the top 0.001 percent of Americans in income and wealth.[38]

But what all these mothers shared was the experience of being Black pregnant women in the United States in their thirties. Kira Johnson, Tahmesha Dickey, and Shalon Irving all came to their birthing experiences without recognizable preexisting conditions. Their tragic stories could be described as some combination of bad luck, acts of God, and medical errors, including ones made as a product of racist ideas.[39] Serena Williams, who did have a preexisting condition, in the form of a history of blood clots, could be seen as just an unfortunate example of a high-risk pregnancy. But were they?

Each of these women could be written off as an exception. But it may not be by individual misfortune that they suffered as they did. It's possible, even likely, that in part or whole, their lived experience as Black women exerted wear and tear on their bodies in a way that predisposed them to highly traumatic birth experiences, which for three of them led to their deaths.

Serena Williams had a history of blood clots before her pregnancy, so it should have been no surprise that she developed blood clots after giving birth. But the fact that she had such a history at all is, at first glance, surprising. Why would a woman as young and fit as Serena Williams have experienced life-threatening blood clots in her twenties, years before her pregnancy? Outside of pregnancy, primary risk factors for blood clots are being middle-aged or older, being obese, being male, and leading an extremely sedentary life—none of which describe Serena.

So, what happened? Media coverage of her blood-clotting disorder chalked it up to a vague notion of "family history," implying it must be an inherited predisposition. But no specifics were given, and in the absence of any proof of a family history, a much more likely cause is weathering. Insofar as "family history" *is* involved, however, Serena and her equally extraordinary sister Venus (who was diagnosed in her twenties with Sjögren's syndrome, an uncommon autoimmune disorder) do share a history—a history of being pioneering Black women in a virtually all white country-club sport who were treated with hostility and subjected to gendered and racist stereotyping throughout their highly visible careers.[40]

In fact, their grit and determination in the face of such barriers was likely one source of their weathering. Serena and Venus Williams have both negotiated systemically racist spaces throughout their lives, whether those spaces were the material, environmental, and physical aspects of their disinvested racially segregated childhood neighborhood, or the racist halls of the elite tennis circuit of their professional lives. Many spectators have commented on the extraordinary levels of hostility Serena and Venus have had to contend with from the media, sports announcers, some tennis fans, and even game officials. As recently as March 2021, in a statement of solidarity with Meghan Markle, whose experience with racism in the tabloid press appears to have reminded her of her own, Serena said, "I know firsthand the sexism and racism institutions and the media use to vilify women of color to minimize us, to break us down and to demonize us. [...] The mental health consequences of systemic oppression and victimization are devastating, isolating and all too often lethal."[41]

Giving Birth while Being Black: "Devastating, Isolating, and All Too Often Lethal"

Having access to a good medical care system does not protect Black mothers from the implicit or explicit biases of clinicians in a systemically racist system. Many have rightly pointed to racism as contributing to the disproportionate number of Black maternal deaths.[42] A frequent refrain is that Black mothers are often not attended to responsively by their care providers when their condition begins to go south, or even once it begins to plummet disastrously. There is compelling evidence that this is true.

The stories of all the women described here suggest that they fell victim not just to weathering, but also possibly to the implicit anti-Black bias in the health-care system. Shalon Irving made several calls and trips to the doctor complaining that things were not right. After being repeatedly turned away, she collapsed and died at home only hours after the last doctor she saw dismissively gave her the "all clear."[43] Kira Johnson spent ten hours hemorrhaging after a physician botched her C-section, in a top-ranked hospital, before she was finally attended to, far too late to save her life. Serena's attempt to call attention to her risk of blood clots was at first dismissed.[44]

Many would say that what separated Serena Williams's outcome— she survived—from those who died was that, as Serena Williams, she was ultimately able to demand that her concerns about the possibility of blood clots be addressed. But it was a struggle, and one she shouldn't have had to make. She had experienced life-threatening blood clots in the past and was familiar with the symptoms. Moreover, the physical demands of pregnancy augment any woman's chance of suffering blood clots, with or without a history of them. Even so, Serena Williams had to fight to be taken seriously. When she told her nurse that she needed a CT scan for blood clots, the nurse assumed she was confused and instead a doctor ordered an ultrasound of her leg, which revealed nothing. When she was finally given the CT scan she had insisted on, her doctors discovered the blood clots that had settled in her lungs.[45] One wonders what would have happened if she had been someone with fewer resources—less wealth, less celebrity, less tenacity. Most likely, she would have died.

The stories of Shalon Irving, Kira Johnson, and Serena Williams certainly raise questions about whether their being Black women had something to do with the slow-to-respond medical care they received. Ignorance on the part of their clinical caretakers might have played a role, too, in theirs and in Erica Garner's and Tahmesha Dickey's pregnancy-associated health crises. Did any of the medical personnel know that, as Black American women in their twenties and thirties, all of them were at high risk for severe maternal morbidity and mortality despite their financial security and success? Or did they assume that they were low risk, given they were not teenagers, high school dropouts, or over age forty?

Long before they entered the medical profession, the doctors and nurses in the delivery room may have been primed to be unaware of the lifelong health erosion of Black women, even the wealthy and educated ones. That ignorance is yet another result of life and work in a racist society where the reality of weathering is simply not seen or acknowledged. For the women in those delivery rooms, the result can be that their medical team makes life-threatening errors.

The role of racism, whether implicit or explicit, in shaping the response of health-care providers and health-care systems must be called out and addressed. Health-care providers need to understand that how they treat Black women prenatally, during delivery, and in the postpartum period can make a life-or-death difference for the mothers and their babies. However, they also need to understand the role weathering plays in making childbirth a life-or-death situation for too many Black mothers and babies in the first place.

Society needs to take Black women's health seriously, not only when they are fighting for oxygen or their pulse is fading or they are bleeding out in the prenatal, delivery, or postpartum period, but during the decades before they land, in extremis, in the maternity ward. If we don't, the consequences will continue to be "devastating, isolating, and all too often lethal."

Since 1991, the rates of teen pregnancy have dropped by roughly 75 percent.[46] In 2013, the CDC reported that birth rates for US teens fifteeen- to nineteen-years-old dropped to a low not seen since 1946.[47] Nonetheless, even now, after the enormous decrease in teen motherhood in America, it is rare for poor or working-class Black mothers to postpone childbearing beyond their early twenties. Whether consciously or culturally, they know better. Culturally, they know postponing childbearing is risky and not well calibrated to their personal needs or those of their child, their family, or their community. But what is it that they know that the rest of us do not see?

5.

Collectively Weathering Weathering

For members of oppressed groups who cannot count on range or generosity of government safety nets that just about every other affluent country in the world offers its citizens, the secret to surviving hardship is hiding in plain sight: their own extended families and friends. These constitute the reciprocal and mutually affirming networks that allow them to piece together some kind of economic security, and that help to buffer them against the worst consequences of weathering.

To see this in action, I can look to my own multigenerational working-class immigrant family, both sides of which immigrated to the US to escape horrific genocidal pogroms in the Russian Empire, and then had to endure fierce anti-Semitism and poverty in their new country. My maternal grandfather, Isadore, fled the pogroms taking place in his Ukrainian shtetl in the early twentieth century when he was only sixteen. He never saw his family again. My older sister was named for Grandpa Isadore's mother and sister, who survived the pogroms only to be killed in the Holocaust. While still in his teens, my grandfather served in the US armed forces in World War I. Family lore has it that he began his adult working life in the upper boroughs of New York City as a banana peddler, keeping company with the pet banana spiders he rescued from his import crates. Eventually, he kept company with my grandmother Annie, who was also a Ukrainian

Jewish immigrant whose family had come to the US to escape the violence of the pogroms. Annie and Isadore married, and together they raised three first-generation American children, including my mother, Miriam, her older brother, Henry, and her younger sister, Riva.

My grandma Annie was what is known in Yiddish culture as a balabosta. A balabosta is a woman who commands respect in the family and within the broader community. She takes great pride in making a home, raising children, sustaining the spiritual life of the family, keeping the financial accounts of the household, and doing good works in the community. She is also likely to engage in income-generating activities, whether in the paid labor market or from her home. In my grandmother's case, she worked long hours in a sweatshop.

To protect her family and carry on all her many disparate duties successfully, a working-class balabosta is required to have what we call a *yiddishe kop*—literally a Yiddish head. A *yiddishe kop* has the mental agility to think fast when her back is up against the wall and the stakes are high. My grandmother had to use her *yiddishe kop* every day to help her family survive and thrive. (When, at age three, my daughter offered her observation that "men can do some things, and women can do everything," I imagined that she had channeled this perspective from the spirits of her balabosta ancestors.)

With time, my grandfather was able to develop his own small banana-import business. He and my grandmother saved and invested in a truck and rented storage space at the Bronx Terminal Market. In this era before supermarkets, he delivered bananas to small fruit-and-vegetable markets in the Bronx and in Harlem, within a short radius of where they lived. It was a living, but such a modest one that the family was often unable to pay their rent. So they were perpetually on the move from one apartment to another. This helped them reduce their housing costs because they could take advantage of "first month free" promotions, but moving every year must have put quite a strain on everybody.

By age forty-two, my grandpa developed a heart condition that left him physically disabled. While he could still drive the truck, he could no longer lift and pack the crates into the truck or unload and carry the crates to customers. To help out, his son, Henry, quit high school after the ninth grade. This multigenerational all-hands-on-deck approach was expected of members of working-class immigrant families, as it always has been and continues to be for many marginalized groups with precarious incomes and little wealth. Had my uncle Henry not stepped in, the family would have descended into greater poverty and, possibly, homelessness.

Henry fought in World War II and got married shortly before the war ended. He and his wife lived with her parents for a time before they could move into a home of their own. Multigenerational households are one way working-class families stretch dollars (although the value of this form of family organization goes beyond the financial). While living with his in-laws, Henry continued to deliver the bananas his father imported, thus continuing to be a major provider for his family of origin even as he was working toward becoming the primary supporter of the family he had formed with his wife.

Neither Henry nor Riva rose professionally far above their working-class roots. But one member of the family—my mother, Miriam—would, against all odds, find her way into the professional class. Rushed to the hospital with a burst appendix at age eleven, she was so impressed by the doctors who diagnosed her condition and the surgeons who operated on her that this daughter of a fruit vendor and a sweatshop worker set her sights then and there on becoming a physician. Never mind that female doctors were a rarity at this time, or that medical schools actively discriminated against not just women applicants but Jewish applicants too, my mother believed in her balabosta-daughter's heart that she could do anything.

Just as they rallied to my grandfather's aid when he would otherwise have lost the small banana business, my mother's family rallied to make her dream a reality. Not only did they keep the family afloat day to day, but Henry and my grandmother also contributed to a family fund to support Miriam's dream of attending medical school.

Miriam certainly did her part. She quickly dispatched with her high school education, taking advantage of the "rapid advance" program in New York City public schools to graduate at age fifteen. She proceeded to attend night school at Hunter College, a public, tuition-free women's college she could reach by subway, living at home and working a full-time job during the day to make her own contribution to the family coffers. It took her six years to graduate on a night school schedule.

After first being rejected by the few US medical schools that admitted women, Miriam was ready to move to Switzerland, where women doctors were not so unheard-of. However, at the last minute, with her bags packed for Switzerland, she got word that the Women's Medical College of Pennsylvania had granted her admission. My grandmother was so committed to helping my mother achieve her goals that she hid some of her meager sweatshop earnings from the household accounts until she had saved enough to buy my mother a car so she could live at home and commute to her medical school classes in Philadelphia—two hours each way. I don't know who named the car Gorgeous, but the name reflected the excitement and gratitude Miriam felt at having been gifted it. I could still hear those feelings of excitement and gratitude in her voice when she spoke the name decades later, long after Gorgeous was retired to the junkyard.

Miriam realized her dream, completing medical school and her residency, to become a board-certified pathologist. Hired to work as a pathologist in a Veterans Administration hospital, analyzing biopsies and conducting autopsies on veterans, she never came close to matching the earnings of her male colleagues (or what she might have made in private practice). Such jobs were hard to come by for female physicians. The prevailing ideology at the time was that men were breadwinners who should be paid a "family wage," and women, should they work at all, worked for "pin money"—with no exceptions made even for women who became physicians and continued to contribute to the support of their parents as well as their own households.

My hardworking balabosta grandmother died of a stroke at age fifty-eight after suffering minor strokes and complications of diabetes for at least a decade. Her last year of life was my first. During the final days of Annie's life, when she needed round-the-clock care, Riva and Henry and their families, who lived close to my grandparents, did both the literal and the figurative heavy lifting for them. And although my mother had by then moved to Boston, she spent many of her weekends in New York taking her turn caring for her dying mother and disabled father. This was before the Massachusetts Turnpike had been built; the tedious drive took her six stop-and-start hours each way—quite a burden for a woman who at that time had two children under five and a full-time job.

My mother died of an aggressive cancer at the age of forty-five, even younger than her mother had been at her death. She left behind three small children, my sisters and me. Our father, who was at that point living in an affluent suburb where nuclear families were the rule, had none of the multigenerational familial help that characterized the homes that both he and my mother had grown up in, so he raised us on his own. But even as he was supporting us, he continued to send money to his mother and one of his sisters—and even to my mother's father and, occasionally, to her sister, Riva, my maternal aunt, as long as they lived. Being accountable to a multigenerational and extended network of kin was how he himself had been raised, and that's what he felt was expected of him.

It would be easy to frame my mother as Horatia Alger, proof that anyone can succeed in this country if they just work hard enough and keep their eyes on the prize. But although that is how our individualist culture would probably view her, that would be wrong. Yes, my mother worked hard, and she never allowed the many societal barriers to deter her from achieving her professional goals. Yet the willingness of her mother and her teenage brother to roll up their sleeves to support her in her ambitions was critical to what she was able to achieve. Her social mobility was a cooperative venture.

Rather than acknowledging my uncle Henry's important contribution to his sister's success, popular culture would probably brand him a high school dropout, lacking in ambition and self-regulation. After all, if his sister could defy the odds and become a female physician, what was wrong with him that he couldn't even graduate high school? Comparing Miriam to Henry through the prisms of individualism and the American Creed might suggest that he was just a loser, someone unable to rise above his station in life because he did not take personal responsibility, while she succeeded because of her single-minded determination to do so. But this characterization of my uncle's role and of my mother's unlikely academic journey fails to capture the reality of their lives.

Whether or not he had a sister who dreamed of becoming a doctor, Henry needed to work full time in order to rescue his family from potential disaster once my grandfather became disabled. That he could also contribute to Miriam's improbable medical school aspirations was icing on the cake. But without the contribution he made, those aspirations would almost certainly have come to nothing, a pipe dream that my mother could never have realized on her own. And the family recognized that contribution. Uncle Henry was never held in any less esteem by his family than my mother was. Although the dominant culture might value a medical school education over a ninth grade education, no one in the family ever seems to have forgotten that what my mother achieved was possible only because of what my uncle sacrificed.

My mother's childhood family was resilient in the face of its challenges, thanks to its members' willingness to share responsibility for the economic well-being of all, and to be flexible about reassigning roles when, as in the wake of my grandfather's disability, it became necessary. Like members of all marginalized groups, this family of immigrant, working-class Jews developed and maintained strategies — in effect insurance policies — that allowed them to at least mitigate the adverse impact of systemic prejudice and entrenched poverty. Such strategies, which are deeply embedded in the respective cultures of the various groups that employ them, are almost automatic. They become what the Harvard anthropologist Robert A. LeVine calls "tested commonsense formulas that embody a folk wisdom."[1] This folk wisdom is woven from the facts of people's lives—the resources and opportunities available to them, the constraints operating against them, and the particular cultural values they hold, given their history and their traditions.

Many of us, including legislators and policy makers, dismiss or are completely unaware of the importance of these "commonsense formulas" because, in light of our greater opportunities, financial resources, and privileges, they don't seem like common sense to us. Why would a son quit high school in the ninth grade, or a widower feel himself responsible to contribute to the family of his dead wife? But for those who have lived precarious lives, which may be cut short or made difficult by the early onset of disabilities such as that experienced by my grandfather, they are critical to maintaining some kind of stability and security. Acknowledging the survival value of such strategies, however, doesn't mean that we should minimize the profound and often painful trade-offs and sacrifices that have to be made in the absence of a reliable social safety net, secure employment, and a living wage.

Early Death and Prolonged Disability in Marginalized Families

I never knew my mother well enough to know whether her cancer and early death might plausibly be attributed to weathering. Given a childhood spent in poverty and uncertainty about the future, the anti-Semitism and sexism that she faced in making her way into the profession of her dreams, and the hard work, tenacity, and logistical heroics required to get her there, her life certainly shows all the earmarks of weathering. My grandparents' lives do, too.

My grandfather's youth was hard, even traumatic; the losses he sustained at a young age are unfathomable. The same could be said of my grandmother. And both had to work extraordinarily hard to feed, clothe, and house their children. My grandfather's early disability from heart disease (at forty-two), my grandmother's decade of minor strokes and diabetes culminating in her early death from a stroke (at fifty-eight), and my mother's even earlier death from cancer (forty-five), are all diseases and conditions in which weathering can play a part.

If you are a member of the dominant culture, it is safe for you to assume, as the English writer Ronald Blythe wrote, that your death will likely fall in its "logical position" at the end of a long and healthy life.[2] However, those in culturally oppressed and exploited populations can make no such assumption. My research team calculated the age trajectories of disability and mortality across a number of disinvested urban and rural areas, as well as for white people nationwide.[3]

According to our calculations, populations that are among the poorest, most marginalized, and culturally oppressed—whether Blacks living in disinvested neighborhoods in the urban North or whites living in disinvested areas of Appalachia in the rural South—die and incur disabilities at ages that are much younger than the national average among whites.

Two examples of the populations we studied are Black residents of segregated, high-poverty neighborhoods on the South Side of Chicago and white residents of high-poverty counties in the Appalachian region of Kentucky, including Owsley County, which is among the poorest counties in the nation. What characterizes these two groups is not their entrenched poverty alone, but also their long histories of economic exploitation, cultural oppression, and political marginalization. Today, these populations serve as the canaries in the coal mine, so to speak. In the face of macroeconomic restructuring, globalization, automation, and the evolving high-tech and green economy, they are becoming less employable than ever—and unhealthier than ever, too.

The table on the next page shows the dramatic disparities in the percentage of men and women who can expect to die before age sixty-five in each of these two communities compared to the average among white Americans in the US.

Probability of Dying Between Ages Sixteen and Sixty-Five, as of 2000

	United States (All Whites)	Appalachian Kentucky (Poor Whites)	South Side, Chicago (Poor Blacks)
Men	20 percent	29 percent	50 percent
Women	12 percent	18 percent	32 percent

As of 2000, the average white sixteen-year-old in this country could reasonably expect to live until at least their sixty-fifth birthday. (Eight out of ten white men and almost nine out of ten white women were estimated to do so.) But for poor whites in Appalachian Kentucky, nearly a third of the men and nearly a fifth of the women could have no such expectation. The corresponding probabilities for poor Black residents of the South Side of Chicago were even worse. About a third of sixteen-year-old girls and fully half of sixteen-year-old boys could expect to die before their sixty-fifth birthday. Bear in mind that in these impoverished, oppressed populations, life expectancy has gotten lower since 2000, so there's every reason to suspect these numbers are now worse.

The media likes to point to existential despair and the abuse of opioids as the main causes of early death in poor and working-class areas of Appalachia, and to the violence of the drug economy and the frequency of overdoses as the main causes of early death in poor and working-class areas in disinvested urban communities like South Side. But as we saw in chapters one and two, such claims are much exaggerated. For example, for every Black man between the ages of sixteen and sixty-five killed by homicide on the South Side, four Black men in the same age range suffer deaths attributable to circulatory disease and cancer. Among Black women on the South Side, nine times more excess deaths are due to circulatory disease and cancer than to homicide. The disproportion is even greater for poor Appalachian whites: seven times more excess deaths in men and twelve times more excess deaths in women are attributable to circulatory disease and cancer than to homicide. In short, we found that the primary causes of excess deaths in these and other similar populations are chronic diseases associated with weathering. (In Appalachia, workplace accidents also contribute, especially for coal miners.)

But death is only the tip of the iceberg. For those who do not die from disease or a workplace accident, the probability of being disabled at an early age looms large. We compared health-induced disability rates by various ages for the same three groups portrayed in the table on the previous page. A health-induced disability is defined as a functional limitation that results from a health condition of at least six months' duration that hampers one's capacity for work, mobility, or personal care. My grandfather's heart condition is an example of such a disability because it limited his capacity to work.

As shown in the table, the results of our study were sobering. For example, the disability rates for thirty-five-year-old male Black residents of South Side (26 percent) were similar to the national average of whites twenty years older (24 percent), while thirty-five-year-old male white residents of Appalachian Kentucky suffered a shockingly high 36 percent disability rate.

Estimated Prevalence of Any Health-Induced Disability by Age, Sex, Race, and Population in the Year 2000

Age	United States	Appalachian Kentucky	South Side, Chicago
Men	All Whites	Poor Whites	Poor Blacks
35	15 percent	36 percent	26 percent
55	24 percent	50 percent	41 percent
75	44 percent	71 percent	57 percent
Women	All Whites	Poor Whites	Poor Blacks
35	13 percent	28 percent	27 percent
55	21 percent	42 percent	44 percent
75	43 percent	67 percent	64 percent

With a quarter to more than a third of the men and women in these two high-poverty areas suffering a health-induced functional limitation by the age of thirty-five, and 41–50 percent of the fifty-five-year-olds suffering health-induced limitations, families face prolonged disability of the kind that weakens their economic prospects and may call for adaptations like those in my own family, in which my young uncle had to drop out of school when my grandfather could not continue his banana business without help.

When we looked at the most severe health-induced limitations, like those my grandmother suffered in her last years—those that interfere not just with the ability to work but with the ability to leave home alone or to perform personal care activities, such as bathing or dressing—we found even worse disparities. The rates for disabilities that require constant care are two to three times higher for thirty-five-year-olds in the Chicago and Appalachian populations than for the average fifty-five-year-old white person in the US. Rates for fifty-five-year-olds in the two local areas were as high as or higher than those for seventy-five-year-old whites nationwide. And the data for seventy-five-year-olds in the two local areas show that more than half of those who survive to this age are disabled, with up to about 40 percent—twice the national average for white people—suffering disabilities severe enough to require 24/7 care. Imagine the burden these disability rates place on families!

Both of these populations—one Black, one white—show evidence of severe weathering. Along with other similarly high-poverty urban and rural populations we've studied, the bulk of the health disadvantage among these groups occurs in those of working and reproductive age. A substantial percentage already suffer from stress-related chronic diseases in their mid-twenties and early thirties, and the proportion increases rapidly through their forties and fifties. Those affected may be unable to work or limited as to the kind of work they do, may require caregiving, and may face an early death.

With such high rates of death and disability, only about 50

percent of Black youth residing in the South Side's disinvested neighborhoods or white youths residing in Appalachia's pockets of poverty and exploitation can expect to survive and be able-bodied at age fifty. In both places, those who survive to their fifties can expect to spend about a third of their lives disabled.

Taking death and disability together, families in populations subject to weathering need to be prepared for the very real possibility that one or more family members will experience prolonged disability, and that one of their main providers may die at a young age. These considerations are overlooked by popular age-washed narratives that assume everyone of working and reproductive age will be able-bodied. Poor and culturally oppressed families know otherwise.

For families living uncertain paycheck to uncertain paycheck, anticipating the potential impact of weathering is tricky, because weathering does not mean that *every* member of a poor, culturally oppressed, or politically marginalized community will get sick, become disabled, or die young. It means that *anyone* could—but predicting who will is no easy task. In my mother's family of origin, she along with her mother and sister all died relatively young (between the ages of forty-five and sixty-one). Meanwhile, her father lived with his disability for forty years (half his life), and her brother survived to just shy of his ninetieth birthday, suffering severe chronic morbidity and functional disability only in his last decade. Without a crystal ball, some flexibility in family roles and responsibilities is required as preparation for a whole range of plausible scenarios of weathering. Not knowing who will be in need, or how much need, or when, but having every reason to believe that need will come sometime, people in these communities cannot leave the outcome to chance, nor can they hope to depend on the kindness of strangers—or on the weak and unreliable American social welfare safety net.

As we've seen time and time again, weathering lays bare the myth that working-age adults are by definition able-bodied. This myth underlies so much of the dominant cultural disdain for the oppressed, whether they are stigmatized as hillbillies in Appalachia or as inner-city Black people in the North. It also helps to explain why Americans look down on those on welfare. As Martin Gilens reported in his book *Why Americans Hate Welfare*, Americans interpret welfare as "cash benefits paid to the working-age, able-bodied poor."[4] As the statistics just cited make clear, a very substantial percentage of working-age adults who receive government benefits (or don't but desperately need them) are not able-bodied. They are suffering from weathering-related disabilities that afflict them at far too early an age.

Commonsense Formulas for Configuring and Protecting Poor and Marginalized Families

Weathering is cruel and unforgiving. Because it increases the chances of widowhood, orphanhood, and prolonged disability in the family, weathering enlarges the scope of caretaking needs in a community even as it simultaneously depletes the pool of caregivers and economic providers. It means that there is a lower chance of both parents surviving and being well enough to care for their children. It also means that many working- and reproductive-age adults, plenty of whom have disabilities of their own, will be sandwiched between caring for their children and their parents and extended families—a challenge that is hard enough for the affluent, and can be overwhelming for those living in poverty.

To anticipate their chances of becoming sick or disabled or dying at a relatively young age, today's poor and marginalized groups do not need to calculate probabilities or refer to tables that provide the relevant statistics. They have only to look at the evidence around them. In an earlier ethnography of a Black high-poverty population, Burton noted that 91 percent of the women interviewed estimated their life expectancy to be sixty years.[5] A twenty-one-year-old mother in the study commented, "I've been seeing people die when they are around fifty-eight all my life. I'm surprised that my grandmother (age sixty-two) is still around." I saw evidence of this, too, in the interviews I did with teen mothers from disinvested urban and rural areas. And Dr. Karida Brown's ethnography of an Appalachian coal-mining town showed that the possibility of death and prolonged disability loomed large in the minds of people of any age, not just the chronologically old.[6] For example, several of the children she interviewed

> were hyperaware of the possibility that a mining accident could befall their fathers any day. [...] The unspoken under-standing that their family could be the next one to get "the call" is the tie that binds all mining families. Memories of the ambulance sirens, broken and dismembered parts, and gur-neys and hearses were just as everyday as the sound of the red robins chirping and the sight of the blackberry and apple orchards blossoming.

How do twenty-first-century families who are poor, culturally oppressed, and marginalized cope with the formidable threat that weathering poses to their family economies and caretaking systems? Such hardships and caretaking challenges can be met only if one looks beyond the nuclear family—i.e., two married parents and their children—to a much larger universe of adults who can take responsibility for financially supporting and caring for dependents, both old and young. Growing ethnographic scholarship of and by members of these communities, as well as memoirs written by some who were raised in these circumstances, paint a vivid portrait. Their commonsense formulas for resilience and resistance include some version of the following features.

Kin Networks

Ethnographic and survey evidence shows that African Americans and rural poor whites often view family as a multigenerational network of kin who may or may not be biologically or legally related, but who share a mutual understanding that they are part of a familial network of reciprocal obligations. Acting in accordance with this perception, they fulfill economic and caretaking functions that are often thought by the dominant culture to be the responsibility only of the parents in nuclear families. As the anthropologist Carol Stack first elaborated in her classic work of ethnography, *All Our Kin*, kin networks are dynamic systems that help to shore up scarce material and caregiving resources among members by pooling risk: today I will take care of your sick mother and children while you go to work; tomorrow you will take my family in when I am evicted.[7] Household boundaries and practices are, as Stack termed them, "elastic." Whether families need to double up, send children or disabled elders to be cared for by others, or have members migrate to greener employment pastures than are available nearby, it is critical that they acknowledge as central members of their network people who may or may not be blood relatives or part of their immediate household, and indeed may live at a considerable distance from them.

In order to maximize flexibility in the face of necessity, kin networks also operate within relatively more fluid gender role norms for the division of labor than the dominant (and contested) American ideal, and less-rigid developmental understandings of what the capacities and responsibilities of older children and youth can be.[8] As a whole, this commonsense kin network formula increases the number of potential "hands on deck," as well as the pool of resources to draw upon. As Stack explained, "in times of need the only predictable resources that can be drawn upon are their own children and parents and the fund of kin and friends obligated to them."

The obvious value of multigenerational kin network systems does not mean that they are uniformly positive for or without costs to their participants. The costs can be very high indeed, involving considerable sacrifice and a willingness to put off or forego personal goals. Of course, that is true of other family structures, too, including the nuclear family. In a 2020 commentary in *The Atlantic*, David Brooks made the case that, as a headline-writer put it in an article subtitle, "the [nuclear] family structure we've held up as the cultural ideal for the past half century has been a catastrophe for many."[9] A 2022 Pew Foundation report found that the population living in multigenerational households in the United States had quadrupled since 1971, showing the weakened strength of the 1950s nuclear family norm, even among white families.[10] When assessing the value of various family arrangements in specific contexts, the only relevant question is whether they work. Are they, on balance, and in the absence of any other realistic options, better or worse than the alternatives in terms of serving the needs of those who have to be cared for and supported?

Collectivism

Different groups or societies thread the needle differently between the human desire for independence and the human need for interdependence. For culturally oppressed groups, however, the collective ethos is an essential pillar of survival, resilience, and resistance. Child-rearing goals and social expectations and sanctions must center cooperation, interdependence, mutual responsibility, and a willingness to suppress personal goals when necessary for the group. Collectivism is the normative glue that makes the fulfilling of obligations as a member of an extended, multigenerational, cross-household kin network possible and a source of pride. As the psychologist and professor Janie Ward recalled from her childhood, "For many summers our home was like a Black folks summer camp, with my family informally adopting kin and friends, all focused on nurturing our collective survival, fostering cooperation, interdependence, and responsibility for one another."[11]

In addition to material resources and opportunities, this sense of collectivism and community provides an affirmation of the cultural values, practices, affective ties, and beliefs that give life purpose and meaning. And it offers members of the community a counternarrative to the dominant culture's image of them as morally marred or culturally deficient. These psychosocial resources may be especially important in mitigating the stress-related diseases that are weathering.

Childbearing at an Early Age

As discussed in chapter four, my research shows that in populations subject to weathering, the probability of adverse pregnancy outcomes increases with a mother's age. The disability statistics listed previously also suggest that any adult's ability to offer care and support, rather than to require it, is uncertain. To maintain the collective functions of kin networks, weathering places a premium on at least some women having children before the onset and progression of chronic diseases. As one fifty-eight-year-old participant in Linda Burton's ethnography of a Black semirural, high-poverty community said, "The best way to make sure that you have enough able bodies to take care of the needs in the family is to start the women having children as soon as they can."[12]

Shocking or surprising as this may sound, because of the impact of weathering on fertility, birth outcomes, early and prolonged disability, and premature death, some (maybe many, but not all) mothers will have their first children between the ages of sixteen and twenty-two. (Most of these mothers are at least age eighteen.) Doing so can be a well-calibrated adaptation to the realities of life in culturally oppressed, exploited, and poor communities. This is not deterministic. Even among sisters in the same family, the age at which young women bear children can vary widely, and each can be supported for their actions and recognized within their family for the contributions to the network their disparate paths provide.

Individual young people may have personal agendas that do not include early childbearing. Moreover, young people who show promise as economic providers, or have other talents that give them the opportunity to overcome structural barriers to social mobility, may actually be discouraged from early childbearing.[13] Peers and elders who themselves have little chance at social mobility may rally around and invest in supporting these exceptional youth, just as my grandmother and uncle did for my mother, playing an important role in their eventual social or economic success.

Women-Centered Networks

The concept of a balabosta may seem quaint or folkloric and sexist to people in the dominant culture today. It *is* sexist, and it is a sexism that is systemically imposed. The critical onus placed on American women in working-class and culturally oppressed populations to ensure collective survival existed before balabostas immigrated to the US, and continues to this day to be a feature of life in low-to-moderate-income and marginalized communities. To call a network women-centered neither denies the contributions that men make nor implies that women fall into the stereotype of the emasculating matriarch. Instead, it refers to the ways their structural position at the intersection of class, race, ethnicity, and gender places women in unique positions to contribute to kin networks in critical ways.

There are no pedestals to honor the effort and sacrifices of women in Black or Appalachian families or other oppressed populations. But like my grandmother, these women are essential contributors who assume extraordinary duties in order to foster the survival of their families and communities. In reference to the history of Black women carrying such responsibilities, the late anthropologist Leith Mullings described the ubiquity of the "Sojourner syndrome," named after the abolitionist and women's rights activist Sojourner Truth, who epitomized resilience and activism in the face of racist and material adversity.[14]

Damon Young's tribute to his mother provides one example. In attributing his mother's cause of death to "living while Black," Young, a highly successful writer and public intellectual who grew up in Black, working-class Pittsburgh, describes the lengths his mother went to and the hardships she endured to support their family, given his father's chronic unemployment in the face of racist discrimination. Young recalls "the multiple buses Mom would catch to and from work [...] and the (overfilled) work bag [...] and the purse she'd lug with her, and how the weight of each would make her left shoulder lean like a tree permanently bent by wind." She struggled quite literally under the weight of supporting her family. Drawing on his lived experience, Young writes in his book, *What Doesn't Kill You Makes You Blacker,* that "Black women are socialized to be enduring and steadfast and forgiving and giving giving giving so much that there's nothing left of them but dust."[15]

As is the case for too many weathered and medically underserved Black women, Mrs. Young died in late middle age, having been diagnosed with stage-4 cancer. Young muses: "I wonder if the stress and pressure from existing as our family's only stable income for a decade permeated, consumed, and overwhelmed her." He also notes his closeness to his father during his younger days, when his father was more available to him than his mother because "during this time he wasn't working. [My] Dad-specific nostalgia might not exist the same way without the bricks laid by mom."

Cassie Chambers, now an Ivy League–educated lawyer, grew up in Owsley County, Kentucky, in a multigenerational, extended family of white sharecroppers so poor that a splurge for her family after church on Sundays was to buy one single Happy Meal at the local McDonald's for the entire family to share. She describes the unyielding women in her extended family who played central and critical roles in their survival. In her memoir, *Hill Women,* she writes that these women "modeled independence, hard work, persistence. They took care of me, of one another, and their communities. They embodied the strength and security of the mountains that surrounded them."[16]

Both Cassie Chambers and Damon Young credit their mothers and other female elders in the family for the upward mobility they each achieved. Like my mother, they got ahead in life thanks to the investments and support they received from their family members, not because they simply pulled themselves up by their own bootstraps. And like Damon Young, Cassie Chambers saw the physical price these women paid for their efforts.

The hill women young Cassie Chambers most relied on were her mother, Wilma, and her aunt Ruth. Wilma Chambers developed a debilitating autoimmune disease during her working years—a possible outcome of weathering—and was functionally limited for the rest of her life as her immune system attacked and killed her nerves, causing her horrific and exhausting pain.

Aunt Ruth kept their family of tobacco sharecroppers afloat when her aging parents could no longer manage. As Chambers described it, Aunt Ruth spent her life "breaking her body to contribute to her family." Ruth developed arthritis early in life and suffered bilateral breast cancer at a young age. Chambers notes that Ruth also suffered multiple skin cancers by her mid-thirties and "would cut them off herself with a pocketknife because she didn't have health insurance."

In Chambers' opinion, the backbreaking physical labor endured by both men and women in Appalachia, whether in the fields or in the mines, was a precursor to the opioid epidemic. She concludes that the opioid epidemic hit Appalachian Kentucky hard precisely because "there was so much physical pain there," not because of character weakness or despair.

Wanda and Donnie

The ethnographer and University of Chicago sociologist Sharon Hicks-Bartlett tells the story of Wanda and Donnie, two members of a high-poverty Black urban community she observed.[17] Their story encapsulates all four features of the commonsense formulas for resilience and resistance: a reliance on kin networks, collectivism, early childbearing, and women's central contributions to economic and caretaking support. It also encapsulates the weathering effects of poverty and cultural oppression.

Wanda and Donnie were siblings whose parents raised them along with their two sisters and two male cousins who were taken into the family after the early deaths of their own parents. By middle age, Wanda and Donnie's mother was severely weathered and needed constant care; their father was away from home, having had to migrate to find employment. Wanda, who at this time was a young mother herself, qualified for Aid to Families with Dependent Children (AFDC—the precursor to today's TANF, commonly referred to as welfare), while her sisters had working-class jobs, one in a factory and one clerical. Since her benefits allowed her to stay home, Wanda took over the care of her invalid mother, while also watching her own small child and sometimes her sisters' children, too, as part of the patchwork they cobbled together in the absence of reliable, affordable childcare or eldercare resources. Wanda's ability to shoulder these multigenerational caretaking needs enabled her father and her two sisters to remain employed and provide the family with income. Like a balabosta, or, to be more culturally appropriate, a Sojourner, Wanda also engaged in income-generating work from home, selling snacks to her neighbors.

Wanda's brother, Donnie, and her male cousins were unable to obtain steady employment. So Wanda opened her home to any of them whenever they could not afford a place to stay. Just as Donnie was set to migrate south for a job, Wanda was felled by a serious and debilitating brain aneurysm. Instead of taking the job, Donnie stayed, moved in with Wanda, and took care of her and her children. However disappointed Donnie must have felt to pass on his job in the South, he understood that "he couldn't get another sister," and he contributed selflessly to Wanda's care. Once she had fully recovered, Wanda went to school to become a teacher's aide. Donnie continued looking after her young children while she went to class. Once certified, she was able to obtain gainful employment.

Racism, poverty, and weathering place their indelible imprints throughout this story. Wanda and Donnie's aunt and uncle died prematurely when their kids were small. Their father had to migrate for work. Their mother became disabled at an early age, and Wanda took care of her mother. Wanda had a sudden aneurysm. Donnie had to give up his own opportunity for work in order to take care of Wanda and her children, first while she recovered and then while she trained for a skill that would allow her to get a job.

Ignorant of the constraints imposed by weathering, and focused on nuclear family self-sufficiency rather than collective networks, someone from the dominant culture might easily conclude that this extended family, which comprised so many people and a household that was constantly expanding and contracting according to the needs of its various members, was "disorganized" or chaotic. Through the prism of dominant cultural ideas about individualism, family support, and what constitutes work, along with racist stereotypes about laziness and welfare dependence, it is easy to miss the high-effort coping, hard work, and positive contributions of the many members of Wanda's extended family. Through that same prism, her father's migrating for work would earn him the label of "absent father." Likewise, Wanda would be viewed as a "welfare queen" once she became a young single mother and started accepting aid. Worse yet, if her income-generating work at home had come to light, she would have been identified as a welfare cheat. The father of her child would be presumed absent, even though we are supplied no information about his whereabouts, employment, or possible remittances or in-kind contributions. And Donnie would be seen as an unemployed loafer who mooched off his sister by moving in with her. That Wanda recovered from her illness and went on to be trained for a paying job might be characterized as her finally standing straight and flying right, overcoming her humble beginnings, escaping her multigenerational family's constraining demands. In fact, it was Donnie's presence and willingness to suppress his personal goals indefinitely that enabled her to get her assistant teacher's certificate.

Meanwhile, their two sisters, who held down working-class jobs while Wanda cared for their mother and provided day care for their children as needed, would be seen as "deserving" poor. The contributions made first by Wanda and then by Donnie, who made it possible for their father and sisters to work, would not be acknowledged. As Hicks-Bartlett observed, in many families the working poor are able to hold down jobs only because those who are not working watch their children. Hicks-Bartlett concluded, "the symbiosis between working and 'nonworking' welfare moms makes it impossible to draw moral and ethical distinctions between the two."

Today, weathering thrives as a by-product of the synergies of racism, classism, cultural oppression, macroeconomic restructuring, neoliberalism, austerity urbanism, and autonomous efforts to be resilient in the face of all these. Weathering is the missing and too-long-ignored piece in the puzzle of entrenched inequity. While it behooves us to see more clearly and admire the contributions made by the balabostas, Sojourners, and hill women, it would be wrong to romanticize their resilience and resistance as producing equity of any kind. Their steadfast efforts, along with the financial and in-kind contributions of their fathers, brothers, partners, cousins, and uncles, keep them afloat where they would otherwise drown, but the undertow of systemic racism and classism keeps them from swimming to shore. Like wearing a mask in a pandemic, their efforts provide a degree of protection, but are neither as effective as a vaccine nor a substitute for a societal commitment to eradicate the virus. Instead, as will be elaborated in chapter eight, an ill-thought-out, underfunded, completely inadequate, and in many ways destructive collection of social policy programs were put into place during the 1990s.

6.

Killing Us Stealthily: The Weathering Effects of Racialized Social Identity

On May 12, 2008, Rosa was only ten minutes into her first shift at Agriprocessors when the helicopters began to circle.[1] Supervisors told employees to run, while ICE agents threatened to shoot. One mother, afraid of losing her children if she was arrested, slipped into a freezer alongside the slaughtered chickens, hoping she wouldn't be discovered.[2]

That morning, 900 ICE agents armed with military-grade weapons and backed up by a UH-60 Black Hawk helicopter descended without warning on Agriprocessors, a slaughterhouse and meat processing plant in the small rural town of Postville, Iowa. In an unnecessary show of force, costing the US taxpayers more than $5 million, ICE agents arrested 389 employees on the spot.

Although ICE had good reason to believe some, even many, of the workers were undocumented, none of the 389 workers ICE arrested were known by name or known specifically to be undocumented at the time of arrest. Nor were any of them—including the undocumented—guilty of the crime with which they would be charged. But in deciding whom to arrest, the agents relied on two assumptions: first, that they could actually identify who was Latinx by sight, and second, that anyone who was Latinx was undocumented. "I don't think it's right the way they came busting in," said a maintenance support supervisor. "They took every Hispanic person out in cuffs until they're proved to be a US citizen."[3] Not every citizen had proof on the spot. The original arrests, then, were made not on the basis of individual identity but on the basis of presumed Latinx ethnicity, the racialization of Latinxs as undocumented, and the racialization of undocumented Latinxs as criminals—the current widely circulating Latinx stereotype was that they were criminals who stole jobs that rightfully belonged to American citizens. In other words, the individual arrests were made on the basis of racial profiling.

Of the 389 workers who were arrested in Postville as presumed undocumented Latinx workers, most were of either Guatemalan or Mexican heritage. The rest, again of unknown status, were from Israel and Ukraine. All were rounded up, handcuffed, and chained together at the waist. Female arrestees were detained in county jails. Mothers of small children were allowed to return to Postville with ankle monitors but were barred from working. Male arrestees, however, were packed into buses with blacked-out windows and herded into the National Cattle Congress in Waterloo, Iowa, which was eighty miles from Postville and, according to one witness, "had been transformed into a sort of concentration camp."[4]

There, the men were arraigned in groups of ten on felony charges of aggravated identity theft—a charge that the Supreme Court later ruled could not be levied against undocumented immigrants unless they knowingly stole an authentic Social Security Number, which none of the arrested slaughterhouse workers had done. (Most had no idea what a Social Security Number was, and their employment paperwork, including SSNs, had been filled out by their employers.) Nonetheless, the arrested workers were coerced into guilty pleas en masse. Instead of being deported directly, as was the norm at the time for arrested undocumented immigrants, most of the workers, who financially supported their families and were never arraigned as individuals, were sentenced to five months in federal prison before deportation. A severe punishment carried out by unnecessary, expensive, militarized methods—all due to a presumption of criminality based on presumed social identity.

Everyone in Postville was affected. Postville's population was small, and its economy was heavily dependent on Agriprocessors. Asked for her reaction, Sister Mary McCauley of St. Bridget Catholic Church, where many families of the arrested slaughterhouse workers congregated, replied: "Look at the pain on their faces. The pain is palpable." One Guatemalan woman named Ana broke down when she listened to her husband's voice mail notifying her of his arrest. "He said to take care of myself," Ana said, as she fielded endless cell phone calls from friends and relatives, some calling from Guatemala.[5]

In reality, no more than five of the originally arrested workers had any kind of prior criminal record. Of the five with records, none had committed a violent crime. There was nothing threatening about them. Consider this eyewitness account by Erik Camayd-Freixas, a Spanish interpreter for federal courts retained by ICE for the post-raid arraignments:

> Driven single-file in groups of ten, shackled at the wrists, waist and ankles, chains dragging as they shuffled through, the slaughterhouse workers were brought in for arraignment, [...] before marching out again to be bused to different county jails, only to make room for the next row of ten. They appeared to be uniformly no more than five feet tall, mostly illiterate Guatemalan peasants with Mayan last names, some being relatives, some in tears; others with faces of worry, fear, and embarrassment. They all spoke Spanish, a few rather laboriously. [...] They stood out in stark racial contrast with the rest of us as they started their slow penguin march across the makeshift court.[6]

Also, by way of reality check, the horrible jobs these immigrants performed under dangerous working conditions were ones that US citizens would not abide, as the slaughterhouse managers soon learned when the temporary American workers they hired to substitute for the arrested immigrants quit within a week. As for "stealing" from citizens, the fact is that undocumented workers' payroll tax deductions are added to the Social Security Administration's Earnings Suspense File for payers with mismatched Social Security Numbers. Those dollars then are credited to the general SSA Trust Fund. In this way, undocumented workers subsidize the retirements of US citizens and legal residents, while undocumented workers who pay into the system never see a dime in benefits. The Earnings Suspense File is estimated to have accumulated about $2 trillion, most of it since the so-called war on terror enabled ICE to conduct raids such as the one in Postville.[7]

Rather than operating based on facts or evidence, ICE agents were operating on the currently widely publicized and understood "social identity" of Latinx immigrants to the United States. A social identity that is racialized as criminal, even though being undocumented is a civil infraction. Moreover, if Congress had not obstructed comprehensive immigration reform for decades, it would almost certainly have included a temporary work permit provision for just these types of workers—a benefit to them and the American economy. In crafting the narrative of criminality to include being undocumented, Latinx immigrants were racialized as dangerous.[8]

When we think of our individual identity, we think of something we've autonomously developed that is deeply personal. We understand it is influenced by where, when, and with whom we've grown up. Yes, it is also informed by our religion (or lack thereof), our ethnic background, etc. But on some essential level we own it. It's not something imposed on us from outside.

Social identity is different. It *is* imposed on us from outside, on the basis of our perceived membership in a socially defined group that might mean nothing to us. And depending on how much or little the dominant culture values, stigmatizes, or exploits our designated group, social identity can have a significant impact on our health (and on virtually every other aspect of our life).

Social identity categories can correspond to society's constructs of race, class, ethnicity, gender, religion, ancestry, language, sexual orientation, immigrant documentation status, place of residence, and other currently or historically salient nodes of racialization and social classification. These various categories link people—often very different kinds of people—together and can determine their fate. Such categorizations are initially formed and then reinforced by what social groups know—or think they know—about people from other backgrounds, often based on stereotypes or political propaganda that substitute for firsthand knowledge.

For example, in March 2022, many Americans cheered Ukrainian grannies throwing Molotov cocktails at Russian soldiers seen on the nightly news. If the televised pictures were of grannies in burkas doing the same, the image would have more likely aroused contempt, panic, and fear, not cheers. Yet, in neither case is the character, predicament, or motivations of the respective Molotov grannies known firsthand. Their placement in different racialized social identity groups provokes opposite reactions in the dominant culture. As Bulgarian prime minister Kiril Petkov declared to a reporter based on only the sight of Ukrainian refugees flooding his borders: "These people are intelligent, they are educated people. [...] This is not the [Syrian] refugee wave we have been used to, people we were not sure about their identity, people with unclear pasts, who could have been even terrorists."[9]

How people experience, treat, and regard one another, and the raw power and privilege they have in relation to one another, all flow from these racialized social identity categories. As a result of this kind of profiling, on the basis of how one looks or sounds, what their name is, how they dress, where they live, and how they are depicted in the media, not on any personal knowledge of them as individuals, certain people may be targeted or looked on with suspicion. Or, as we can see from what happened as a result of the Postville raid: arrested, deported, and, as we'll soon discuss in more detail, exposed to serious health consequences. As the law professor Cesar García Hernández observes, the nature of the profiling depends on who gets to decide whether immigrants are publicly portrayed as "deserving individuals in need of safe harbor [and] as morally upright people coming to the United States to work and perhaps reunite with family or, instead, as criminals who endanger the law-abiding public."[10]

Birth Outcomes Based on Social Identity

As we might predict, based on what we know about the effects of stress and weathering on pregnancy, pregnant women who were either arrested in the Postville raid or had loved ones arrested in the raid experienced increased chances of poor birth outcomes—including babies born too early, too small, or both. As we've seen, these are not trivial effects. In addition to these human costs, we all bear the exorbitant health-care costs.

The impact on the pregnancy outcomes of Latina women at the Agriprocessers plant alone would illustrate how social identity can affect health, at least in direct and extreme conditions. However, the health consequences of the raid went far beyond the women immediately affected, in ways that may surprise you.

In studying the Postville raid's impact on pregnancy, Nicole Novak, Aresha Martinez-Cardoso, and I discovered that there was a ripple effect on pregnant Latinas throughout Iowa, who experienced an increase in adverse birth outcomes after the raid.[11] The percentage of babies born too small or too early to Latina mothers throughout the state was higher from May 2008 through January 2009 than in any other nine-month May–January period (the length of a full-term pregnancy) from 2003 to 2013. Iowa's Latina mothers experienced a dramatic uptick in their rates of delivering low-birth-weight babies in the nine months immediately following the raid, whether they were US or foreign born.

Undocumented immigrants would account for some of the foreign born—others were legal residents or naturalized citizens (by definition, none of the US-born Latinas were undocumented). Even though "documented" Iowa mothers and those born in the United States were legally protected from deportation, the stress they felt at learning of the Postville raid was sufficient to retard their babies' growth or cause their preterm birth. In comparison, the rate of low-birth-weight babies born to white non-Hispanic Iowa mothers had been trending down at least since 2006 and continued to do so through the nine months after the raid. It's also notable that foreign-born Latina mothers had lower rates of poor birth outcomes than non-Hispanic white mothers in both 2006 and 2007, but by thirty-eight weeks after the raid, they had surged dramatically higher.

We evaluated possible alternative explanations and found that the increase among Latina mothers could not be attributed to changes in other known risk factors such as smoking or lack of pre-natal care, or to any change in the socioeconomic composition of Latinxs in Iowa over that time period. Furthermore, the percentage of poor birth outcomes among non-Latina mothers in Iowa did not change during the same time period; only that of Latina mothers changed. In the wake of the raid, something affected the pregnancies of Latina mothers that had not affected them prior to the raid, and whatever it was did not affect white mothers at all.

How could this be? Though the Postville raid centered on the Agriprocessers plant, news of the raid quickly spread throughout Iowa, including through Spanish-language media, stoking panic among Latinxs living in other Iowa cities. "I was on the radio after the raid, and I got 125 calls," radio host Olga Sanchez said of a Spanish-language program on St. Ambrose University's KALA. "When you get that many calls, you know people are fearful. Many of them wanted to know what they could do to help in Postville, but a lot wanted to know if ICE is coming here."[12] In interviews across the state, Latinxs likened the profoundly stressful impact of hearing about the raid to the experience of going through a flood or an earthquake, experiences many of them or close relatives had had in their home countries—and experiences that social epidemiologists have found hurt birth outcomes among affected pregnant women.

News of the raid, even hundreds of miles away, placed Latinxs on high alert for weeks and even months afterward. In cities and towns across the region, churches and advocacy groups were flooded with immigrants desperate for help. This included documented immigrants who feared—for themselves and their children—that they could be detained before they could get their paperwork in order.[13]

Because public discourse frequently made the same set of assumptions that the ICE agents did, conflating apparent Latinx identity with undocumented status, and undocumented status with dangerous criminality, Latinx Iowans experienced increased discrimination and racialized exclusion. All across the state, Latinx Iowans understood that their social identity group was deemed threatening and "other," and they felt their own safety at risk. Furthermore, to the extent that the raid scared employers away from hiring Latinx workers, the livelihoods of Latinx people throughout the state were also put on the line.

Business owners across the state described "panicky" and "traumatized" communities who stopped going outside for fear of being detained and stopped spending money in order to save up emergency funds should the worst-case scenario play out.[14] Journalists and researchers who interviewed Latinx individuals and families in Iowa after the raid reported that many prepared for the possibility of further immigration harassment by avoiding public spaces and restricting their spending to save for a quick departure, if it became necessary. Nearly one-third of Postville's elementary and middle school students stopped showing up to class, causing even non-Hispanic white American parents to complain that "their children were traumatized by the sudden disappearance of so many of their school friends [and were] having nightmares that their parents too were being taken away."[15]

As we discussed in chapter four, complex immune, inflammatory, and hormonal pathways link a mother's psychosocial stress to the health of her baby. For pregnant Latinas, just knowing that they shared a stigmatized social identity with those targeted in the raid was enough to activate their physiological stress response, and to affect their children at critical periods of their fetal development.

This raises a further possibility: if pregnant Latinas throughout Iowa showed such palpable evidence of stress reactions to the raid, even when they were not part of it, we can surmise that other Latinx Iowans—men and women, children and adults—likely also experienced physiological stress reactions when they heard about the raid, fomenting weathering—although we had no way to measure such effects in our study.

The Postville raid and its aftermath is an extreme example of the kind of weathering stressors that Latinxs throughout the US face as a contingency of their social identity, at a time when, thanks to the actions of many politicians, including the forty-fifth US president, Latinx immigrants have been vilified and criminalized. Our immigration policies and the militarized enforcement of those policies exacerbate the effects of this prejudice on Latinx in the US, compromising their freedom of movement, their ability to participate fully in the society around them, and their feelings of safety. This may contribute to a cumulative health burden for immigrant and US-born Latinx alike.

Latinxs are of course not the only ethnic or racial group whose social identity puts them at risk in various ways. The epidemiologist Diane Lauderdale looked at birth outcomes for women in California who had Arabic names during the six months after the attacks of September 11, 2001. She found that they had a significantly elevated risk of preterm birth and low birth weight compared both to Arabic-named women in the six months before the attacks and to all the other racial/ethnic groups who were studied. Since an Arabic name indicated a high chance of Muslim social identity at a time when Muslims were being targeted as the enemy, it didn't matter whether the women were actually Muslim—they understood that they were being identified as such, and, although they lived clear across the country from where the attacks had taken place, they experienced heightened levels of stress arousal as a result, and that stress impacted their babies.[16]

Another example that shows how even vicarious stressful experiences can adversely affect birth outcomes comes from the social epidemiologist David Curtis and his colleagues. In 2022, they reported that Black women—across class—who were in the early stages of pregnancy when incidents of anti-Black violence were highly publicized were more likely to have preterm births than Black women who were not. Here, too, the pregnant women studied were not women who were, themselves, the object of these violent acts; they simply heard about them in the media.[17] Being a Black American at times of publicized incidents of anti-Black violence that trigger anxiety, fear, vigilance, rage, horror, and grief may be another biopsychosocial contributor to weathering.[18]

What we see in the instances described here is the measured physiological effect of racism and racialization on women (and, by extrapolation, probably men and children, too) socially identified as Latinxs, Muslims, and Black people. Social identity, when it is stigmatized by the dominant culture as inferior, threatening, other, or in some way undesirable, shapes the lived reality and health of each person who is defined by it.

Social Identity: A Group Project

But what exactly is social identity? Each person has multiple, intersecting social identities, the biopsychosocial relevance of which changes according to situations and settings. For example, knowing my gender identity is as a woman may matter more or less depending on whom I am with and where I am. In some situations, it doesn't register in my consciousness at all; in others—for example in a roomful of male colleagues—it is my defining identity.

Which of our social identities are salient at any moment depends on what cultural assumptions we share with those around us, on how they view us, and on the power dynamics at play. As the Stanford social psychologist Claude Steele describes:

> If you are in a setting where there is nothing that you have to deal with specifically because you are a woman, or Black, or old, or have a Spanish accent, or whatever, then these characteristics will not be important social identities for you in that setting. They won't much affect how you see things, whom you identify with or easily relate to, how you react emotionally to any events that occur, and so on. They won't become central to who you are there.[19]

But if in the course of the same day you find yourself in a completely different setting, you may become acutely aware of other aspects of your social identity. The degree of that awareness can impact how safe or threatened you feel—and, in turn, whether or not a physiological stress response is activated in your body. When you are in a setting where you fear that you are being profiled as threatening, inferior, or an outsider in some way, the stress arousal in response to that fear can foster weathering.

To illustrate, consider how a young Black man may experience his Blackness when at home with family and friends compared to when the same man is pulled over by the police for a minor traffic violation. Although his skin color doesn't change, the impacts of his social identity as Black certainly do.

In this example, he may not even be consciously aware of being

Black when with family and friends, or he may feel something positive and affirming about his Black social identity. His encounter with the police officer, on the other hand, may activate an acute awareness of being Black—and the associated dangers—resulting in psychosocial distress and vigilance, which trigger the physiological stress response before any words are exchanged with the officer. This stress response will last for at least the duration of the encounter, and likely beyond. No matter how professionally the officer behaves, even if he is doing his job without any malice or racism or ill will, the young man's fear is nevertheless reasonable in light of the US history of over-policing Black people, racial profiling, and police brutality—and it is physiologically damaging.

Remember, when a potential predator is nearby it's better to react to a false alarm than miss a true one. But that does not mean there is no physiological price to reacting to false alarms. That the Black man has been taught strategically to suppress any automatic urge to fight or flee in order to stay polite and look nonthreatening adds to the physiologic toll of his experience.

A person's vulnerability to being stereotyped, stigmatized, or profiled stems from a society-wide understanding of the racialized characteristics associated with their social identity. Perceived social identities are reinforced by widely shared stereotypes that social groups substitute for firsthand knowledge of one another. For example, Latinx people are suspected to be undocumented, people with Arabic names are seen as potential Islamic terrorists, Black men are viewed as dangerous, and teen mothers are interpreted as promiscuous and irresponsible. Black or white, rich or poor, immigrant or native-born citizen, none of us can individually declare or fully define our social identity. That's done by others. And just as we cannot autonomously invent our perceived social identities, we cannot avoid their consequences or fail to benefit from any associated privileges.

I remember that even my infant daughter was treated differently by passers-by on public outings depending on whether she was dressed in her red jumpsuit or her pink one. In the red jumpsuit people would call her slugger or buddy—one particularly effusive man even punched her in the stomach to punctuate his male-bonding greeting. In the pink jumpsuit, she was treated delicately, spoken to softly, addressed as sweetheart. Her social identity as male or female was based entirely on the color of her outfit, not on her behavior or biology, or any gender identity she "claimed." She obviously had no say in the matter (or in how I dressed her, either).

In *Stone Butch Blues*,[20] Leslie Feinberg's protagonist recounts brutal police raids on gay bars in upstate New York in the 1970s. The difference between whether a Butch lesbian or a trans-man was arrested in the raid could come down to whether those assigned female sex at birth were adjudged by the officers to be wearing at least three pieces of "women's" clothing. If not, they were immediately subject to arrest and brutal abuse on the basis of their clothing alone.

Weathering is a product of the nature and intensity of such contingencies of social identity over the course of each day—day after day, year after year. These contingencies are structurally rooted and potentially harmful to health, not just because of the activation of physiological stress responses that have both short- and long-term effects, but also because social identity groups deemed undesirable are likely to suffer disinvestment in their communities and from limited employment opportunities. More directly, social identity can get them punched in the gut. Or detained or deported. Arrested. Or shot by the police.

And members of racialized groups are vigilant to such threats. Research in social psychology tells us that members of stigmatized groups enter new situations with uncertainty about whether those they interact with will judge them according to the stereotypes related to their social identity. If they know they are members of a stigmatized group—or could be seen or "outed" as one—they automatically become vigilant for cues indicating whether or not they belong, can trust others, can be authentic, or will be treated fairly.

An example of this comes from Arthur Ashe, the first African American man to become a Grand Slam tennis champion. As he wrote in his memoir:

> I am almost always aware of race, alert to its power as an idea, sensitive to its nuances in the world. Like many other blacks, when I find myself in a new public situation, I will count. I always count. I count the number of black and brown faces present, especially to see how many, if any, are employed by the hosts.[21]

Marginalized people are always searching for situational cues in their environment, cues that are actually clues to how they can expect to be sized up and treated. In Mr. Ashe's case, he took the number and station of people of color around him as clues to what his race would connote to those in the room with him, and whether he belonged there.

Mr. Ashe also recounts a telling story of a time he was taken to the emergency room at New York Hospital with a heart attack—when he was only thirty-six! (One might surmise his cardiovascular system was weathered.) What do you imagine you would be thinking if you were being rushed into an acclaimed hospital with a massive heart attack? Would you be consumed with the physical pain? Scared that you might be about to die? Feeling momentary relief that you'd made it to a hospital where you would be in good hands? Arthur Ashe counted. He counted the darker faces in the emergency room, taking note of the few Filipino nurses, the even smaller number of Black nurses, and the one Black medical resident among a sea of white faces. He noted that most of the people with Black faces he'd seen in the hospital were cleaning the floors. This act of vigilance was so automatic that it occurred even as he was having a heart attack so serious that it necessitated an immediate quadruple bypass surgery.

In the midst of an existential health crisis, he looked for cues to let him know whether his physicians could be trusted. How safe would it be to put his life in their hands? Would he matter to them? It's also worth noting that, like Serena Williams, Ashe was a model of the kind of discipline, physical fitness, and grit that make a champion. Yet he, too, had been victimized by racial hostility as he rose through the ranks of a mainly white, elitist sport. And he, too, was suffering a major health crisis in his thirties.

In everyday settings such as schools or workplaces or stores, a stigmatized social identity can have adverse effects on cognition and emotion, undermining self-confidence and diminishing performance. This impact reduces opportunities for social mobility, while ensuring that those who "beat the odds" pay a physical price for their positive efforts. Differences in life experiences shaped by the prevailing beliefs about what can be expected of, and is deserved by, specific population groups translate social inequality into health inequality.

Othering

In a structurally racist society that privileges some groups as dominant and marginalizes others through cultural oppression, the dominant culture "others" those they profile as members of undesirable social identity groups. Othering results in marginalized groups being discriminated against in access to material goods, employment opportunities, healthy residential and work environments, nutritious food, and quality education, all of which can lead to negative health impacts. But even those members of marginalized groups who are not wanting for any of the material benefits of the good life—like Arthur Ashe or Serena Williams—experience the health impact of weathering.

No member of a marginalized group fully escapes othering experiences. How damaging those experiences are will vary from person to person, from setting to setting, from something that is immediate and in their face to something that is perpetrated, society-wide, by people in power, and even by our legal system.

You might be bullied in school because of your social identity, or profiled, followed, and surveilled as you shop in a store. Othering can seem benign, as when a white girl touches her Black classmate's hair "to see how Black hair feels"—an example of the kind of reminders of difference and microaggressions marginalized people experience in everyday life. Othering can also be blatant and vicious, for example when a sitting US president refers to members of your social identity group as thugs, criminals, barbarians, terrorists, or citizens of "shithole countries."[22]

Othering can be expressed through laws and policies, for example: laws against same-sex marriage that prevent LGBTQ+ people from enjoying a basic human right; voter identification laws that make it difficult for members of certain social identity groups to vote; anti-trans bathroom policies that invalidate trans and nonbinary social identities, or construe them as pedophiles. This list goes on and on. These are among the many ways of signaling to those affected that they are other, lesser, to be looked down upon and even despised or attacked.

Othering can be perpetrated through the media, for example when the "good guys" in movies resemble the dominant group, while those from a marginalized group are portrayed as inferior—less moral and law-abiding, less articulate, less talented, less attractive, less worthy of being kept safe or guaranteed rights that the good guys take for granted. But othering can also occur through sins of omission, as when, for example, members of your social identity group aren't portrayed at all, rendering your group invisible.

This lack of representation is an insidious form of othering that occurs in many different contexts, ranging from the news media to scientific research. For decades, medical institutions issued authoritative guidelines for how to diagnose and treat serious, life-threatening illnesses such as heart disease—guidelines based on studies whose participants were all white men. Now that the National Institutes of Health has made aggressive efforts to include women in such studies, it has become clear that women with heart disease often have different risk factors, present with different symptoms, and require different treatments or different dosages than men do. In my own field, my former student and current colleague Jay Pearson, now a tenured professor at Duke University, convincingly argues that although it has long been a basic tenet of public health that there is a strong and direct relationship between socioeconomic status and health, with high status benefiting health and low status harming it, the research supporting this thesis over the last century was based on population samples that were predominantly and often exclusively white, Northern European men, and therefore not comprehensive enough to be definitive.[23] Now that factors such as race, ethnicity, gender, place of residence, and other vectors of social identity have begun to be taken into account, the strength of the relationship between socioeconomic status and health has been found to be much more variable than was previously understood and contingent on gendered or racialized social identity.

Of course, to be affected biopsychosocially by othering, you need to sense, even unconsciously, that you're *being* othered or could be subject to othering in the setting you are in. For most members of marginalized groups, this is not a challenge. They are well aware of having a social identity that constitutes the "other" in the culture surrounding them. But occasionally, a person being othered is unaware of it. If they don't have the same fluency in dominant cultural racializations or associated stereotypes and valuations, it can take them a while to catch on.

Think of the subplot in the *Seinfeld* episode "The Understudy."[24] In this episode, Elaine gets a manicure. The manicurists insult her in Korean, all the while smiling at her. Elaine is none the wiser and stays perfectly relaxed because she does not understand Korean. Later, however, she starts putting two and two together when she notices that the manicurists use the same Korean word to greet another customer's dog that they had used when referring to her.

Once Elaine suspects the manicurists are making fun of her, she is visibly distressed and becomes obsessed with the idea. Eventually, she takes her friend George Costanza's father, Frank, who is white and happens to be fluent in Korean, to "spy" on the manicurists and translate their words. Frank Costanza confirms that the manicurists are, indeed, insulting her. Elaine spends the rest of the episode trying unsuccessfully to convince them that she's a good person, going to great lengths and losing sleep in her attempts. The stress this causes her is palpable and can be seen clearly in her facial expressions and other body language.

Presumably if Elaine were a living and breathing person this is an experience that will not have long-term weathering consequences for her. As a white, educated, cisgender female, she will not be other outside the nail salon, and in most of the settings in which she finds herself. For those who are perpetually other, the need to be sensitive to what is being said about them is instinctive, can be strategic, and does have consequences.

The Health Consequences of Othering

Sometimes, however, even for those who routinely experience othering, it may take time to catch on. This is sometimes the case with newly arrived Mexican immigrants, for example. All immigrants to the US will at one point or another get slotted into racial stratification categories that they may not have been familiar with in their land of birth and primary socialization.[25] These taxonomies are socially constructed and not always easy to discern for a newcomer. Before they crack the American racial/ethnic or class code, recently arrived immigrants may, for a while, escape the full biopsychosocial force of othering because they can't decipher many of the microaggressions that target them. You're unlikely to be triggered by the US president's referring to your home country as a "shithole country" if you don't understand English. Newly arrived Mexican immigrants often live in ethnic enclaves where everyone shares their cultural framework, everyone speaks Spanish, and many people are not (yet) fluent in English. The cues to their being othered are all Greek to them (or Korean).

This changes over time, as people of Mexican origin become long-term residents and learn that here in America, they and their descendants are considered other, and are stigmatized accordingly. My colleagues and I wondered whether their increasing awareness of othering might be relevant to some interesting findings about what happens to the health of Mexican immigrants during their years living here.

Numerous studies have found that the health of Mexican immigrants in the United States is better when they first arrive than it is after they've resided in the US for a decade or more. It's also better than the health of their children who are born in the United States. This is particularly noteworthy because immigrants who have lived here longer, and their children who are born here, tend to be more assimilated and to have higher levels of education and income than newly arrived immigrants.

The decline in health is often believed to be caused by immigrants' and their children's becoming Americanized and adopting an unhealthy diet and lifestyle—eating fast food, taking up smoking, being sedentary, etc. But is that really the reason? What does the evidence suggest?

To answer this question, my colleagues and I analyzed data from the National Health and Nutrition Examination Survey (NHANES) to estimate what we in the sciences call allostatic load scores—a fancy term for the measurable indicators of the impact of chronic stress on physical well-being. These indicators include levels of stress hormones and inflammation measured through blood or saliva analysis; waist circumference as a measure of the distribution of fat in the body (belly fat is linked to stress as well as to health harms); and the presence of stress-related conditions and diseases, such as high blood pressure, and so on. From here on out I'll refer to the allostatic load score as the Stress Impact Scale, since all of the factors it measures are related to stress. Having a high score on the Stress Impact Scale is an indicator of weathering.

Using biological data collected by NHANES from a sample of Mexican immigrants in the US and a group of same-age non-Hispanic white Americans, my colleagues and I classified sample members according to whether they had a high score on the Stress Impact Scale. Higher scores indicate greater stress-mediated wear and tear across body systems than would be expected at a given chronological age—i.e., weathering. We then compared members of both groups in the NHANES sample—the Mexican immigrants and the same-age non-Hispanic white Americans—to see whether the length of time the Mexican immigrants had resided in the US increased the odds of their having a high score, and to find out who was more likely to have high scores.

Focusing on people forty-five to sixty years old, we found:[26]

Mexican immigrants who had lived in the United States for less than ten years were no more likely to have a high score than same-age non-Hispanic white Americans.

Mexican immigrants who had lived in the United States for eleven to twenty years were more than twice as likely to have a high score as same-age non-Hispanic white Americans.

Mexican immigrants who had lived in the United States for at least twenty-one years were almost four times as likely to have a high score as same-age non-Hispanic white Americans.

In other words, the longer they had resided in the United States, the more likely it was that Mexican immigrants would have a higher score on the Stress Impact Scale than their non-Hispanic white counterparts. But why?

To help answer that question, we controlled for the adverse effects of smoking, inadequate fruit and vegetable consumption, lack of health insurance, and low levels of physical activity. If adopting unhealthy Americanized behaviors was the reason immigrants who had been here longer had worse health than those who had recently arrived, then controlling for the effects of smoking, diet, exercise, and access to medical care should have reduced or removed the difference in health outcomes.

But that's not what we found. Controlling for the negative health impacts of unhealthy behavior, we found that:

Mexican immigrants who had lived in the United States for less than ten years still had the same odds of having a high score on the Stress Impact Scale as white non-Hispanic Americans.

Mexican immigrants who had lived in the United States for eleven to twenty years were twice as likely to have a high score as same-age non-Hispanic white Americans.

Mexican immigrants who had lived in the United States for at least twenty-one years had even higher odds—5.5 times the odds—of having a high score than same-age non-Hispanic white Americans.

Controlling for health behaviors clearly fails to explain the disparity in Stress Impact Scores between the Mexican immigrants and their non-Hispanic white counterparts. If unhealthy diet and lifestyle don't account for the fact that the scores of the immigrants increase the longer they live in the US, what does? Answer: weathering.

It is also worth remembering, as I noted above, that the immigrants who had been in the US longer had higher incomes and more education as a group than the more recently arrived. Yet, as we have seen in other contexts, and as Jay Pearson analytically observed, education and income are not equally protective across groups. This finding is consistent with the possibility that the immigrants' lived experience of advancing their education and increasing their income was so stressful that it may actually have exposed them to more severe weathering—an effect I have alluded to in chapter four and will explore in more detail in chapter seven. This could happen as they spend more time interacting with members of the dominant group, who see them as other, and less time living or working among people like themselves, who affirm rather than deny their worth.

Weathering in Detroit

Research my colleagues and I have done comparing the health effects of upward mobility on Black, white, and Mexican-descent residents of Detroit further supports the idea that upward mobility among Mexican Americans is harmful to their health. As you will see, this is the exact opposite of what we found in white people.

Life in Detroit has become increasingly hard and racialized since the 1970s, especially in the wake of the 2008 financial crisis. The massive flight of residents and capital from Detroit to the surrounding suburbs over the past five decades significantly eroded the city's tax base and reduced its population, from 1.85 million in 1950 to just 640,000 in 2020.[27] White flight has been particularly pronounced, with the result that Black residents, who made up about 30 percent of the total population in 1960, constituted 85 percent by 2010.[28] Since the 1940s, the Mexican immigrant population has maintained a significant presence in Southwest Detroit, and grew by approximately 45 percent between 1950 and 2010, due to the post-1965 upsurge in immigration, especially during the 1990s.[29]

Detroit's resources have been progressively depleted, and although the city was once home to the nation's most affluent Black population, most remaining residents now have low-to-moderate incomes. They and their elected officials face deep obstacles to improving their circumstances. After the economic collapse of 2008, chronic revenue losses imposed constraints on the city's government and reduced its ability to deliver basic public services. Between 1990 and 2013, Detroit lost nearly half of its municipal workforce.[30] After racially targeted subprime loans flooded Detroit's housing market in the 1990s and early 2000s, 28 percent of Detroit's mortgageable properties underwent foreclosure between the years 2005 and 2014, causing property values to decline precipitously, with such a rash of evictions that something like 78,000 buildings were abandoned in their wake.[31] As of 2014, about 60 percent of Detroit's children lived below the poverty threshold—a greater proportion than in any other large US city.[32] The cumulative effects of all these problems resulted in the filing of the largest municipal bankruptcy in US history, in 2013. Funding for public services then dropped even further, evidenced by the scarcity of working streetlights and widespread water shutoffs in residential neighborhoods.[33]

Was the impact of all this misfortune felt equally in the bodies of white, Black, and Mexican populations in Detroit? If not, how did the health impact of living in poverty affect each of these three communities? Did those living in poverty always suffer the most physiologically?

To begin to answer these questions, I spearheaded two studies in collaboration with the Healthy Environments Partnership (HEP), which brought together academic researchers and Detroit community stakeholders. We augmented data collected between late 2008 and 2011 through a HEP survey with data we collected pertaining to blood pressure, height, and weight, as well as fresh blood and saliva samples we collected from each participant. We performed the range of laboratory tests and measurements needed to arrive at a score on the Stress Impact Scale. We also extracted DNA from the blood samples in order to measure telomere length, which as you'll recall is a way of assessing biological aging.[34]

In our statistical analyses, we broke down our Detroit population sample by race and ethnicity, and each racial/ethnic group by whether they lived beneath the official poverty line. Looking at the weathering indicators among only the impoverished members of our Detroit sample, we found that white residents were the most likely of the three racial/ethnic groups to have high scores on the Stress Impact Scale and to have shorter telomeres. Among the relatively more affluent, the white residents had lower Stress Impact scores and the longest telomeres—that is, they were the least weathered—of the three. That white people living in poverty were more likely to have high Stress Impact Scale scores and short telomeres compared to white people with more economic resources is exactly what most would expect. For Black residents of Detroit, we found a smaller difference in Stress Impact scores between the poor and more affluent Black residents and no statistical difference in telomere length. In other words, having greater economic resources did not spare Black residents in Detroit from weathering as measured by telomere length, and made a smaller difference to their Stress Impact score than it did for white residents.

For the Mexican population of Detroit, we found slightly higher Stress Impact scores among the relatively more affluent compared to the impoverished. And we also found that poor Mexican Detroiters had longer telomeres than those above the poverty level. That is, the more affluent Mexicans in Detroit were biologically older—had weathered more—than those living below the poverty level.

This finding that poor Mexicans fared better than more affluent Mexicans is not what most people would expect. And conventional age-washing wisdom to the contrary, neither smoking nor being overweight contributed to the differences we found.

As a group, our findings suggest something surprising: higher income improves health among white people in Detroit; makes a smaller difference, if any, among Black people in Detroit; and actually impairs health for Detroit Mexicans. How could this be?

Some call such findings a paradox.

Paradox Lost

This apparent paradox makes sense if we take seriously the impacts of biopsychosocial stress responses triggered by othering. While higher income provides a household greater access to certain privileges and services, it also likely indicates that a Black person or person of Mexican descent spends a fair amount of time negotiating white spaces, and therefore spends more time being vigilant to real or possible othering. By putting our quantitative research in conversation with studies based on firsthand observation, the case becomes much stronger. Fortunately, thanks to ethnographic work done by the late Latina/Latino Studies professor Edna Viruell-Fuentes, we have qualitative evidence of the impacts of othering on health in Detroit. A Mexican immigrant who received her doctorate in my department, Viruell-Fuentes conducted a "participant observation" study in Detroit with Mexican residents, some of them immigrants, others native-born citizens of the US. Participant observation is a type of research strategy whereby the researcher is embedded within a community for a period of time, during which she gains trust and becomes intimately familiar with the everyday activities and practices of a group through observing and participating in those activities.

In interviews with immigrants and second-generation Mexican women in Detroit, Viruell-Fuentes found consistent evidence that second-generation Mexican Americans experienced more instances of discrimination and othering than did their immigrant parents. She attributed this in part to the protective effects that living in ethnic enclaves had for the immigrant generation, but also to the second generation's "frequent, cumulative, and ongoing burden of exposure to 'othering.'"[35] She saw, and heard them describe, the ways in which the need to "become American" entails learning and interpreting the racial dynamics of the US and finding their place — too often a low and stigmatized one — within society's hierarchy.

In Detroit, Viruell-Fuentes found that the second generation was more likely to have regular contact with mainstream institutions, which exposed them to more pervasive and cumulative experiences of othering, than the first generation. As Diana, a second-generation woman from Detroit describes:

When I went to high school and college, that's when I became aware of more, you know, racism, more—prejudice and different things. [...] I always knew I had to prove myself. [But] when I got to [college,] speaking the [Spanish] language, some people would get offended. You know, one time I was talking to one of my friends and I had someone come up to me and say, you know, "I don't understand what you are saying. That's so rude that you're speaking Spanish," and I turned around and said to the person, you know, "Do I know you?" And they were like "No." I said, "Well, I'm sorry, but I'm having a conversation with my friend; I am not talking to you, or about you, and you shouldn't be offended." [...] I was upset, you know. I said, "Why should I have to justify this?"

Moreover, the second generation grew up with a deeper sense of stigma than their parents, because unlike their parents, they learned in their early childhood to, in effect, "speak Korean." This early exposure made their sense of otherness a core part of their identity. Many described school as a daily reminder that they did not belong. Roxana, a Mexican American native of Detroit described:

To a certain point, you know, the only people you know are your family: your home, your parents. It's a little world, you know, and everything seems to be perfect or fine. And it's when your world meets the other world that there are clashes and problems. You know, there were three of us [my brothers and I]. When we were, the three of us, going to school, it was like, almost like the three musketeers because it was us against everybody else.

In contrast, first-generation immigrants spent less time in spaces where these two worlds could clash. As Viruell-Fuentes explains, first-generation immigrants in Detroit did not have to defend or contend with their identity as other as frequently because they "were able to replicate, within their small social circles and the neighborhood, many aspects of their lives in Mexico." One first-generation immigrant, Ernestina, said:

Everything here is the same [as in Mexico]. I think because here [in this neighborhood] we are all from Mexico. And the same things that you used to do there, you can do here. Like the same way of throwing a party, the same foods, the same pastimes, everything, everything is the same.

If we put Viruell-Fuentes's qualitative observations together with our quantitative findings about the health of Detroit residents of Mexican descent, we get the following picture: The longer new immigrants live in the United States, the more aware they become of the racialized hierarchies and ideologies that apply to their social identity in this new context. The same goes for their children, whose awareness begins at a much earlier age. Through that socialization process, both the parents and their children become more vulnerable to the physiological impact of the profiling and prejudices that target them, such as the assumption that they are not legal residents of the US, or truly American. Navigating such prejudices and stereotypes in daily interactions in integrated settings can chronically activate their physiological stress processes. And the more aware they are of being othered, Viruell-Fuentes's qualitative study suggests, the worse the biopsychosocial health impacts of that othering.

As our own findings on Stress Impact scores and telomere length suggest, Mexican immigrants and their children become weathered not only despite their extra years of education and higher incomes, but possibly because of them. The stress of trying to "better" themselves socioeconomically takes a toll, as does the time spent in the kind of environments that their education and income allow (or require) them to enter.

I first saw this close-up in my father.

7.

Weathering for Success: Age against the Machine

As children, my sisters and I learned not to talk to my father when he first came home from work. As he described it, he was ready to interact with us only after he had the chance to "take off his armor." What armor? I always wondered. He worked a desk and laboratory bench job: supervising lab technicians, planting cultures, peering through the microscope to determine which infectious agents were making patients sick and which antibiotics would vanquish them, completing paperwork, and interacting with physicians and hospital administrators. It was demanding work, with life-or-death consequences for some patients, but it wasn't physical combat.

It wasn't until much later that I understood the intricate ways in which decades of trauma, coupled with ongoing othering, were taking their toll on him day by day.

As with Italian and Irish immigrants in the 1800s through the mid-1900s, Eastern European Jewish immigrants were seen as nonwhite when they first arrived in America.[1] (Remember, from our earlier discussion of diabetes, that Jews were considered Asiatic or Mongoloid; sometimes even Negro by powerful white members of the dominant culture.) It's difficult for many Americans today, who tend to assume that all Jews are highly educated and affluent, to understand the depth and threat of cultural oppression my father and his parents faced. It was only in the second half of the twentieth century that Jewish Americans were invited into the privileged space known as whiteness—to the point that now Black Jews and working-class Jews can feel erased or excluded when people refer to Jewish Americans. But this was not the case for my father's generation of working-class Eastern European immigrants. Both my parents lived at a transitional point in American Jewish history, with the racialization of Eastern European Jewish people changing over the course of their lifetimes. But during that transitional time, anti-Semitism and the experience of being othered had an impact on both of them.

My father grew up in a Yiddish-speaking immigrant ghetto in Brooklyn before World War II. His parents fled horrific pogroms in Russia after witnessing unspeakable genocidal atrocities against their family and community—gruesome, sadistic, and violent deaths at the hands of their anti-Semitic oppressors. Escaping gunfire with babies in tow, my father's twenty-something-year-old parents arrived in the US in the early 1900s. I don't know many specifics about what they endured in Russia, but those that my bubby (grandmother) told me were horrifying.

My father was born during the great flu pandemic of 1918. He was the youngest of eight children, one of whom died in infancy and another in early childhood. He told us how deeply affected his mother was by the deaths of her two young sons and by the slaughter of her parents, who had remained in Russia. She had learned of their murders through the mail. As a toddler, my father heard his mother cry so often after reading letters that came in the mail that he bit the postman who delivered them. My father credited his mother's intense overprotectiveness of him throughout his youth to her desperate fear that she would lose him, too. Her fear was not unfounded. As a young boy, he suffered from a severe case of diphtheria, an often fatal infectious disease that was so horrific it was characterized as "the strangling angel of children," for there were no vaccines to prevent it or antibiotics to treat it at that time.

My father's "upward mobility" began as he entered college. A first-generation college student, he commuted ninety minutes by subway each way from the tenement in Brooklyn where he lived to City College of New York in uptown Manhattan. After serving in the army during World War II, he attended graduate school and joined the ranks of the highly educated and professionally employed, ultimately landing a job directing the bacteriology lab of a major hospital affiliated with Harvard Medical School in Boston. Compared to his parents, he was socially mobile and had acquired white privilege, no question. (It bears noting that he was able to achieve his college education thanks to the existence of City College, the first free public institution of higher education in the United States, and his graduate degree with the financial assistance of the GI Bill, a type of government funding not available to his older brothers, who were sixteen and fourteen years older than he and just above draft age when the war started, or to very many women or Black Americans, even if they had served.) As such, he was a member of the first generation of Eastern European Jews to "become white." But being white, male, highly educated, and professionally employed was not enough to erase the stigma of being from an immigrant and working-class Eastern European Jewish family. That his degree was from a public commuter college that had been branded as Communist after his classmate Julius Rosenberg—whom my father did not know—was convicted of and executed for espionage in 1953, didn't help matters either. During the McCarthy era, my father, along with more than four thousand other City College grads, was blacklisted in the job market just for being in the same CCNY graduating class as Rosenberg.

After graduate school, even as his professional status gave him entrance to an upper middle-class income and lifestyle, the contingencies of his early, formative, and oppressive social identities remained with him. He spent his workday among Boston Brahmins as well as Jewish Americans of a "lighter color"—that is, those whose immigrant ancestors were middle-class or wealthy assimilated Jews from Western Europe. These families came to the US fifty to a hundred years earlier than his own family, and unlike his family, who came seeking asylum from the violence and persecution they suffered in their Russian shtetl, their families came because the US was a land of opportunity where they could expect to expand their fortunes.

As a telling aside, many people may be unaware of this "colorism" among different waves and geographic origins of Jewish immigrants during the first half of the twentieth century, but it existed and was palpable, especially for my father's generation. This was a time when working-class Jewish children from Eastern Europe—along with first-generation Catholic immigrants from Ireland and Southern European countries—were still striving to join the ranks of the middle and upper middle classes, even as Jews from earlier waves of Western European immigration had already ascended. Before they became upwardly mobile, Eastern European working-class Jewish immigrants were racialized as Asiatic or Oriental, in an era when Chinese immigrants were deplored and subject to the Chinese Exclusion Act. In some quarters, Eastern European Jews were described as "essentially Negro in habits, physical peculiarities, and tendencies."[2] Meanwhile, the more assimilated and affluent Jews were seen as Western, European, and even, for a short period in the mid-1800s prior to the waves of Eastern European Jewish immigration, as Teutonic Aryans, the group believed to be of the highest racial caste during the eugenics movement.[3]

These distinct and inequitably stigmatized social identities within groups whose members we would now simply call Jewish, or even white, were widely accepted in the first half of the twentieth century, particularly among the Protestant elite. For example, when trying to limit the percentage of Jewish undergraduates admitted to Harvard, President Lowell (the university's president from 1909 to 1933) made distinctions between the "better class of Jews" (those of German background) and the "undesirable Jews" (those from Eastern Europe). And to maintain their status among the Protestant elite, the more assimilated and well-off American Jews often did their best to distance themselves from the Eastern European Jewish political refugees. For example, in his book about the anti-Semitic treatment of the Jews by elite college admissions offices, Jerome Karabel notes that at about the same time as President Lowell was working to solve Harvard's "Jewish problem," Jewish alumni of Dartmouth College expressed their (self-serving) pleasure that Dartmouth was admitting "only the better type of Jews and not the Brooklyn or Flatbush crowd."[4]

Returning to my youth: In the suburban Massachusetts town in which I grew up, my native Yiddish-speaking, Brooklyn-bred, highly educated father never felt at home except when he was literally at home. He spent his white-collar workdays cognitively and emotionally engaged in actively managing his social identity, "thinking Yiddish, acting British"—an Eastern European Jewish version of code-switching. He was perpetually alert to the possibility of being stigmatized, discredited, or humiliated if his ethnic immigrant working-class roots or City College education were exposed. Where the other professional men had Ivy League pedigrees, dressed in Brooks Brothers, and spoke like Endicott Peabody, he spoke like Bernie Sanders and sported the same hairstyle. In light of these social identity differences, my father went to work every day steeling himself for psychosocial combat. He lived a *Groundhog Day* scenario where he felt the need to establish his worth anew day after day. His vigilance never waned.

Now I understand that the "armor" he referred to during my childhood was the heavy psychological weight that came with managing his social identity at work, always defending himself against being viewed as an undesirable when interacting with the physicians and upper-level hospital administrators. Even as he ascended the ranks of American privilege, he was forced to navigate his work environment with a constant sensitivity to being othered. His self-conscious and ceaseless need to keep up appearances suggests he may have been in a prolonged state of chronic physiological stress arousal.

My father died in his sixties of sarcoidosis, an inflammatory disease that affects multiple organs in the body, including the lungs and heart. The physician who performed my father's autopsy told me that his lungs, heart, spleen, and brain were so damaged that he must have had undiagnosed and untreated sarcoidosis for decades, and that, given the widespread damage to his vital organs, it was surprising he was even able to remain upright toward the end of his life. For years before his death, his body was a Jenga tower one move away from collapse.

Though this appeared nowhere in the official cause of death, one could certainly speculate that my father's premature death was the result of unrelenting social pressure on top of childhood trauma— or, in other words, weathering. And there was a generational legacy of weathering to contend with, too—not just his own, but the weathering that was passed down to him from his family, whose uphill battles began in the shtetl and continued after their escape from persecution in Russia, when they came to America as poor immigrants and settled down to a difficult life in a working-class urban ghetto. Being targeted for genocide, and suffering the losses of two of her children and the slaughter of her parents, plunged my father's mother into depression and left her desperately anxious about the health of her youngest son.

In current parlance, we would speculate that my father was affected by adverse childhood experiences (ACEs), a type of trauma that is associated with diminished health in later life.[5] Examples of ACEs include losing a family member to death or to prison, being depressed or having a primary caregiver who is depressed, going hungry for long periods, and suffering neglect or abuse. Today, scientists have found evidence that if you were subject to ACEs during critical periods of your brain development, your brain architecture may be affected such that your threshold for physiological stress arousal is permanently lower (meaning it is triggered more easily).[6] To the extent that you will live your life in similarly adverse circumstances, having this lower threshold can be adaptive. But what if the adversity you actually face is entirely different from the circumstances in which you were born?

Imagine what it would be like if your brain architecture was calibrated by a world rife with ACEs, yet, as you grew up, you entered an environment that contained none of the kinds of threats or stressors your brain had prepared you for. You went to school with, worked with, or lived next to members of communities whose neurological threshold for stress arousal was shaped by enjoying lives of privilege and safety. Your hair-trigger reactions to perceived threats could get you dismissed as uncivil, touchy, hot-tempered, a troublemaker, or a snowflake. Your more privileged classmates or coworkers or neighbors could feel superior as they patted themselves on the back for remaining civil and calm, letting verbal provocations roll off their back or, worse, being happily unaware that the substance of their civil discourse could, in fact, be a verbal provocation to race-conscious ears. They would not understand that your brain and body were adapted for responding to a world filled with threats and that you had been primed to be in a continuous state of vigilance. Or you knew that when the privileged performed civility, that alone did not imply they weren't proliferating racist ideas. This appears to have been my father's lived experience as an adult. He probably lived in a permanently sustained or easily escalated state of physiological stress arousal, which over time weathered his body.

For my father, achieving an advanced education conferred real material benefits and privileges. These were important prizes, and they offered my sisters and me a degree of financial security and opportunities he never had in his youth; yet, for my father, this alone was not enough to heal his early and intergenerational traumas, or to prevent the physiological damage that led to his early death.

My Armor: Othering in the Second Generation

While I took him at his word, I didn't have a personal feel for why my father chose the metaphor of wearing armor at work until I had my own firsthand experience of being othered as a contingency of my own social identity: a female member of the first generation of US Jews born on the white side of the color line. My identity allowed me greater access to privileged spaces than my father had at my age, but also exposed me to some pressures similar to those he felt at work. I was admitted as an undergraduate to Princeton University in its early years of coeducation, when it was self-consciously working to increase cultural diversity. I was an ethnic public-school girl trying to navigate a kingdom of high WASP tradition and inherited wealth, marinated in centuries of testosterone. I had book smarts, a good work ethic, even a dash of intergenerational street smarts, but the currency at Princeton at that time was old-money elite smarts.

I entered Princeton naively believing that its prestigious reputation was owed entirely to its academic excellence. Luckily, there was enough of that to keep me distracted, and, to a point, validated. I owe my professional academic career in no small measure to my academic experiences at Princeton. I am eternally grateful for that. Yet, I also suffered from APEs—adverse Princeton experiences—beginning on day one.

Let me be clear: I do not mean to suggest that my uncomfortable experiences at Princeton have any equivalence to the racism or classism experienced by people of color throughout US history. I relay my experiences only because they provided me some degree of personal insight into the high-effort psychosocial coping that members of culturally oppressed groups spontaneously engage in when they enter a world that was not made for them. For Black people in a fundamentally white-supremacist and racist society, that experience pervades many aspects of their lives from day one. While the Princeton of my vintage had clearly not been made for me or people like me, many other places I navigated were, and I certainly did not live every day of my life in a state of perpetual vigilance.

Nonetheless, there was a lot of vigilance, which got jump-started at the very beginning of my time at Princeton when I met the parents of one of the girls in the dorm—a second-generation Princetonian—and saw the look of horror they registered when they realized I—with my Star of David necklace—was who their daughter would be living with. I overheard them referring to me as "that Jew girl." I was beginning to learn that my acceptance letter from the Office of Admission was no guarantee of acceptance into the broader Princeton community. Another roommate was an Upper East Side of Manhattan girl—also a legacy—who expressed her great social consciousness and frugality in our very first conversation by boasting that she had not let her parents spend more than $1,000 (about $6,000 in 2022 dollars) on her debutante ball gown, as she "could not see them spending more than that on a dress [she] would wear only once." I didn't know what a debutante ball was. The nicest piece of clothing in my wardrobe was last year's $5 dress (about $25 in 2022 dollars) from Filene's Basement. As another point of comparison, note that $1,000 covered about a third of a year's tuition at Princeton at that time. And then there was the constant anxiety of feeling that there was a hidden social curriculum that I wasn't privy to, that I was the only one who hadn't gotten the memo on how to behave or pass social muster according to dominant Princeton culture. For example, the dining halls opened at 5 p.m., yet some of us were mocked for eating dinner before seven, a sure sign that we had no class.

We've all had our "Toto, I've a feeling we are not in Kansas anymore" moments. Sometimes we are over the rainbow, seeing Technicolor for the first time. Sometimes we land on a battlefield. Sometimes, we're in a hologram, simultaneously experiencing the thrill of breathtaking new vistas and the anxiety of falling off the mountain ledge. For me, Princeton was that hologram.

I quickly learned that the recruitment brochures advertising Princeton as a welcoming place for women, students of color, and public-school students were, shall we say, aspirational. And hearing about the university's presumably well-meaning, if misguided, gesture of providing a sewing machine to each female member of the first coeducational class, which had arrived on campus just a few years before I did, was not reassuring, though it certainly spoke volumes about how women were seen (and struck me in particular as an odd gesture, since I was the granddaughter of a sweatshop worker).

Indeed, coeducation was actively contested at 1970s Princeton. A fervent alumni group formed in protest of the school's increasing diversity: the Concerned Alumni of Princeton, or CAP. As T. Harding Jones ('72), cofounder and executive director of CAP and editor of its magazine, *Prospect*, opined in the *New York Times* my first year at Princeton, "Coeducation has ruined the mystique and the camaraderies that used to exist. Princeton has now given into the fad of the moment, and I think it's going to prove to be a very unfortunate thing."[7] I guess T. Harding Jones worried he wasn't in Kansas anymore, either. Princeton was no longer his "safe space." In his eyes, Princeton had become a battlefield, not a rainbow coalition.

On that symbolic battlefield, I often spontaneously donned my "armor" as I walked from my dorm to the lecture hall, to the dining hall, or to rehearsals for the annual Triangle Show. The Triangle Club is a Princeton undergraduate musical comedy troupe that dates back to the 1880s. All it took to trigger my vigilance was to see fellow students wearing Concerned Alumni of Princeton swag—hats, T-shirts, even protest buttons that said "Bring Back the Old Princeton"—as they played Frisbee on the lawn. I could only take off my armor in situations that allowed me to unself-consciously assume that I had a legitimate claim to a place at Princeton, such as in the classrooms for the subjects in which I was intensely engaged, inspired by professors like James MacPherson, in American History, or Sheldon Wolin, in Political Theory, whose exciting and intricate lectures coaxed my brain to think at new levels; or at the dinner table where I could self-select to sit with other interlopers like me. When my social identity as an undeserving gate crasher, an *other*, was foregrounded, the armor went back on.

Being a cast member in the Triangle Club was meant to be a fun extracurricular activity, and it was for me—sometimes. But I spent much of my time there on spontaneous guard. If I had had elite smarts, I might have noticed that calling Triangle a club rather than, say, a theater group, had social implications. I was quite aware that the Triangle Club's board of trustees was made up of wealthy white alumni who had attended Princeton before it had admitted any Black people or women, and when its quota of eleven Jewish admits per year was drawn only from the "better kind," descendants of German immigrant businessmen, not Eastern European political refugees like my grandparents. I did not know if any of these men were sympathetic to CAP, but it certainly seemed plausible to think they might be, so whenever I was around them, my armor automatically enveloped me. Although the troupe was of course coed when I joined it, it remained steeped in wealthy-white-Princeton-male tradition. Hearkening back to the "good old days" of notable Triangle alumni like F. Scott Fitzgerald and Jimmy Stewart, the signature number in every show featured a chorus line of male cast members in drag. It was hard for me not to wonder how—or whether—I fit in.

Early Death Among Black Alumni of the Ivy League

In summer 2020, I received word that eleven of my Princeton classmates had died over the preceding year. Three were Black men, although Black men made up only 3.4 percent of the class. Their names were Ronald Shepperson, Stanley Reeves, and Krishna Singho. Up to that time, only about seventy-three of the 1,124 classmates, just over 6 percent, had died. However, 32 percent—a little less than one out of three—of the Black male members of the class were already deceased, more than five times the rate of white male members. Twelve percent of the Black women had died to date, four times the rate of white women. As for the white men from the class who had died, they mainly died from freak accidents and, in a couple of cases, of AIDS. (Ours was the generation that was blindsided by HIV, and with no available treatments, AIDS was a uniformly fatal disease.) In stark contrast, the women and men of color who were deceased, died disproportionately of cardiovascular and autoimmune disease or cancer, where weathering plays a role. Can this be just a coincidence?

Of the three Black classmates who died that year, we were told Stanley died after a "valiant fight with cancer"; Ron "lost his long fight with colon cancer"; and Krishna died of multiple myeloma, a type of blood cancer that affects the immune system. In the US, Black men have higher prevalence of colon cancer than white men and die from it at earlier ages. Oscar-winning actor Chadwick Boseman died of colon cancer in 2020 at age 43, and the anti-racist public intellectual Ibram X Kendi was diagnosed with stage-4 colon cancer at age thirty-six. Recent research has found that the excess prevalence of colon cancer among young Black men appears to be related to premature epigenetic aging of the cells in the walls of their right colons. The same cells do not age as quickly in white men.[8] Black men also have twice the rate of multiple myeloma as white men, and with an earlier onset.[9] My classmate Krishna Singho was diagnosed at age fifty with a cancer that is mostly associated with the elderly.

Not only were these three men Princeton graduates, but all went on to become highly accomplished professionals. Ronald Shepperson went to medical school and served as the chair of the anesthesiology department at the medical center where he worked. Stanley Reeves attended Harvard Law School and worked for many years in one of Manhattan's elite law firms. Krishna Singho worked at the

Department of Justice, where he was recognized with numerous honors and commendations. By the end of their lives, all three men could be assumed to have grit, privilege, and affluence. Their obituaries described them as brilliant.

Why did these men die in their early sixties? The life expectancy of white men in their age sixty cohort and social class is ninety-two years. The national average for Black men in their age cohort across all educational and income levels is well into the seventies. It could certainly be a coincidence, although their overrepresentation among early deaths in our class mirrors findings about their peers at Yale, suggesting otherwise.[10] A more likely possibility is that they suffered severe weathering, having spent large portions of their adult years wearing psychosocial armor, just as my father had.

Krishna, in particular, appeared to have been a well-assimilated and certainly well-known member of our class during our college years. I still remember him for his engaging smile and beautiful singing voice. More than many Black undergraduates at the time, he traveled in campus "high society." He auditioned for and became a member of Princeton's signature, storied, all-male and preppie-clad a capella group, the Tigertones, and was chosen to join one of the exclusive eating clubs whose invited members were rarely people of color. However, despite living within driving distance of Princeton for the rest of his life, he attended only one class reunion (out of forty since we graduated), while other nearby alumni members of his social circle attended annually. Even the class officers who notified us of his passing remarked that he was "surprisingly absent from most reunions and other events." I can't help but wonder: was he avoiding something? Was spending time at Princeton stressful for him, despite his apparent social successes there? Maybe having assimilated into the highest social circles at Princeton had exposed him to so many othering encounters that he chose to sidestep them in his postcollegiate years.

Reading the obituary of Stanley Reeves, the elite Manhattan

lawyer, I was struck by this description: "Personal and engaging during the workday, he retreated home at night, content with a glass of wine and C-SPAN."[11] I wondered, was that the only time he was able to take off his armor?

These are only speculations, of course, but what is not speculative is the tragic fact that these men all died relatively young, of diseases connected to weathering.

The Weathering Effects of Integration and Upward Mobility

Historically, we have been concerned with the damage marginalized groups suffer as a result of being segregated into underfunded school systems and disinvested neighborhoods. We know and now espouse as a truth championed by the Supreme Court in 1954— when it ruled on the *Brown v. Board of Education* case — that separate is not equal. But as the stories of my father, my Black Princeton classmates, and even, to a lesser extent, my own Princeton experience suggest, integration is not equal either. When in-groups and othered groups sit at the same table, members of the latter group are more likely to be subjected to the biopsychosocial stress arousal response that triggers weathering than when they spend time only with members of their own group.

A new study led by one of my former students, Cynthia Colen, and her colleagues at Ohio State University, illustrates this strikingly.[12] Colen and her team analyzed data from the Add Health study—a nationally representative sample of more than twenty thousand adolescents who were in grades seven through twelve during the 1994/95 school year, and who have continued to be followed into their thirties. The researchers compared the risk of developing metabolic syndrome by the early thirties among two groups of Black Americans: those who attended historically Black colleges or universities (HBCUs), and those who attended predominantly white institutions (PWIs). Metabolic syndrome is a cluster of conditions that occur together, increasing one's risk of heart disease, stroke, and type 2 diabetes. These conditions include increased blood pressure, high blood sugar, excess body fat around the waist, and abnormal cholesterol or triglyceride levels—all factors implicated in weathering. Colen and her colleagues found that Black American college graduates who had attended HBCUs were 35 percent less likely to develop metabolic syndrome by their early thirties than Black American college graduates of PWIs, an indication that they were less likely to have demonstrably weathered as young adults.

Findings such as these raise difficult questions. Have we taken too shallow an approach to integration? Are our expectations of integration infused with the racist, white supremacist notion that Black people will benefit from gaining access to white institutions because those institutions are inherently superior? Have racist ideas about substandard intelligence or character in Blacks led us to believe that Black institutions are necessarily "lesser"? We are seeing that some of the highest-achieving African Americans are HBCU graduates, including Kamala Harris, the first woman, not to mention the first woman of color, to serve as vice president of the United States. Colen's study tells us that HBCUs not only foster socioeconomic achievement in their graduates, they also promote their physical health. That racialized social identity becomes central to students of color when they attend a PWI is suggested as far back as 1928 when Zora Neale Hurston wrote:

> I remember the very day that I became colored. Up to my thirteenth year I lived in the little Negro town of Eatonville, Florida. It is exclusively a colored town. . . . But changes came in the family when I was thirteen, and I was sent to school in Jacksonville. I left Eatonville, the town of the oleanders, a Zora. When

I disembarked from the river-boat at Jacksonville...I was not Zora of Orange County any more, I was now a little colored girl...

I do not always feel colored...I feel most colored when I am thrown against a sharp white background. For instance at Barnard [College]. "Beside the waters of the Hudson" I feel my race. Among the thousand white persons, I am a dark rock surged upon, and overswept.[13]

A strong argument could be made that in the current racialized environment, high-achieving Black students should give serious consideration to attending an HBCU even if they have access to a top PWI like Princeton. However, over the long term, if we want to find a solution to the issues that prompt such a recommendation, it would be worthwhile for all of us to deepen our understanding of what happens to the bodies of high achievers from culturally oppressed communities who attend PWIs, and then to investigate what would be necessary to make these institutions places where members of marginalized groups would feel welcome and thrive without a serious cost to their health. HBCUs will always have a valued place in the Black community, but students considering their educational options shouldn't have to take their physical health or life expectancy into account when they make their decisions about where to go to school.

Stereotype Threat

Whether on the savanna or in a classroom, physiological stress processes are set in motion when any kind of threat is perceived. The threat does not have to take the form of a raging beast. In the education literature, the eminent social psychologist Claude Steele and his colleagues have demonstrated repeatedly that racial stereotyping constitutes a threat that can be so powerful that social identity becomes "the center of a person's functioning, powerful enough to make it more important, for the duration of the threat, at least, than any of the person's other identities."[14] This, in turn, through the neuro-endocrine impact of the stress responses, can undermine a person's performance on a high-stakes academic test.

Since social identity stereotypes permeate the air in our age-washed and race-, ethnicity-, class-, and gender-conscious society, the fear of seeming to confirm a negative stereotype is always a potential problem for members of marginalized groups. But there is a body of research suggesting that there are ways of manipulating the cues to stereotyping in order to neutralize the threat it presents to stigmatized group members. Experiments have shown that these strategies can work to benefit not just the academic performance of Black students generally but also that of girls in math, science, and engineering classes, and even the athletic performance of young white men.

For example, when Black American college students were told beforehand that performance on a standardized test would be diagnostic of their intellectual ability, this cue made them alert to the stereotype that Blacks are innately less intelligent than whites. The result: Black students who took the test performed significantly worse than those who were *not* told the same test was diagnostic of intellectual ability.[15] Women's experiences in science and math are also significantly shaped by cues pertaining to their social identity.[16] While investigating the power of both racist and sexist stereotypes, for example, researchers found that Asian American girls performed better on tests of mathematical achievement when they were cued to remember they were Asian (the relevant stereotype being that Asians are good at math). Asian American girls did worse on the same math tests when cued to remember they were girls (the stereotype being that girls are bad at math).[17] This impact has been observed experimentally in Asian girls in the US as young as five years old!

Regarding athletic performance, when white male college golfers were asked to perform a task they were told measured "natural athletic ability," they performed worse than a control group that was not told that. When Black male college golfers were assigned a task they were told would measure their "sports strategic intelligence," they performed more poorly than their control group. By contrast, the same experiments showed that Black performance was *not* undermined when athletes were told they were being tested for "natural athletic ability"—the relevant stereotype here being that Black people are by nature athletic. Likewise, white performance was *not* undermined by the "strategic intelligence" cue because the relevant stereotype is that white people are smart.[18] Another stereotype threat experiment involved older people who were given a memory performance task after being cued that old age impairs memory. You won't be surprised to learn that they remembered measurably less than their peers who were not reminded of that ageist stereotype.[19]

No matter your social identities or privilege, you have probably bought into various stereotypes about yourself—both positive (I'm Asian, so I must be good at math; I'm Black, so I must be good at sports) and negative (I'm female, so I must be bad at math; I'm old, so I must have memory problems)—that have the potential to affect your performance.

Researchers who are trying to address this issue have found that certain kinds of carefully designed cues in classrooms or other performance settings may be able to improve the engagement, aspirations, persistence, and performance of members of various marginalized social identity groups.[20] Other stereotype threat researchers found that even small and seemingly cosmetic changes in classrooms could profoundly affect the appeal of the subject matter being taught to members of marginalized groups. For example, experiments showed that undergraduate women in computer science classes were more engaged by the subject matter when their classroom was decorated with nature posters than when it was decorated with *Star Trek* posters. Being in a room with nature posters boosted their interest in computer science to the same level as men's. Undergraduate men's interest was unaffected by which posters were displayed.[21]

Just as Arthur Ashe always counted the number of Black or brown faces in settings where he felt his racial identity could be a factor, always hoping to find safety in numbers, one study that manipulated the number of male test-takers present in a testing room found women's math performance was directly related to the number of male peers in the testing environment. The more men, the worse their performance. But there was no such effect observed for men when women's representation was manipulated.[22]

A growing body of evidence from brain-imaging studies helps to explain how stereotype threat operates to impede performance by recruiting the neural mechanisms of emotion in the brain while short-circuiting the cognitive ones. This is but one strand in a complex web of the physiological processes that will, over time, trigger weathering.

For example, one study found that African Americans completing a test in a stereotype-threat situation exhibited higher blood pressure and worse performance than when they took the same test in a nonthreatening environment. Their blood pressure remained elevated during a rest period and at least through completion of a second test. No such effect was found when white American study participants took the test.[23]

In another study, the social psychologist Mary Murphy and her colleagues found that a group of women who were shown a male-dominated video advertising a leadership conference for math, science, and engineering students experienced faster heart rates, enhanced skin conductance, and greater sympathetic activation of the cardiovascular system (all signs of physiological stress arousal) than a comparison group of women who were shown a gender-balanced video. Women who watched the video with a predominance of men in the room were also less interested in attending the conference than the other group, which was mostly women.[24] Having such experiences on occasion is unlikely to cause lasting harm to health. But encountering them time and time again over a long period, even a lifetime, can be immensely damaging.

Stereotype threat is particularly pernicious among those who face it repeatedly in their daily rounds. And it can be all the more so when they are in situations where their ability to perform or their livelihood is at stake. For example, think of a woman in a predominantly male engineering company, an older person navigating a tech start-up headed by a twenty-five-year-old CEO, a white person on a predominantly Black basketball team, or a Black person in a predominantly white college. All of these are high-stakes settings where the contingency of social identity can activate harmful physiological stress processes that impede performance.

The Cost of Ambition and Grit

What we learn from stereotype research literature is that the exact same setting can be experienced differently by members of different social identity groups. This is why the traditional narrative of upward mobility—that if you work hard to earn your seat at the privileged table things will go smoothly for you thereafter—does not hold true for everyone. Different people will have different experiences at the same table. Those from the dominant culture feel quite comfortable in privileged spaces; the marginalized, however, are likely to experience such spaces as othering. In fact, if you are a member of a marginalized group, being in one of those privileged spaces can constitute an ongoing source of stress, as it did for my father.

My colleague Jay Pearson, whose work on socioeconomic status and health I described earlier, seems in many ways to be the ultimate modern success story. In his twenties and thirties, I watched him navigate a doctoral program and early postdoctoral career to the heights of early academic success. Such achievement is exceedingly unlikely for a guy who spent the first decade of his life without indoor plumbing, did grueling farm work as a child, worked in a meat processing plant in his teens, and attended a public school where fewer than one in four students performed at grade level. His tenacity and intelligence were always impressive. Yet, during the decades of his meteoric rise, I watched his health deteriorate as he suffered a series of chronic and acute health events one would typically associate with someone decades older. His morale deteriorated in pace.

In early 2017, Jay sent me a distressing email. By that point in his forties, he had just suffered a significant cardiac event, the capstone — to date — of a series of dramatic health problems I had seen him endure for as long as I had known him. Still, he was thinking affirmatively about what he could do to turn the tide. The message he sent me read:

I am not currently well, pretty bad actually, but have insight into the fundamental changes that may move me in a positive direction. In short, I need to get a handle on reducing distress and increasing sleep. I didn't really appreciate how much those two matter and assumed that my broader healthy lifestyle was protecting me. As you know I have never drunk alcohol, done drugs, or smoked. I eat healthy, exercise regularly and work hard to avoid dramatic social relationships.

My ambitious journey has come at a cost that, despite my best efforts, is starting to (has) impact(ed) my well-being. Much of it is exactly what I learned from you and now aspire to teach my students. I should also say that is the most disconcerting of all things to realize that I am being impacted by the very phenomena I study and teach.

From an aerial view, Jay Pearson's biography looks something like a fairy tale, the American dream personified: a Black and Native (Haliwa-Saponi tribe) man born in the depths of southern rural poverty who worked his way against strong headwinds to a tenured faculty position at Duke University. His success is the type that might make you think that anything is possible if you just buckle down and work for it—and Jay certainly worked extremely hard. The more we zero in, however, the more we see how closely Jay's story resembles that of my father, and of my prematurely deceased Black Princeton classmates.

Let's start from the beginning...

Born in rural North Carolina, Jay was ten years old before he lived in a home with running water, which happened only once his family moved from the country to a trailer park closer to town. At the same age, he began working in the watermelon fields. At age twelve, he, his brother, his cousins, and his neighborhood friends were recruited to the fields to pick cucumbers. They agreed to take on this physically demanding farm labor after being told they would be paid each day by the number of bushels they picked. However, after the first full day of picking, no pay was forthcoming. In response to this exploitation, the other boys lost faith and did not return the next day.

Jay, however, did go back, and he continued to work through the whole week. Each day he received no pay; each day he was told he would be paid the next day...and the next...He essentially worked for no payment for the better part of five days, yet persevered doing heavy labor in the searing sun, picking as many bushels of cucumbers as he could.

When he was finally paid at week's end, he was stiffed. The check was written out for $17 when, according to the piece rate he had been promised per bushel, it should have come to $92. He was paid for less than one day of labor after working five.

No one contested the number of bushels of cucumbers he had picked—and the pay was supposed to be purely a function of that number. Hoping this was an honest mistake, Jay went to ask for his full pay from his boss, Mr. Parsons, a white man he had never met.

Sitting at his desk in an air-conditioned trailer, Mr. Parsons told him: "If you want to get paid more, you are going to have to work harder. This is good work for people like you, and I am not giving you any more money. I say it's good work because if you weren't out here working in my fields, you would be at home on welfare with your mother collecting my tax money."

Jay's worth in Mr. Parsons' eyes was contingent on Jay's social identity as a poor Black youth, not on his actual performance. Based on similar stereotyping, Mr. Parsons assumed Jay's mother was a welfare recipient, when he had no knowledge of whether she was or wasn't. She wasn't. As Jay described it, "Mr. Parsons had determined my market value and I was going to be paid that rate, completely independent of how hard I had worked. The power dynamics of the position Mr. Parsons occupied in relation to the one I occupied in the community made it such that there was nothing in any practical sense that I could do to defend myself."

Jay notes he felt enraged and that his first impulse was to attack Mr. Parsons, but he didn't. Instead, Jay viewed what had happened as a learning experience.

> I took that lesson with me and held on to it. It guided my commitment to do well in the classroom and, frankly, influences the work now in my research, teaching, and advocacy, this notion of a hierarchy of human valuation and what happens when someone relegated to an inferior position performs beyond their position.

Jay has told me about this defining experience many times. Although the incident occurred decades ago, each time he tells it, the urgency in his voice and demeanor makes it feel like it happened yesterday. He moves to the edge of his seat, his eyes widen, his throat tightens—all signs that the memory still has the power to activate physiologic stress arousal in his body several decades and countless tellings later. He sometimes chuckles during the most horrendous parts of the story, as if to reassure me they were not as painful as they clearly were.

Many would have assumed that Jay's professional success and everything that has come with it—income, prestige, connections, a home in a well-resourced neighborhood, a sense of mastery—would have dimmed the memory of that long-ago week in the cucumber fields and given him a better health outcome than he could have expected had he remained living in rural poverty, working in a chicken factory like his mother or as a truck driver like his brother. Not so. He may even have become more sensitized to the stereotyping Mr. Parsons directed at him because of the many other hostile stereotyping episodes he experienced during the course of his rise to success. And the cumulative effect of all these traumatic experiences likely set in motion a series of chronic stress arousal processes.

Here, I'm thinking not only about the challenges of navigating privileged white settings while being a Black man from a poor family where he was the first to graduate high school, and the only one to graduate from college and graduate school; I'm also thinking about the qualities he had to have in order to achieve that success against such odds. That's why I recounted the story he told me about being stiffed after a week of grueling labor—labor that the other kids refused to continue doing after one day of being cheated. Jay's going back to work, day after unpaid day, was evidence of grit.

Grit and resilience, as well as self-regulation, impulse control, and high executive function, which allow for delayed gratification, are highly prized attributes in our culture, attributes parents and school curricula seek to develop or enhance in our children, especially in our children of color given pervasive racist ideas that their troubles stem from essential deficiencies in these areas. This is why the so-called marshmallow test has become such a marker for children's potential for success, and why parents keep posting videos on Instagram showing their children taking that test.

In case you have somehow managed to avoid seeing these ubiquitous videos, the test involves a child who is left alone in a room with a marshmallow (or other treat), after an adult has told the child that if they can go fifteen minutes without eating the treat, they can have two treats. The point of the marshmallow test, aside from generating some incredibly cute videos of children devising their own methods for holding out for fifteen minutes, is to see whether the children who participate are capable of self-regulation and high executive function. Children who hold out for two marshmallows are believed to have greater impulse control, cognitive flexibility, and working memory than those who do not.[25]

The original marshmallow experiment was done with children at the Bing Nursery School, which is affiliated with Stanford University. The children came mainly from white, affluent, highly educated families. Bing's curriculum was and is based on the highest levels of expert knowledge in early child development. Follow-up studies suggest that the children from the original experimental study who did well on the marshmallow test were significantly more competent and had higher SAT scores in high school than the children who didn't.

How well the marshmallow test might predict later educational success in children from marginalized groups was not tested in the original study. However, a recent study that drew on a larger and more socioeconomically diverse sample found little evidence of the test's ability to predict academic success in adolescence if the differences in socioeconomic position among the children were controlled for.[26] The authors concluded that the capacity to hold out for a second marshmallow is shaped in large part by a child's social and economic background—and moreover that having a privileged background is a better predictor of the likelihood of success than the ability to delay gratification. In other words, among the highly privileged there may be some "within group" differences in long-term success between those who do and do not hold out for the second marshmallow; but in the big picture these are rounding errors;

the best predictor of long-term socioeconomic success is how privileged a background a child is born into.

For most students from highly disadvantaged backgrounds, impulse control in the context of holding out for the second marshmallow makes little difference to their ultimate socioeconomic success—a testament to the structural barricades impeding their efforts toward socioeconomic mobility. Interestingly, there have been versions of the study that find that whether a child waits for the extra marshmallow depends not only on the predisposition of the specific child, but also on whether the experimental manipulation provides the child reason to trust that the experimenter will keep their word about returning to offer the second treat. In one variation, the children were randomized into two groups: in one group, the experimenter broke a promise to them before starting the marshmallow test; in the other, the experimenter kept a promise before doing so. Children in the reliable tester (promise kept) group waited up to four times longer than those in the unreliable tester (broken promise) group for the second marshmallow to appear.[27]

So, in fact, we might conclude that, far from lacking executive function, children from poor families who eat the single marshmallow are actually making a realistic appraisal, based on their life experience of broken promises, that since there is no guarantee a second marshmallow will be produced, it's not worth waiting for. We are deeply impressed by twelve-year-old Jay Pearson's persistence, but we also can understand his brother's and cousins' and friends' choosing not to return for a second day of grueling physical labor after they were not given the pay they had been promised. "Fool me once," we might say. With only $17 in his pocket after a week of punishing work, many—including Jay—would think that *he* was the chump.

We might wonder whether those who do well on the marshmallow test despite being members of poor or racially excluded groups, like Jay Pearson, are expending a greater effort in coping than more privileged children. The high value placed on the capacity for self-control implicit in the structure of the original marshmallow test does not take into account what effect a child's being malnourished or coming from a food-insecure family might have on the results. Yet the majority of American teachers say they have children who come to school hungry on any given day; government estimates suggest about 50 million Americans, including about 17 million children, suffer food insecurity. We might excuse a hungry child for gobbling up the marshmallow and not conclude that their behavior indicates a lack of executive function.

What does it cost a child who is hungry to hold out for a second marshmallow? What must it have cost Jay to hold on to his faith in an ultimate reward even in the face of each day's broken promises? And might we conclude that children and young adults from marginalized groups who show the greatest grit and perseverance in everyday life are likely to pay a price in their health for their strict, even remarkable persistence in the belief that their efforts will reap future rewards? There is a quickly developing scientific literature that suggests the answer to that question is yes.

Overcoming the Machine: The John Henryism Scale of Active Coping

The John Henryism Scale of Active Coping (JHAC12) is a simple psychometric test composed of the twelve items listed on the next page. The respondent indicates the strength of their agreement with each statement on a five-point scale from "I disagree a lot" to "I agree a lot." As you will quickly realize from reading the items, a higher score on this test indicates a higher psychological predisposition to take personal responsibility, have grit, be resilient, and remain determined to succeed in the face of adversity—all core values of the American Creed.

THE JOHN HENRYISM SCALE OF ACTIVE COPING

I've always felt that I could make of my life pretty much what I wanted to make of it.

Once I make up my mind to do something, I stay with it until the job is completely done.

I like doing things that other people thought could not be done.

When things don't go the way I want them to, that just makes me work even harder.

Sometimes I feel that if anything is going to be done right, I have to do it myself.

It is not always easy, but I manage to find a way to do the things I really need to get done.

Very seldom have I been disappointed by the results of my hard work.

I feel that I am the kind of individual who stands up for what he believes in, regardless of the consequences.

In the past, even when things got really tough, I never lost sight of my goals.

It is important for me to be able to do things the way I want to do them rather than the way other people want me to do them.

I do not let my personal feelings get in the way of doing a job.

Hard work has really helped me to get ahead in life.

This well-validated psychometric scale is the scientific brainchild of the social epidemiologist Sherman A. James, former president of the Society for Epidemiologic Research. Early in his career, James was inspired by the story of John Henry Martin, a Black patient with hypertension in North Carolina whom James interviewed as part of an effort to understand why Black working-class men, on average, suffered the highest rates of hypertensive disease. It was not lost on Professor James that Mr. Martin shared a name with the legendary John Henry who, according to folklore, mobilized his physical and mental capabilities to challenge the steam engine, succeeding at that task but dying of exhaustion at the moment of his triumph. James saw this myth as offering a distinctively African American allegory about the profound physical cost of a Black man's self-reliance and determination in the face of a racist society.

As Professor James tells his story, John Henry Martin was born into a dirt-poor sharecropper family and dropped out of school in the second grade to help farm the small plot of land that the family rented.[28] As a youth, "he vowed that he would not be trapped in a system of labor that kept him perpetually in debt to white landowners." After taking a forty-year bank mortgage to purchase seventy-five acres of his own farmland, he paid off the mortgage in only five years. To do so "he worked day and night." One might guess that John Henry Martin would easily ace the marshmallow test, as he did this much harder and higher-stakes test in the real world.

James observed that both John Henrys were tenacious, self-reliant, and optimistic, both overcame "the machine," and both paid a high health price for their victory. The legendary John Henry died of exhaustion. Professor James noted that Mr. Martin suffered from chronic hypertensive disease and disabling osteoarthritis, and that in late middle age he had to have 40 percent of his stomach removed when it was found to be riddled with severe peptic ulcers. Confiding in Sherman James, Martin said, "I believe the reason my legs are all out of whack, today, with arthritis [is that] I pushed myself too hard."[29]

Clearly, Jay Pearson is a modern-day John Henry as well.

James demonstrated through his research that African American men who score highly on the John Henryism scale (i.e., have a strong internal locus of control and are determined to succeed) but run up against structural impediments to success—as so many Black American men do—are at increased risk for high blood pressure. Those from equally disadvantaged and humble beginnings with low JHAC12 scores are not. It is not their Blackness or working-class status, per se, that causes those who rank high in John Henryism to develop hypertension; it's the interaction of the three. Contrary to the entrenched beliefs about hypertension genes, unhealthy habits, or a lack of economic resources as the explanation for high hypertension rates in Black men, James documented that among poor and working-class Black men, those who evidenced the greatest grit were more likely to develop hypertension than those who had *less* of it.[30]

Many additional studies have since provided evidence that among the Black working class, being high in John Henryism predicts higher mean blood pressure, obesity, and other risk factors for cardiovascular disease and cancer.[31] In other words, in the face of structural adversity, Black working-class people who persevere and strive to pull themselves up by their bootstraps are likely to weather more than others.

Over the last decade, an impressive body of research has emerged that confirms the physiological toll of resilience among people of color and other marginalized groups. Drawing on representative samples from both rural and urban environments, this research bases its conclusions on a variety of objective measures of physical health as revealed by medical diagnoses and laboratory tests. The findings pertain to a wide range of health outcomes, ranging from asthma to hypertension to diabetes. Researchers have also measured levels of stress hormones circulating in the bloodstream, inflammation, metabolic syndrome, and other laboratory indicators of the propensity for the early onset of chronic disease, including cardiovascular disease.

One body of studies followed a representative sample of 489 African American youth living in rural Georgia, many of whom were from socioeconomic backgrounds similar to Jay Pearson's. Following this sample through young adulthood, the researchers found that:

Those who had exhibited higher levels of self-control as disadvantaged youth had higher blood pressure, more body fat, and higher levels of the stress hormone cortisol, compared to peers who were more impetuous and less upwardly mobile. They also found that those who attended college had worse physical health than their similarly disadvantaged peers who did not attend college.[32]

Those who had grown up in persistent poverty and who were reported by their teachers as having high levels of "planful self-control" when they were age eleven were more likely to attend college and were also more likely to have insulin resistance and metabolic syndrome at age twenty-seven. In other words, they were more likely to show signs of weathering before age thirty.[33]

In addition to following their sample's trajectories of disease risk and adverse health conditions, the research team considered differences in weathering at the cellular level. Molecular information was collected on about 300 of the sample members when they were twenty-two in order to measure epigenetic aging, a biomarker that reflects the disparity between one's chronological and biological age, and thus a molecular indicator of weathering. The investigators found that:

Among twenty-two-year-olds from low-income families, those who maintained self-control, resisted temptation, and achieved long-term academic aspirations, were less likely to express aggression or use drugs than their childhood peers. Even so, they showed more rapid immune-cell aging than their peers who had exhibited less resilience and self-control in childhood.[34]

Other studies have come to complementary conclusions.

In a study of Black, white, and Latinx youth with asthma in Chicago, those minority youth who experienced high levels of school stress and also evidenced greater self-control despite the stress, showed worse asthma inflammatory profiles and more frequent physician contacts during the one-year follow-up than minority youth with less self-control. These patterns were not evident in white youth with asthma.[35]

A nationally representative study (the Midlife in the United States study) that collected data from Americans ranging from twenty-five to seventy-five years old found that being a college graduate lowered the probability of having metabolic syndrome for young-to-middle-aged white adults, but it increased the risk of metabolic syndrome among the Black and Latinx adults.[36]

One study based on data from the Add Health study found that white college graduates who came from disadvantaged childhoods had lower rates of metabolic syndrome and better mental health than Hispanic and Black college graduates from disadvantaged childhood environments.[37]

Another Add Health–based study found that Black participants who had shown high-striving tendencies in their adolescence were more likely than others to have graduated college and have higher incomes, as we might expect. However, the high-striving Black participants from the most disadvantaged families had a greater likelihood of developing type 2 diabetes by age twenty-nine than those who were not high-striving as youth. No such pattern was found among whites.[38]

A study analyzing data from the Health and Retirement Study, whose sample only includes Black and white Americans who had survived at least until age fifty (leaving out the Americans most likely to be weathered, namely those who die before age fifty), found that lab measures of accelerated biological aging accounted for up to 95 percent of Black/white differences in health span and mortality.[39]

The burning message of all these studies is that culturally oppressed children of color raised in poor or working-class families who beat the odds through hopefulness, hard work, and perseverance weather young, across many body systems. Evidence of this weathering is found in children, young adults, and the middle-aged and elderly alike. The avalanche of evidence that supports this conclusion cannot be ignored.

Before moving on, please take a moment to sit with these

findings. Let it sink in that, however counterintuitive you may find these facts, they tell us that success comes at a spectacularly high health cost for those who have to fight the hardest to achieve it in the context of a society that doesn't value them.

We are left to ask, along with Larry Davis, dean emeritus of the University of Pittsburgh School of Social Work, "Have we gone too far with resiliency?"[40] In his provocative essay of the same name, Davis construes resiliency as the ability to withstand bad things happening to you without the expected devastating outcomes. He wonders aloud whether those like him in the helping professions are "spending too much of our energies charting and applauding the ability of individuals, families, and groups to successfully sustain societal abuse, hardship, and injustice."

That those suffering hardship or abuse need to be so extraordinarily resilient if they are to have any chance of succeeding is an indictment of our society, which not only sets up a large swath of the oppressed for failure, but also sets up those few who succeed in beating the odds for a lifetime of poor health. The weathering impacts of othering, stereotype threat, and John Henryism tell us that the resilient will not escape scot-free. Their physical health cannot withstand what society asks them to withstand, whether in segregated or integrated settings.

Why should marginalized, oppressed, and exploited people have to be superheroes in order to survive and thrive within this system? And, in the face of systemic injustice and cultural oppression, why do we continue to put so much of our focus on applauding the victims who against all odds succeed at avoiding the natural consequences of a racist system, rather than doing what we can to dismantle the system itself?

8.

Social Policy and the Assault on Black Family Life

Several signature pieces of legislation of the past thirty years—all ostensibly intended to promote better living conditions, higher incomes, better education, safe neighborhoods, and overall improvements in the futures of poor youth and families—have placed new barriers in the way of marginalized populations' efforts to survive and overcome. Among these legislative initiatives were welfare reform, the implementation of school voucher policies for students in failing schools, which took them out of their neighborhoods, and housing policies aiming to "deconcentrate" poverty in racially segregated cities.

To make matters even worse, these policies coincided with other societal trends that reinforced weathering, including the loss of low-skill jobs, declining real wages for blue-collar workers, and skyrocketing housing and health-care costs, as well as the move to a competitive health-care system, which, among other consequences, shuttered hospitals in disinvested urban and rural areas and disproportionately reduced access to health care for the very populations most vulnerable to weathering. The specific policies, whose weathering impact I will describe on the pages that follow, were enacted alongside the War on Drugs, which resulted in the mass incarceration of Black people. Sending all these men and women to prison peeled them away from their kin networks and left them less employable upon release. It also increased the economic, practical, and biopsychosocial burdens on those they left behind, who had to hold down the fort while carrying on in the face of yet more feelings of loss and injustice. As a group, this combination of policies and secular trends added to the burdens of individuals and kin networks, making it harder for them to support their down-and-out members while, in effect, increasing the probability that members of their networks would *be* down and out.

Some of the impetus toward these policies was mean-spirited— designed, for instance, to punish so-called welfare queens. Some was well-meaning yet infused with prevailing age-washed and racist ideas. Most often, the policies were designed by politicians and policy makers who, in considering how limited public resources should best be allocated, did not make social equity a priority. Rather, they tended to attack the problems of cost and scarcity as the result of financial accounting issues and saw the solution as necessary budget tightening, or austerity policies. And they often justified their actions as aimed at encouraging personal responsibility among the poor. But their concept of what constituted responsible action grew out of their own narrow and highly privileged worldview, whether from the right or the left. The narratives they traded on ignored or caricatured the actual needs and experience of marginalized groups, becoming racist in their impact, if not always in their intent. Our research provides evidence that the weathering of oppressed populations worsened, and that overall health inequities were entrenched, in the wake of these policies.[1]

As a general guide, there are three criteria to use in evaluating the degree to which public policies and laws are likely to contribute to weathering:

Do they proliferate demeaning or threatening stereotypes about marginalized communities and their residents?

Do they diminish income or buying power, or degrade housing or environmental or neighborhood conditions?

Do they fragment or impose new burdens on the kin networks that members of marginalized populations depend on in order to alleviate the burdens they face?[2]

How did key social policies of the 1980s and 1990s, which continue in one form or another to this day, measure up in these three dimensions?

The Personal Responsibility and Work Opportunity Reconciliation Act of 1996

The Personal Responsibility and Work Opportunity Reconciliation Act of 1996 (PRWORA), which was signed into law by President Bill Clinton, is most often referred to as welfare reform.[3] Many, however, would argue that a more accurate characterization of it would be welfare *repeal*. PRWORA ended the welfare entitlement program known as Aid to Families with Dependent Children (AFDC), which guaranteed monthly cash assistance along with automatic access to Medicaid for single mothers whose income fell below a conservative federal poverty line. AFDC was imperfect and had its own weathering effects. However, what replaced it—Temporary Assistance to Needy Families (TANF)—is worse.

PRWORA instituted the TANF program in 1996. Among TANF's many drawbacks is that it severed Medicaid from automatic enrollment, which made it harder for the poorest families to obtain health insurance. It also included work requirements even for mothers with preschool-age children and, in some states, infants.

TANF is not an entitlement program, meaning it isn't guaranteed to all mothers who meet the low-income eligibility threshold. The federal government's economic contribution is provided through lump sum block grants to the states, which then administer the program. The block grants come with a federally mandated five-year lifetime limit, regardless of what a recipient's needs are. States have discretion to make the time limit even shorter or to add other restrictions, such as a "family cap" that excludes TANF-assisted families from receiving any additional aid at the birth of another child. About half of all states now have a family cap, and many states have reduced lifetime limits to fewer than five years. Time limits are only one of the provisions in TANF that allow for the involuntary removal of a TANF recipient from the program. Because the grants are not an entitlement, a state can deny assistance to any family for any reason.

Indeed, states are allowed broad discretion to use the block grants for a variety of purposes besides direct cash assistance for families. And since the federal government has moved toward fiscal austerity, allocating fewer resources to states, the states have responded by increasingly shifting the TANF block grants to other needs and services that lacked funding. Perversely, as sociologists Kathryn J. Edin and H. Luke Shaefer have documented, the move to TANF has led to a deepening of child poverty, with many Americans now living on essentially "$2.00 per person a day."[4] Many families who migrated from AFDC to TANF lost much of the meager economic protection they once had.

In conception and practice, PRWORA fulfills all three of the criteria for stoking weathering. Let's evaluate it in more detail.

PRWORA and Racist Stereotyping: The Vilification of the Teen Mother

The personal-responsibility narrative that rationalized welfare reform clearly generated demeaning and demoralizing stereotypes. In fact, its entire logical foundation was crafted from the big lie that urban decay was the result of moral decay in Black families, and that Black poverty was the inevitable and just consequence of their behavior. Ignoring the strengths of the Black family structure, which had historically been flexible and resilient in the face of material hardship, cultural oppression, and severe health challenges, this dominant narrative suggested that motherhood in the teens was proof of moral decay, and was the cause of poverty rather than a response to it. Kin networks, with their elastic household boundaries, were redefined as disorganized and pathological. Men who had to leave their household to find work, or who weren't legally married to their children's mothers, or who suffered early disability, death, or incarceration, were reframed as irresponsible "absent fathers." And young Black men, who faced permanent unemployment for structural reasons, were painted as threatening: sexual superpredators, muggers, and violent drug dealers whose images, as Robin D. G. Kelley, a historian at UCLA, described it, were publicly circulated as "the very representations of race that generate terror in all of us."[5]

This narrative put Black families in general, and so-called teen mothers and absent fathers in particular, at the center of urban poverty, crime, and poor infant health. It ignored the tangible effects of racial segregation and disinvestment in predominantly Black urban centers. Essentially, it reversed cause and effect.

Central to this racist narrative is the unexamined stylized assumption that by the end of the 1960s, the Black family, once strong, had become a "tangle of pathology."[6] Daniel Patrick Moynihan asserted in his now infamous 1965 report to the US Department of Labor, *The Negro Family: The Case for National Action*, that the weakness of the Black family structure was a "principal source of most of the aberrant, inadequate, or antisocial behavior that did not establish, but now serves to perpetuate the cycle of poverty and deprivation" in the Black community. The proximate cause, according to Moynihan and his ilk: Aid to Families with Dependent Children (AFDC), which had originated as a program to provide for white widows with young children but was opened up in the 1960s to unmarried Black mothers, who had until then effectively been denied such welfare assistance. These new Black clients were stereotyped as people who, given welfare, would become dependent on it owing to their weakness of character. The goal of the new social welfare policy that replaced

AFDC with TANF was no longer to ensure every family a decent standard of living, but to cure Black adults of their imagined depraved addiction to being "takers."

The basic mythology was that the availability of AFDC to unmarried Black mothers had let Black men off the hook for the responsibility of supporting their families, which meant they didn't have to get jobs, while incentivizing young Black women to become pregnant in order to receive a welfare check. Riddled with racist ideas, the personal-responsibility narrative was sold as being "evidence based." But if one closely follows the science, the so-called evidence is as flawed as it is racist in its basic assumptions.

The statistical "evidence" for this narrative came from the census and national surveys, which showed that Black American fathers were less likely than white men to reside with or be legally married to their children's mothers; that Black women were disproportionately more likely than white women to begin childbearing in their mid-to-late teens; and that young Black men had higher unemployment rates than young white men. Despite the many conceptual leaps it took to get from these descriptive statistics to the particular interpretations based on them, and despite the fact that the census was particularly flawed in its substantial undercounting of Black men, a wide confluence of media, academics, advocacy organizations, politicians, and various think tanks viewed the data as irrefutable scientific evidence of the ignorance and moral deficiencies of Black youth and adults. Encapsulated in concepts like "female-headed households," "babies having babies," "absent fathers," "welfare queens," and "superpredators," these skewed and error-strewn statistics were spun into systemically racist gold.

In reality, all of these statistics could be interpreted in a number of ways to support a number of disparate theories. In fact, when they have been subjected to careful quantitative and qualitative investigation, the breakdown is found to be in the narrative, not in the morality of Black families. Initial analysis of the census data about "absent fathers" did not take into account a variety of factors, including that fathers might be "absent" when the census taker arrived because of death, disability, work-related moves, mass incarceration, welfare eligibility rules, or just a deep-seated mistrust of the government and its census takers. There was also no recognition of the fact that an unmarried woman giving birth does not automatically imply that she will raise the child alone. The reality is that grandparents, biological fathers, and other extended family members are often on the scene and actively invested in a child's upbringing. Indeed, the whole construct of a "female-headed household" is misleading, totally ignoring the contribution of the extended kin network. For example, a census taker who went to Wanda and Donnie's home would have coded it as "female-headed," as Donnie was not the biological father of her children, even though he was living with them and taking a central role in raising them.

As noted in chapter four, the widely publicized term "babies having babies" was also a major distortion of the statistics. It slotted everyone from thirteen-year-olds to nineteen-year-olds into one category, without acknowledging that most of the teen mothers (three quarters of them, in fact) were eighteen or nineteen — ages at which a woman can vote, sign legal contracts, and go to war. Fewer than 2 percent were younger than sixteen. Obscuring these facts made it easy to cast "teen mothers" as so immature, irresponsible, and deficient in morality and parenting skills that their children had no hope but to grow up in a moral vacuum, thus perpetuating poverty and depravity in new generations.

Then there was the claim that early childbearing would put an end to all chances of the teenager's being able to educate or take advantage of other opportunities to advance socioeconomically — a narrative that had originally been popularized by those concerned about white teenagers. Generalizing from affluent white to poor Black teens presumes that there is a level playing field of opportunities and resources available to all. There is not. As we've seen, the implication that every young woman will categorically be better off if she delays childbearing is simply false. The evidence for this assumption? The early studies of the consequences of teen childbearing that failed to account for the very different life experiences, opportunities, constraints, and health risk profiles of the various populations among whom most teen childbearing occurs. Today, most (though not all) investigators who use state-of-the-art methods to try to account for these differences have concluded that teen childbearing, per se, has few, if any, adverse effects on long-term economic outcomes. There is widespread agreement among social scientists employing the most rigorous research methods that the causal link between early motherhood and long-term welfare dependence simply never existed.[7] (Nor did superpredators;[8] nor did crack babies.[9])

However, politics, as well as an uncritical acceptance of the story that becoming a teenage mother would not only harm the woman and her children but be costly to society as well, prompted President Clinton to sign the new welfare bill into law in August 1996. Explicitly tying its provisions to the age-washed ideology of personal responsibility, President Clinton stated: "Ultimately, what is needed to stop teen pregnancy is a revolution of the heart. We must all work to instill in every young man and woman a sense of personal responsibility. Having a child is the greatest responsibility any person can assume. It is not the right choice for a teen to make."[10]

The Personal Responsibility and Work Opportunity Reconciliation Act (PRWORA) made it much harder for teen parents to receive benefits, eliminated eligibility for welfare altogether for certain segments of the teenage-mother population, and, operating on the unjustified assumption that biological parents alone held the full responsibility for financially supporting their children, reduced cash grants by at least 25 percent for teens who did not identify their child's biological father.[11] While a teen mother could fulfill the work requirements by attending high school or a GED program, they could not fulfill them by attending college—a very strange proviso for an act that was supposed to promote social mobility. As a professor at the University of Michigan, I saw the results of this firsthand. During my first ten years of teaching, I had a number of young mothers who were AFDC recipients in my classes; since the implementation of TANF there have been none.

The law also called for the secretary of Health and Human Services and the attorney general to implement programs aimed at teenage pregnancy prevention and to assure that at least 25 percent of US communities would have teen pregnancy prevention programs in place within a year. Reducing teenage childbearing was cast as a measure of moral necessity. Remedies included punitive measures such as the denial of welfare and a national discussion of religion, culture, and cultural values.[12] PRWORA earmarked $400 million for abstinence-only education programs for teens, but eliminated the mandate that made family planning available to welfare beneficiaries—another entirely misguided and counterproductive proviso.

If we didn't tie personal responsibility so directly to individual behavior and age at childbearing, and if we considered the implications of weathering, we might ask: Is it irresponsible to maximize the chances your babies will be born healthy and survive their first year of life? That they will not be orphaned? That they will have relatively healthy older kin who can care for them while their mother works, or take them in should their parents die? Norms for childbearing age reflect opportunities available as well as values about what gives life purpose and meaning.[13] And if we didn't erase the weathering experiences of populations where teen childbearing is most common, we might understand.

Every rationale and provision of PRWORA proliferated degrading stereotypes about Black mothers, fathers, and communities and was, therefore, ripe to increase weathering through biopsychosocial routes, as well as material ones.

PRWORA and Material Hardship

The fact that PRWORA increased material hardship is hard to debate. When PRWORA replaced AFDC with TANF, the amount of financial assistance to poor families was substantially reduced and also limited to a maximum of five years. The new work requirements added de facto costs of childcare, transportation, and work wardrobes to already strained budgets. They exacerbated rather than mitigated income poverty and created new uncertainties and challenges for kin networks to navigate, both of which can exacerbate weathering.[14]

Sociologists Kathryn Edin and H. Luke Shaefer have done extensive study of the economic impact of PRWORA. They found that mothers living in states in the Deep South and parts of the West have virtually no access to TANF, and that child poverty in those regions has increased precipitously in recent years. After analyzing several sources of government data, Edin and Shaefer concluded that "roughly 3 million American children spend at least three months in a calendar year living on virtually no money."[15] They also found that the number of poor women and children still eligible to get TANF benefits had been reduced by 75 percent since its inception, not because these women had become economically self-sufficient—the stated goal of the legislation—but simply because of the time limits. Meanwhile the need for the safety net has only increased. In the years since PRWORA became law, the US has experienced two great recessions that disproportionately affected low-wage workers who were already caught in the crossfire of automation and globalization. On top of that, since early 2020, we have suffered a massive disruption in the form of a global pandemic.

As for how those without jobs or adequate resources survived, Edin and Shaefer found:

Nearly all had sold plasma from time to time, some regularly. In 2014, so-called "donations" hit an all-time high at 32.5

million, triple the rate recorded a decade prior. They collected tin cans for an average yield of about $1 an hour. They traded away their food stamps, usually at the going rate of 50 or 60 cents on the dollar. Some traded sex for cash or—more commonly—the payment of their cell phone bill, a room to stay in, a meal, or some other kind of help. One fifteen-year-old was lured into a sexual relationship with her teacher on the promise of food.[16]

In effect, for these and many other reasons that there is no space here to explore, PRWORA has meant fewer dollars available to increasingly needy poor families. Material hardship is weathering on multiple fronts—through the stress and anxiety it causes, the toll taken by hunger and malnutrition, the environmental hazards and toxins people are exposed to when living in decayed and overcrowded housing, and ultimately the prospect, and sometimes the reality, of homelessness.

PRWORA and the Disruption of Networks

The third criterion for evaluating the weathering impact of social policy concerns any new burdens it places on kin networks and other sources of help that members of oppressed groups depend on. The work requirements that TANF imposes for eligibility certainly fit the bill. By forcing so many friends and family members who were vital parts of those networks onto the work rolls, TANF made life harder both for them and for the parents and caregivers who relied upon them. And since most of the jobs available to TANF recipients paid barely minimum wage, they didn't do much to alleviate financial burdens, either.

The sociologist Linda Burton's landmark study of working-class primary caregivers who were TANF recipients found that these women experienced chronic biopsychosocial stress from the constant pressure of having to look for jobs and find (and pay for) childcare.[17] Many of the TANF recipients had to improvise "heroic schedules for themselves," working two or three low-wage part-time jobs, often including night-shift work, to make ends meet, all the while trying to function without any reliable source of childcare because, as another researcher heard from one of the women she was interviewing, "Everybody's working now."[18] As we've seen, poor people have historically depended on multigenerational networks of extended kin, among whom responsibilities for keeping their families going could be divided. It was never an easy life. TANF just made it harder.

No Child Left Behind? Promoting School Choice and Closing Failing Schools

Welfare reform was not the only policy change in the past thirty years that failed to take weathering into account and disregarded the lived reality of the poor and working class. Another example is our approach to improving public education.

The quality of US public schools varies widely, usually according to the demographic makeup of school districts, such that poor and working-class students of color are more likely to attend low-quality, "failing" schools with health code violations, while students in predominantly white suburbs enjoy the highest-quality public schools. The inequities in resources that I have witnessed firsthand are huge. One example is that schools in poor neighborhoods often have no textbooks or have textbooks that are outdated, falling apart, and so few in number that they have to be shared by several students. Schools in the most affluent neighborhoods, meanwhile, give each student as many as two copies of the same spanking new textbook for each class: one to keep at home, one to keep in their locker. This is to spare children's delicate shoulders from heavy backpacks that may lead to neck and back strain, poor posture, and future musculoskeletal problems.

I am glad some very wealthy school districts are concerned with children's musculoskeletal health, but the health hazards poor children face in school are far worse, including black mold, lead paint and pipes, and inadequate heating and cooling. Consider these excerpts from two newspaper stories about schools in Detroit. From the *Detroit Free Press*:

> City of Detroit inspections of eleven public schools—conducted as part of a district-wide review in response to mass teacher sick-outs—revealed widespread code violations, including multiple instances of rodents, mold, damaged roofs and broken glass.[19]

And from the *Washington Post*:

> Teachers say they are fed up with working in schools that aren't fit for them or their students. Classrooms are plagued by rats, roaches, mold, ceilings full of holes and unreliable heat. Teachers don't have textbooks or other supplies they need to teach, they say, and they haven't had a raise in ten years.[20]

In the late 1980s, an effort began to be made to address the problem of "failing" public schools through school-choice programs that paved the way for a variety of "free-market" options still offered today. These "free-market" approaches, which include open enrollment policies across local public schools, magnet schools, and charter schools, and voucher programs whereby local governments provide public school students financial assistance to attend private schools, are meant to give low-income parents options beyond sending their children to the failing public schools in their own disinvested neighborhoods. But none of these approaches seeks to equalize resources across public schools—instead they often simply result in the closing of the under-resourced neighborhood schools—and none take into account the weathering effect of such policies, which manifest in numerous ways.

Proponents of school choice argue that these programs improve educational outcomes by expanding opportunity and access for historically disadvantaged students. The results, however, are mixed at best. The evidence suggests that a majority of students whose neighborhood schools were closed do not end up in schools that are any better. Moreover, studies have also found a negative effect on the test scores and graduation rates of redistricted students, and a possibly negative psychological effect, too, because the redistricted students report feeling stigmatized as "dumb" and "failures" in their new schools.[21]

The ways in which school-choice reforms have under-delivered on their promise and, in some cases, worsened academic performance, particularly for Black boys, are well documented. But the impact on girls and on kin networks has been overlooked, as have the implications for weathering-related stressors. But these stressors are quite real, and often overwhelming, as some recent studies have found, including one led by Linnea Evans and coauthored by me and Cleopatra Howard Caldwell, the chair of my department at the University of Michigan.[22] Evans is a former student of mine who is now a faculty member at the University of Massachusetts, Amherst.

Evans wanted to explore the possible weathering effects of this "free-market" approach to education, and she led a study in which she conducted open-ended interviews with a sample of Black girls in Detroit about their high school experiences. We found that these girls sought to invest in their education as a path to college; yet the very reforms that were supposed to clear this path for them created stressors and robbed them of the time they needed to spend on the activities believed to be important to their academic success.

We learned that many of the girls, including a research participant who had chosen to go to a school in the suburbs rather than one of the two high schools near her home in the inner city because she was "looking for the best public education," had to wake early and to endure an arduous morning commute. Some were so exhausted by the ordeal that they had to nap when they got home, sometimes for hours, until dinner. One girl reported that she woke at 5 a.m. in order to leave the house with her mother at six. She got to school at seven, an hour ahead of the eight o'clock start time, because her mother also had to take other family members to work, and this arrangement was the only way she could accommodate everyone's schedule.

Another girl, whose mother was concerned about her safety, had to wake at 4:30 a.m. so that her mother, whose job started early, could drop her off at the home of her father, who lived in a neighborhood that was safer for walking to the bus stop. From there, she caught a 7:30 bus that got her to school at eight.

Other girls explained how relying upon city buses to get to and from school required patience and strategic planning:

Interviewer: What time do you usually arrive at the stop?

Student: At 6:50 a.m. [for the] 6:55. It's about ten minutes [to school] with the stops. I walk in the door and I wait till 7:45 [when school starts]. I'm usually the earliest person — me and twenty other kids.

Interviewer: What time does the next bus come if you don't make the 6:55?

Student: 7:15, but that's full, so I'd have to wait for the 7:30.

Since the lines to clear security at the school entrance took upwards of ten minutes, she risked being tardy if she took the 7:30 bus. So she toughed out the earlier wake time and the forty minutes of dead time waiting for school to start.

Another girl had a morning commute to school that required

walking several blocks, a roughly thirty-minute bus ride, and another eight-block walk from the bus stop to school. But since the bus was often late—"it come whenever it want to"—she had devised a strategy that involved her boyfriend, who lived several stops ahead of her and would alert her, via text, on the bus's timing. Her trip home sometimes took over an hour and a half.

Fears about safety during travel to school, the need to coordinate commuting schedules to accommodate everyone's work, school, and caretaking responsibilities, and the frustration with the failures of public transit were frequent refrains in these interviews, though little consideration was given to such concerns when the school-choice programs were devised.

Of course, transportation to and from school is but one of many obstacles facing Black girls who opt into these programs. The teachers don't cut much slack for students who face difficulties getting to and from these far-flung schools. And the teachers themselves, who are underpaid and overworked, are tasked with the impossible job of integrating these new students into what are often already overcrowded classrooms. When even the most well-meaning teachers don't have the time to get to know their new students, the bonds between teachers and students fray. The result can be a harsher learning environment, which increases the likelihood of the students' being suspended or expelled. The stories and data that emerged from our study also described the social isolation many of these girls felt at their new schools. Even if—and this is a big if—their new schools offer a better education, all these challenges and obstacles may be implicated in chronic activation of Black girls' stress-response systems, contributing to their weathering by early adulthood.

School-choice programs also demand a lot from parents: evaluating different schools; learning about the bureaucratic demands of these programs; filling in complicated paperwork to enter lotteries and enroll their children; developing strategies to help their children get to school safely and on time, all the while balancing their own work and family commitments.[23] All of this likely adds to the weathering of parents, too.

Future efforts at education reform must not only hold the schools accountable for better educational outcomes, but should take into account the way policy design can aggravate or reduce the effects of weathering in those whose futures they aim to make brighter.

Housing Opportunities for People Everywhere (HOPE VI)

The HOPE VI program was launched by Congress in 1992. Like the school-choice programs, the goal of HOPE VI was to "deconcentrate poverty." But like those programs, it's another example of good intentions gone terribly wrong.

Danya Keene, now a faculty member at Yale University, began her deep study of the HOPE VI program and its impacts when she was my student. She led several studies on which I collaborated concerning the weathering impact on those who had lived in the nearly ninety thousand public housing units that HOPE VI tore down.

There is no question that by the 1990s, the physical environments in public housing developments and the neighborhoods around them had suffered from decades of disinvestment, leaving many of them unhealthy to inhabit. However, the policies enacted to improve the situation reeked of denigrating and untested racist stereotypes and assumptions. And there were alternative perspectives and policy approaches to be taken that I'll discuss in Part II. The actual policies implemented in the 1990s were usually premised on the idea that the geographical concentration of poor (especially poor Black) residents inevitably leads to "social pathology"; the implication was that the communities they created in those spaces had no social or cultural strengths. Thus, nothing of value would be lost if they disappeared. Erasure.

HOPE VI called for demolishing public housing projects and replacing them with mixed-income housing funded by public-private partnerships. While waiting for the new housing to be built, the former residents of the demolished buildings would have to relocate, but with no promise that they could return to the mixed-income housing being constructed where they had once lived. In fact, many would be excluded from the new units because of the low numbers of affordable ones planned for the new developments compared to the number in the demolished public housing. While public housing in general is racially diverse, HOPE VI has primarily affected Black public-housing residents. A complementary policy initiative, also aimed at breaking down the geographical concentration of the poor, was the Section 8 housing certificate and voucher program, whose goal was to assist very low-income Americans—including former residents of demolished projects—to rent or buy housing in the private sector.

Some analysts were cynical from the start, arguing that HOPE VI and its attendant programs were a means of revitalizing urban areas for the benefit of gentrifiers and developers. Yet many liberal and progressive social scientists and policy makers were motivated by the belief that the demolition of public housing and the relocation of poor residents would be widely beneficial to the health and economic well-being of low-income families. They expected relocated residents to end up in locations that were better in terms of housing quality, neighborhood resources (like schooling and food shopping and transportation), and various environmental factors, and also in terms of employment opportunities.

Empirical support for these presumptions was anemic when the policies were enacted, and the evaluations that have been done since the policies were implemented have provided scant evidence that those forced to relocate benefited substantially—or at all—from their moves. This is not surprising, given that the policies failed to take into account the systemic racism that prevents Black people from getting good jobs and accessing decent housing in the first place. They ignored the strong possibility that using vouchers to obtain better housing would not be easy for a historically denigrated group. Many suburban landlords simply refused to participate in the Section 8 program, for instance. As for the homeownership program, it largely subjected former public housing residents to predatory lending practices during the housing bubble, leaving many underwater and facing foreclosure on their recently acquired homes when the bubble burst. And in their new communities, their already compromised access to health care was further diminished by living in areas that were less likely to have clinicians who accepted Medicaid or to have qualified health centers nearby.

During the debates about these policies, the voices of public housing residents were largely ignored, though residents of the projects engaged in resistance on many fronts before being literally bulldozed out of their homes. Tenant organizations and other community groups actively (and sometimes successfully) resisted HOPE VI redevelopment, but for the most part their concerns were dismissed. No one asked how HOPE VI might disrupt the networks of friends and family that Black public housing residents had developed in order to mitigate material hardship and oppression. And the cooperative strengths and deeply rooted social ties that had developed within such communities were either ignored or, worse, denigrated.

In one study led by Keene, with Mark Padilla, an anthropologist, and myself as collaboraters, we found that few of the former public housing residents in Chicago whose homes had been demolished had been able to move into "healthier" neighborhoods or achieve any measure of socioeconomic mobility.[24] Many had moved to equally disadvantaged neighborhoods where they had to cope with the same challenges of poverty—but without the networks they had relied on in public housing. When interviewed for the study, many described their former communities as "families," even when no blood ties were involved, and they clearly felt a sense of loss. For example, one interviewee said: "[These are] the people you grow to love. It is like we a family. I was heartbroken when they tore them down. Because you get to know people. And you become like a family. They not your family, but you grow to love them. And when they get taken away from you because of nonsense, it hurts you."

Another observed that things weren't the same without the "big building" that kept people together: "In your own mind it's a tragedy, because you probably don't ever see these people again, because you being put here and here and you all was always like a family when you was there. But now, you guys can't be in a big building together, running house to house getting butter and milk."

Research by Keene and others also indicates that relocated residents faced many challenges with social integration in their new neighborhoods.[25] Two years after being moved, Clampet-Lundquist found the majority of people who had been relocated from one Philadelphia development had not been able to create new local social networks, thanks in part to the widespread stigmatization they experienced from their new neighbors. With old ties lost and few new ties to replace them, HOPE VI relocatees experienced increased social isolation and, in the absence of support networks, faced new day-to-day challenges.

These findings directly challenge the widespread belief that nothing could be worse than living in public housing, or that such concentrations of the poor can only be harmful. Public housing communities contain social resources that are important to both the psychological and physical well-being of their residents, even if those resources are not visible to the policy makers who make decisions that override the desires of those residents.

The demolition of public housing caused a tremendous loss of social support networks. Research suggests that a desire to maintain these networks was one of the primary reasons that residents opposed the demolition of their homes.[26] It also may explain why many relocated residents chose to remain physically close to their original place of residence. According to a national study of HOPE VI relocatees, those given vouchers used them to move into housing that was a median distance of only 2.9 miles from their former homes.[27] However, researchers have found that moving even a few miles can be disruptive to social ties, particularly in the absence of adequate transportation.[28] And rarely have the designers of these policies thought about improving transportation options for inner city residents.

HOPE VI demolitions also disrupted or destroyed the political power and collective agency of the various tenant and community organizations that had advocated for the rights of housing project residents to get their needs met—needs that ranged from garbage collection and working elevators to addressing security issues that put people in danger in their own homes. Until such organizations can be reconstituted, which can take a long time, tenants will be left without any kind of representation to help them deal with their shared challenges.[29]

Seen through a weathering lens, the architects and supporters of the HOPE VI and Section 8 programs should not have presumed that their plans would help reduce the stressors that are a source of poor health for low-income Black Americans. Those who anticipated that these programs would be winning strategies for poor Black people vastly underestimated the deep feelings of grief and loss that would be caused by their relocation/dislocation. And they vastly overestimated the benefits that would accrue to the relocated. Their arrogant assumption that there was nothing of value in the communities they destroyed failed to take into account the possibility that for the people who had lived in them, there were in fact many advantages.[30]

We now have evidence, down to the molecular level, that weathering processes can be mitigated for predominantly minoritized people living in racially or ethnically dense settings. In this section I describe two different strands of research that suggest that living near kin may protect health: one related to the prevalence of a particularly virulent form of breast cancer, one to the shortening of telomeres.

The Biological Evidence

Another of my former students, Erin Linnenbringer, now a faculty member at Washington University Medical School in St. Louis, led a study on which I collaborated that found biological evidence to support the idea that living in segregated neighborhoods, even disinvested ones, provides some important health protections, likely due to the importance of kin networks for practical coping and psychological affirmation.[31]

We analyzed data on all women diagnosed with breast cancer in California between 1996 and 2014—both triple negative breast cancer (TNBC) and Estrogen Receptor Positive breast cancer (ER+). TNBC is distinct from ER+, which is the much more common, less aggressive, and more treatable form of breast cancer. Numerous population-based studies have found that in the United States, Black women are two to three times more likely to develop the more deadly TNBC than white women.

Much of the existing research that attempts to understand the reason for these racial disparities in breast cancer has focused on the possibility of a genetic predisposition to TNBC associated with African ancestry. Our own study, by contrast, was guided by weathering theory, so we were interested in assessing the possibility that environmental and social factors might be implicated. Looking at the data on women in California, we did a neighborhood-by-neighborhood comparison of the incidence of TNBC to see whether the racial composition of the neighborhoods where women diagnosed with TNBC lived might be associated with the probability of having this more virulent form of breast cancer.

Conventional wisdom would suggest that the "concentration of poverty" characteristic of living in highly segregated Black neighborhoods would place women at increased risk of TNBC. But knowing what we knew about weathering, we postulated that the ghettoization of racial minority neighborhoods might also provide some protective resources for their residents, just as ethnic enclaves do. We wondered whether these neighborhood-level resources, which often include greater access to social support networks, might be health-promoting enough to reduce breast cancer risk and/or improve outcomes, despite the many socioeconomic disadvantages of living within such neighborhoods.

We found that for Black women diagnosed with breast cancer, living in a neighborhood with a high percentage of Black residents was associated with a lower risk of TNBC. Neither those who assume that Black women's propensity for the TNBC form is driven by African ancestry and genetics, nor those who see concentrated poverty as a breeding ground for social pathology, would have predicted our findings.

In another study, conducted in Detroit, for which I was the principal investigator in collaboration with the Healthy Environments Partnership, my collaborators and I found that the stressors of living in Detroit below the poverty line shortened the telomere length of both white and Black residents relative to national averages.[32] These findings confirm that weathering will occur in any population that suffers the living conditions and stressors most often experienced by poor Black residents of disinvested urban areas. But of particular interest was our finding that these conditions had substantially more adverse effects on poor whites than on poor Blacks. That is, poor whites in Detroit were biologically older—as measured by telomere length—than equally poor Blacks of the same chronological age. This might be related to the fact that, in a reversal of more typical situations, low-income white residents in Detroit are the ones most likely to experience othering and the resulting stress arousal because they are in the minority there. Another possible explanation is that poor whites in Detroit, who are fewer in number and more geographically dispersed than low-income Black residents, have not developed the social and communal network strategies that buffer the negative health effects of material deprivation and stigma. This possibility is supported by the study's finding that Black residents thought more positively of their neighborhoods than did white residents. The social ties they had developed in their communities had helped them cope with oppression and material hardship. White residents aspired to leave the neighborhood, not invest in social ties there.

While Black residents of Detroit have suffered the longest history of poverty and marginalization of all the racial/ethnic groups we examined, they may have benefited in some ways from living in neighborhoods where they were in the majority. Such racial density minimizes the possibility of othering encounters, enhances identity safety, and fosters the kind of togetherness that enables a community to shoulder their challenges collectively. For population groups that have not developed such protective networks, being in poverty would have worse health consequences.

Taken together, these breast-cancer and telomere-length studies underscore the importance of kin networks and social ties for the poor and culturally oppressed. Policy makers should be careful not to create programs that disrupt these adaptive and deeply meaningful strategies. They should always take into account the factors that might either exacerbate or mitigate weathering processes, and the availability of social support is certainly one of them.

After decades of weaving the age-washed personal-responsibility narratives into government policy, the result has been ever more severe weathering among Black Americans. We've also seen its increasingly adverse impact on infant and maternal health in the Black population, despite its stated goal of eliminating such health inequities. We must ask ourselves why the most harmful increases in weathering indicators have appeared in Black women in their twenties and thirties and forties—their working and reproductive ages, when they should be at their healthiest and most vital. There is reason to believe that this is because their central role in kin networks has become so much harder to sustain in the face of the social policies enacted in the late twentieth century.

The problem is not simply that these highlighted and coincident policies were ineffectual. They were and are actively harmful. They became yet another set of challenges for weathered communities to withstand in their efforts to survive and overcome. Based on a racist narrative about the pathology of the Black family, the "teen mother," and high-concentration Black neighborhoods, these policies eroded the already minimal safety net supplied by the federal government, while simultaneously undermining the community and kinship-based safety nets.

Challenging the Black Family Pathology Narrative

For decades now, all but the most draconian versions of the Black family pathology narrative have been impervious to public critique. That may finally be changing, although it is too early to be sure. The first evidence of cracks in this entrenched mischaracterization of Black families came in March 2021. In a last-minute attempt to prevent passage of President Biden's COVID-19 relief package, Glenn Grothman, a Republican congressman from Wisconsin, appealed to a racist trope that would almost certainly have killed it any time in the previous fifty years. "I bring [this criticism of the bill] up because I know the strength that Black Lives Matter had in this last election. I know it's a group that doesn't like the old-fashioned family."[33]

While Grothman is far from alone in this belief, what would once have been a dependable argument for shredding the social safety net backfired on him. Not only did it fail to gain any momentum but it was also quickly and passionately shut down by Congresswoman Stacy Plaskett. "How dare you?" she demanded from the House floor.

> How dare you say that Black Lives Matter, Black people do not understand old-fashioned families? [...] We have been able to keep our families alive for over four hundred years [...] How dare you say that we are not interested in families in the Black community? That is outrageous—that should be stricken down.

Plaskett was calling bullshit on a racist idea that has been sustained at least since the 1970s by Democrats and Republicans, conservatives and liberals alike. It's an idea that has rationalized the extreme stinginess of social programs related to welfare, public housing, health care, and education, most of which remain in place to this day.

Many still do not question the narrative underlying these programs, and some, like Grothman, are seeking actively to perpetuate it. Others, like Senator Rick Scott, are trying to give it new life by shape-shifting the problem from one inherent to Black Americans to a threat from the political left. In his eleven-point plan to rescue America, he states: "The fanatical left seeks to devalue and redefine the traditional family, as they undermine parents and attempt to replace them with government programs. We will not allow Socialism to place the needs of the state ahead of the family."[34]

But Plaskett's blistering evisceration of this racist and specious narrative provides some reason to be hopeful that, along with Confederate statues, it may yet go the way of the Stone Age. If, like Grothman and far too many others, we fail to see its flaws, and continue to enact policies based on it, we will only continue to add to the weathering burdens on marginalized communities that are now strained almost to the breaking point.

Are we ready to do something about it? If so, we must first acknowledge and respect the value of the family support systems developed by marginalized populations, then figure out what policies we can enact to maximize their effectiveness—the very opposite of our current policies and programs. We need to reimagine guidelines and goals for social movements and policy measures, employing a rubric that centers equity and takes weathering into account.

Part II

The Way Forward

If they don't give you a seat at the table, bring a folding chair.

—Shirley Chisholm[1]

We have seen throughout this book that there are dire consequences to presuming that good health and longevity are equally available to all Americans. Because age-washing narratives of personal responsibility take into account neither the structural impediments some groups systemically encounter in their tenacious efforts to support and care for their families, nor the weathering implications of the cumulatively toxic stressors they face every hour of every day, they result in policies that exacerbate rather than reduce health inequity. These policies may (or may not) be well intentioned, but at best they do little to disrupt weathering—and at worst they are deadly.

The pandemic revealed more vividly than ever the health gap between dominant and minoritized groups and between the impoverished and working class compared to the rest of us. Highly publicized police shootings of unarmed Black men, women, and children have made denying systemic racism untenable. Certainly, broad social movements are needed to enact and institutionalize significant action and garner the political momentum to promote health equity. The focus of this section of this book is meant to complement and supplement movement activity. Social change can sometimes be presented as something that happens all at once when, in reality, there are usually decades of tireless behind-the-scenes organizing that builds toward the "moment" that becomes visible to the majority.[2] These moments are met with ideas, evidence, and frameworks that also do not appear overnight—I hope the following section can contribute to the bank of evidence and shared understanding that helps social movement builders be prepared for the moment we find ourselves in today.

The need for change has become so urgent that more and more activists, policy makers, politicians, think tanks, and government bodies are joining the fight for racial justice. Several cities (including Seattle; Washington, DC; and Takoma Park, Maryland) and states (including California, Connecticut, Florida, Iowa, New Jersey, and Oregon) have passed provisions to mandate racial impact statements before a policy measure is passed. At the federal level, President Biden issued executive orders in 2021 calling on heads of federal agencies to review their programs and policies to assess equity with respect to race, ethnicity, religion, income, geography, gender identity, sexual orientation, and disability.

But who will have the authority to define or assess racial impact and ensure racial impact statements do not become performative, or, worse, add to the weathering stressors that surround us in everyday life? Necessary as these developments are, they will only validly assess "equity impacts" if a holistic understanding of the fundamental causes of population inequities—including in weathering—is applied, with all stakeholders having recognized seats at the table.

As defined across this book, weathering is the result of repeated or chronic activation of the physiological stress response over years and decades. This means that a person's health and life expectancy emerge and change throughout their life, reflecting their cumulative experiences as members of racialized social identity groups.

These experiences are shaped by how others treat them based on each actor's racialized social identity, and what their environmental exposures are given the material, political, and geographic constraints systemically imposed on their assigned social identity group, more than their individual DNA or lifestyle. In my view, we must understand that the relationship between age and health is mutable, at least from the womb through middle age, and that it is subject to efforts and commitments we make as a society. Such efforts open up opportunities for social changes — both small and large — that can disrupt and ultimately eliminate weathering inequities.

Any measure that takes meaningful steps to improve the quality of everyday life for the exploited and oppressed will disrupt their weathering. Any measure that makes society more equitable merits doing for that reason alone, and will also disrupt weathering. Disrupting weathering is, itself, a critical step toward making society equitable. There can be no real equity where some populations face substantially shorter healthy life expectancies than others, especially when those same populations have the fewest economic resources and the least political power and are viewed as stereotypes with contempt, fear, or resentment. As the marginalized work to carry on and make positive contributions to their families and society in defiance of the obstacles, exploitation, and indignities they face, their bodies are harmed. Only when we are willing to recognize weathering can we hope to understand the predicament of the exploited, marginalized, and maligned, and only when armed with that understanding can we hope to effect genuine and equitable change.

We've seen that late-twentieth-century policy proposals and legislation erased or ignored the lived experience of oppressed, working-class and racialized groups, defaulted to solutions that worked for the dominant elite, and failed to acknowledge that the fates of dominant and marginalized groups are dynamically linked outside of a "makers and takers" framework. Having seen how badly those in power in the 1990s failed in promoting health equity, it is important that we do better as we fight to address the critical social challenges of the twenty-first century. Today the social problems that many recognize as high-priority on the policy agenda, such as addressing climate change, are existential for all people.

When thinking through the weathering implications of new social policy proposals, we must always ask: when placed in the real context of everyday life for those whose health we are trying to improve, to what extent are these proposals likely to address their actual needs? We need to remain mindful, as discussed in chapter eight, that many such initiatives may increase the stresses on marginalized groups while failing to make real improvements in their lives. And, as discussed in chapter seven, we must be aware that sometimes the coping efforts needed to earn an income or advance one's education in a racist and classist system chronically activate biological weathering processes.

As we consider what kinds of policy, programs, practices, and political actions can help level the playing field for all Americans, a serious look at the causes and potential remedies for weathering cannot help but enrich the social change conversation. Yet it promises no silver bullet or one-size-fits-all solution. It requires each of us in positions of authority or as voters, activists or advocates to step outside our own lived experience and question whether what we see as common sense—even our most deeply held beliefs about family structure, the best way to raise children, the ideal life course— makes good sense for everybody. Chances are it doesn't. Chances are that even with all the good intentions in the world, we are failing to account for the different experiences and histories, different degrees of access to power and economic resources, and different sources of joy, meaning, and purpose that signify that what works for one group of people may be maladaptive for others.

People on different sides of social, racial, and class divides have very different short-term needs and expectations. But just because those in the dominant culture don't have firsthand experience of the worst consequences of social inequity or ignore them doesn't mean they are unaffected. When a Jenga tower falls in the forest and nobody with power and goodwill hears it, that doesn't change the fact that it existed, had value, and fell. Or that its collapse is a loss to us all.

Systemic problems call for systemic change, but structural, even revolutionary changes can happen short of a revolution in the classic sense; in fact, they have to. There is no reason those most subject to weathering must wait for a political revolution, and even less reason for them to have confidence that a new government—if that's all that changes—will better or more permanently safeguard their needs. To achieve that goal requires a collaborative process in which the communities most affected have a respected voice. Short of such a process, we are bound to do more harm than good, because any social policy decision intended to improve everyday life must reflect the lived reality of the people who are meant to be its beneficiaries. The revolution that is required is in how we identify our gravest social problems, how we widen the frame of possible responses, and who we see as having the authority and claim to participate in addressing these problems.

Prioritize Equity Equity Equity

To address racialized injustice and the weathering it causes, we must prioritize equity.

Currently, the default in politics, policy, and program development is to center privilege; instead, we can work to "center at the margins," namely center, not erase, the socially situated challenges from the perspective of the populations who experience health eroding oppression.[3]

To disrupt weathering, we must evaluate any policy or program proposal on the basis of whether or not it will create equity for the most underserved stakeholders. Ideally, any public policy proposal aimed at disrupting weathering will benefit every stakeholder, but if there are conflicting needs and priorities, the greatest benefits must go to those who suffer the most from weathering, and who have the fewest options for combating it. To achieve equity it is necessary to work collaboratively and in mutual solidarity, rather than competitively.

As part of this shift, cultivating empathy as well as respect and solidarity is the just and caring thing to do. It is also strategic because it fuels motivation and political will toward implementing policies from a social justice point of view rather than a "makers and takers" vantage point. Unfortunately, privileged Americans have become so disconnected from the vastly different everyday experiences of the exploited, oppressed, and marginalized that we have no idea how challenging their lives can be—or that we make them so. This ignorance leads to a kind of judgment that results in contempt rather than empathy. If we allow policy makers to frame investments in our marginalized communities as undeserved, wasteful giveaways, it will be because we have failed to portray members of these communities as they really are or, even better, to hear from and partner with them. Our government will then default to the usual opportunistic budgets that benefit the privileged at the expense of everyone else. It is essential for powerful members of the dominant culture to move from hubris to humility.

Guidelines for New Approaches to Disrupt Weathering and Promote Health Equity

In order to move toward equitable and weathering-informed social change and policy, I suggest engaging the following five principles, which I developed as guidelines for deliberation, health impact analysis, and action:

Think biopsychosocially: address the stealth inequities that surround us.

Think holistically and ecologically.

Do not erase oppressed stakeholders: do "nothing about us without us."

Pay attention to the needs of working- and reproductive-age adults.

Recognize all our fates are linked.

In the remainder of this book, I will expand on these guidelines, chapter by chapter. I will begin with examples of simple, scalable changes aimed at neutralizing cues to the lesser valuing of marginalized groups that can activate their physiological stress response in everyday settings. In subsequent chapters, I will move toward ways at arriving at just, caring, and efficacious approaches that will have larger systemic and structural impact.

Along the way, there will be examples of people going astray in their well-meaning or incomplete efforts. As we have seen throughout this book, policy that does not take weathering and equity into account is often counterproductive. My intent in offering contemporary examples of bad policy is not to discourage you but rather to reinforce the importance of prioritizing the five guidelines. Indeed, there will also be success stories, demonstrating the efficacy and possibility of the approach I am suggesting. These examples are far from exhaustive or even fully complete in each of their specifics. They are meant to show that learning about weathering, prior and current policy misdeeds and well-meaning mistakes, need not leave any of us in a state of paralysis or defaulting to the age-washed personal-responsibility narrative to guide action. The examples are varied in scope and content as a way to implore you to accept that no matter your social position, expertise, resources, or areas of interest, there are promising actions you can imagine taking or advocating for in the immediate, short, and long terms if you view health inequity and related social inequities through a weathering lens.

9.

Think Biopsychosocially: Address the Stealth Inequities That Surround Us

Weathering can seem like an incredibly daunting and intractable problem to solve, and it has taken a broad social movement galvanized by grassroots activists to enact widespread demands for health equity. To start, there are immediate, easy changes we can make today that will have a positive impact. These are approaches that address the full range of biopsychosocial stressors that are "in the air" in the daily rounds of the poor, working-class, racialized, and other stigmatized populations.

As discussed earlier in this book, members of dominant groups benefit from the fact that their own values and life experiences are considered the norm throughout society, and institutional structures and priorities are shaped accordingly. Members of dominant groups need not expend bandwidth on being vigilant for cues that their social identity is putting them in harm's way, or on trying to disconfirm negative stereotypes. Members of marginalized groups do not have this luxury. Rather, they live their daily lives in settings where they must be aware of their stigmatized social identity, requiring persistent vigilance and coping. Whether they are stigmatized as "teen mothers" or "welfare queens," "superpredators" or "illegal aliens" from "shithole" countries, and racialized or gendered as inferior or threatening, they all suffer from negative distortions of their social identity.

These distortions show how dominant culture encodes their social identities. Cues to such coding prime the stigmatized to be on their guard, to put on their armor. We may understand the importance of dismantling and condemning some of the most obvious symbols of prejudice—for example, statues of Confederate soldiers, the noose left in someone's locker room—while still being unconscious of the more subtle racist symbols and cues that pervade our culture. They're just "in the air," spontaneously activating adverse physiological processes that contribute to weathering. They are endemic. Like microbes, they may not be visible to us, but they colonize our minds and bodies and can make some of us dreadfully ill.

This chapter is about what we can do to become more conscious of these cues, and to change them. There are strategies that we as individuals can employ, changes we can make in the social-identity cues that occur in everyday settings that can help minimize these distortions and the health harms they effect, even prior to—or in the absence of—sweeping societal change. This alone will not eliminate weathering, but it is something we have the power to do now as part of a harm-reduction strategy. It is scalable and applicable across many settings, with measurable positive effects on equity. If we want to start doing things *today* that will have immediate benefits, this chapter presents some possibilities. We can't stop here, but it's a good place to start.

I call this approach to promoting equity Jedi public health (JPH).[1] If you've seen any of the *Star Wars* movies, you'll recall that the Jedi masters are a network of wise individuals; they are teachers as much as they are warriors. Jedis are bound to one another by their allegiance to a positive force. And so should we be. Although comfortable with space-age technology, they primarily use the most accessible of technologies—their minds—as a force for good. As such, anyone can be a Jedi. The JPH philosophy asserts that if all of us collaborate in changing our environments with the aim of disrupting the physiological stress they trigger in the most marginalized and vulnerable members of our community, we can help combat weathering. We can co-create a culture of identity safety discursively, symbolically, materially, politically, digitally, and practically—in communities, classrooms, online social networks, workplaces, doctors' offices, and hospitals—in short, everywhere we live, think, imagine, and act.[2]

JPH recognizes that health inequity emerges from widely circulated core cultural beliefs that privilege some identities and ways of being in the world while marginalizing and devaluing others. In turn, it recognizes that the policies, practices, and attitudes of community institutions intended to serve citizens (schools, government, economic, legal, and health systems, etc.) may not be a good fit for the marginalized groups who must navigate these systems.[3] Navigating institutions under conditions of misalignment itself can trigger physiological stress responses that increase health vulnerability.[4] We can change this in many integrated settings. As we've seen time and again, hurt feelings are not all that is at stake because of this stereotyping; a negatively stereotyped person has reason to be concerned that aspects of their identity will be used against them, threatening their chances at success, their employability, their financial well-being, their health, and even their life.

The goal of JPH is to ensure that cues to stigmatized social identities are not allowed to become central and defining in the psyches of marginalized people in everyday life, particularly not in high-stakes performance settings, like tests and interviews that influence their access to jobs and schools and various community institutions, or in potentially life-or-death situations like childbirth or medical emergencies. The goal is to level the playing field, setting by setting, so that social identity ceases to play a critical role in how people are seen, treated, and valued, and, therefore, in how identity-safe a person feels in institutional and other everyday settings. This approach provides concrete first steps toward the broader imperative that society destigmatize social identity. By depriving stereotypes of their power, JPH sets in motion processes that will allow diverse people to succeed and stay healthy.

There's evidence in several domains that eliminating harmful environmental cues can make a real difference in people's lives, minimizing physiological stress responses and starting a virtuous cycle toward increasing equity in health and in other realms. Such evidence comes from the maternal and child health literature on reducing the risk of delivery complications when birthing while Black. It comes from the educational literature related to strategies for closing the achievement gap between Black and white students generally, and between male and female students in STEM subjects. It comes from what we know about how characters we see on TV and in movies and video games send messages that reinforce gendered and racialized stereotypes of beauty and power; from our understanding of how computer coding and machine-learning algorithms can perpetuate bias—and how they can be changed to do the opposite. In the following sections, I will offer a few examples of evidence-based strategies that are effective in the aforementioned contexts.

Diffusing Threatening Cues in the Birth Setting

The hypermedicalization of childbirth, due to the fact that the doctors who typically preside over the labor process are likely to view childbirth as not a natural process but a medical problem, increases risks to mothers who do not experience the delivery room as a safe space. The high-profile deaths of a number of Black mothers, which have gotten a lot of publicity in recent years, make this risk clear. And if anything, this has made Black women all the warier of what might happen to them during childbirth. Some are terrified. I have received many questions and emails from women I do not know asking me whether it is safe for a Black woman to give birth in the

United States. The following, from a Black woman writing on behalf of her pregnant daughter, is typical:

> Based on the media reports discussing Black maternal mortality, my daughter has drawn the conclusion that it is "not safe" for a Black woman to have a baby in the US, that [it] is safer for a Black woman to have a baby in [Europe], and that no [B]lack woman who has access to [Europe] should ever have a baby in the US. These articles have left her "terrified" at the prospect of having a baby here.

Clinicians, policy makers, and decision-makers in health-care institutions must be helped to understand how alien and identity-threatening—even terrorizing—a hospital delivery can be. The hospital delivery room is in multiple ways a sterile environment—for good and for bad. And to those laboring mothers who feel that their birth attendants are not listening to their concerns, not taking them seriously, it can be a threatening one as well. No snowflakes here: we've seen multiple examples of the negative, in some cases life-threatening, impact of this kind of dynamic between women and their doctors. Simple alterations in the composition of maternity-care providers and the power dynamics between ob/gyns and other providers at the time of delivery can make a big difference.

Midwives are likely to be more responsive to birthing women than physicians, and they tend to be perceived as less threatening. Better yet, many women have concluded, is to have a personal doula who will provide the continuous care and attention that doctors and nurses don't. The kind of support a doula offers can include teaching, reassurance, and motivational coaching as well as touch, eye contact, and the simple fact of always being there, both literally and figuratively, which can be soothing and confidence-building. The presence and actions of a personal doula can prevent or quell physiological stress responses and remind a laboring mother that she matters, her concerns are valid, and someone has her back. Having an attentive doula can help a woman let down her guard and concentrate on her labor rather than being vigilant to threatening cues in her environment. It makes her feel safe.

In her landmark *New York Times Magazine* article on Black maternal mortality, Linda Villarosa spoke with Dána-Ain Davis, a doula and the director of the Center for the Study of Women and Society at the City University of New York.[5] As Davis explained, the doula serves as "another set of ears and another voice to help get through some of the potentially traumatic decisions that have to be made" during labor, an intense period of stress and vulnerability. Based on her experience, Davis concludes that doulas "are a critical piece of the puzzle in the crisis of premature birth [and] infant and maternal mortality in [B]lack women."

Villarosa provides this example of an interaction between Landrum, a Black mother, and her doula, Giwa, during Landrum's labor. Landrum was agitated by having been given the wrong type of anesthesia after the anesthesiologist required all visitors—including Giwa—to leave the room while it was administered. Villarosa describes Landrum's interaction with Giwa when Giwa was allowed to return to the delivery room:

> As Landrum loudly complained about what occurred, her blood pressure shot up, while the baby's heart rate dropped. Giwa glanced nervously at the monitor, the blinking lights reflecting off her face. "What happened was wrong," she said to Landrum, lowering her voice to a whisper. "But for the sake of the baby, it's time to let it go."
>
> She asked Landrum to close her eyes and imagine the color of her stress.
>
> "Red," Landrum snapped, before finally laying her head onto the pillow.
>
> "What color is really soothing and relaxing?" Giwa asked, massaging her hand with lotion.

"Lavender," Landrum replied, taking a deep breath. Over the next ten minutes, Landrum's blood pressure dropped within normal range as the baby's heart rate stabilized.

In resolving Landrum's elevated blood pressure and her baby's distress, Giwa, in effect, invoked JPH principles. She relied on nothing more technological than her training, emotional intelligence, compassion, resolve, and a Jedi mind trick: "These aren't the droids you are looking for. Move along, move along." It worked.

Randomized controlled trials have shown that doula-accompanied births are associated with significantly lower C-section rates, less use of anesthesia, and more positive experiences of childbirth overall, as reported by mothers of newborns.[6] Having a doula in the delivery room is perhaps the most promising model for diminishing the biopsychosocial risks of birthing while Black. But there are a number of obstacles to making this happen on a large scale.

Although many affluent and well-insured women have been hiring doulas for some time, women with little discretionary income will find it hard to afford their services, as doulas are rarely covered by insurance and are generally paid for privately. Only three states (New York, Minnesota, and Oregon) currently allow Medicaid coverage of doula support, albeit at low reimbursement rates. Another problem with expanding access to doulas on a large scale is that there are currently too few trained doulas in the US to accommodate such an expansion. Programs incentivizing and increasing the accessibility of doula training could ameliorate this problem. More and more people are responding to this need in specific locations. One example is Shafia Monroe, a midwife herself, who also founded the Oregon Doula Association and the International Center for Traditional Childbearing (ICTC), now a training program affiliated with Portland State University. ICTC is a nonprofit, African-centered organization that trains Black women aspiring to become midwives.[7]

Changing Situational Cues in School Settings

In the school setting, stereotype-threat researchers have shown positive results in improving test performance of students of color and women in STEM classrooms through simple methods that focus on altering situational cues.[8] These methods include:

- Avoiding identity-threatening prompts by placing demographic questions (e.g., about gender, race, ethnicity, income) at the end rather than the beginning of high-stakes tests. Placing them at the beginning primes the student to their stigmatized social identity and adversely affects their test performance as the physiologic stress arousal the prime initiates actuates their affective brain segments, while disassociating the brain's cognitive centers needed to perform one's best on the test.
- Removing classroom or workplace decorations such as posters that signal gendered or racialized belonging or exclusion. These serve as a continuous threat to the stereotyped identities of stigmatized group members in the setting.
- Increasing a minoritized group's representation in integrated settings. This diffuses primes related to being the "other" or not belonging, while providing social support.
- Training teachers, including university faculty, to endorse a growth rather than a fixed mind-set through their presentations, syllabi, and student-feedback practices. This approach handles the insecurity and performance anxiety of those stereotyped as inferior or unintelligent.

Some of these are straightforward and could be implemented immediately, at virtually no cost. Placing demographic questions that remind people of their social identity at the end of tests, not the beginning, is a perfect example.

Another low-cost, low-effort intervention might involve decorating a science classroom with nature posters instead of *Star Trek* posters. As we saw in chapter six, doing exactly this led to increased engagement of women in computer science classes.

Some strategies, such as ensuring real diversity in classrooms, require organized, administrative buy-in and effort. Others, such as educating teachers in how to promote a "growth mind-set" in the minds of their students, require training, commitment, and resources.

While some items on this list make greater demands on resources and time than others, all are relatively modest in their requirements, all are scalable across schools, and all have the potential for long-lasting effects. Consider, for example, how teachers can encourage students to develop a growth mind-set—the belief that abilities are not inherent or immutable and can be enhanced and strengthened with the right kind of effort.

In second grade I was paraded around the school district to show how well "average" students took to what was then called New Math. I loved math and excelled at it, and I was actually at the very top of my class. But those teachers and administrators who were lobbying to make New Math a permanent fixture of the elementary school curriculum could still pass me off as average, no questions asked, because I was a girl. To this day, I do not know whether this was the school personnel's conscious strategy or whether they, themselves, were bamboozled by sexism into believing that if a girl could do so well in this math curriculum, any student could. Years later, I took twelfth grade AP Math in eleventh grade and never took math again until I was required to in graduate school. Why? Because, despite my eleven-year history of excelling in math, my teacher could only respond to my scoring the highest grade in the class on the first quarterly exam by humiliating me. He always posted student grades publicly (a questionable practice, all around), and as he posted them this time, he glared at me and mused aloud to the class, "You will never believe who got the top score; it was Arline. Can you believe it? I can't." I soon learned that his statement wasn't just a figure of speech. When, on the midterm exam, I once again got the top grade, he accused me of cheating and took the case to the principal. As when my intelligence had been dismissed in the second grade, my teacher's only evidence for his accusation was that I was a girl (there were only two girls in the class). I was exonerated, but I dropped the class. It was a decade before I walked into a math class again, and then only under duress.

Clearly, my teacher ascribed to a fixed mind-set, believing that ability in mathematics requires a Y-chromosome. Those who ascribe to a fixed mind-set believe that people either are or are not endowed with the abilities necessary for success in, for example, math or athletics. In contrast, people who endorse a growth mind-set believe that ability is dependent on learning, effort, and practice, and not determined by social identity or genetics.[9] Not everyone is able to be Einstein, but everyone should be able to succeed in physics class, and those potential Black Einsteins should be able to excel unimpeded by racist stereotypes "in the air" that diminish their performance or limit their opportunities.

The psychologists Mary Murphy and Carol Dweck examined how fixed and growth mind-sets affect people when they are held and communicated by institutions and those in positions of power, like teachers and workplace supervisors—in other words, when mind-set beliefs become part of the very atmosphere in the room.[10] Teachers communicate a fixed mind-set when they say things like: "You're either born with a talent for this subject or you aren't." "You either have the kind of mind that can understand math or you don't." "If you're having trouble in this course early on, you probably won't do well in it and should consider dropping out." Such pronouncements set students up for failure. They are cues to members of marginalized groups, who may be stereotyped as less intelligent or incapable of excelling in certain subjects, to give up before they even try. They take up so much bandwidth with self-doubt, concerns about failure, anger at the teacher for underestimating and dismissing them, or passionate determination to prove the teacher wrong, that they make it difficult to learn, which then converts the mind-set into a self-fulfilling prophecy.

What if, instead, the instructor started the class by saying: "You are all smart enough to get an A in this subject; however, some of you might find a few of the topics difficult, and if this is the case, please come to my office hours so we can discuss them in more depth"? Murphy and Dweck found that the performance of members of marginalized groups improves in school settings where the ability to meet an academic challenge is framed by educators as learnable and expandable rather than something carved in stone. And they found that there are clear patterns of instructor language and behavior that signal fixed or growth mind-sets to students. Even grades can act as such signals. In a TED talk, Dweck said that she heard about a high school in Chicago that required passing a certain number of courses in order to graduate.[11] But instead of giving an F to students who didn't pass a course, the teachers would give a grade of Not Yet, which communicated to the students that they were on a learning curve, one that would eventually get them where they needed to go in the future, even if they weren't there yet. A grade of Not Yet is a quintessentially Jedi move.

Murphy is developing a low-cost and scalable intervention to mitigate the effects of the stereotyping of girls in STEM classrooms. Instead of communicating, as my teachers did, that girls couldn't possibly excel at math, this intervention will assist STEM faculty in communicating growth mind-set messages through their syllabi, lectures, interactions with individual students, and other classroom practices. Similar interventions can be developed for other subjects and groups to address adverse stereotyping not just by gender but also by class, race, ethnicity, immigrant status, sexual orientation, and religion, for example.

Note that these highly successful and often stunningly straightforward strategies for improving the academic performance of marginalized students focus on changing the learning environment, rather than changing the individual student's behavior. There is now a body of evidence demonstrating that if a teacher's interactions with her students free them to learn the material and perform on tests unencumbered by negative stereotypes, they are much more likely to succeed.

The more settings in which a person experiences identity safety instead of stereotype threat, and the fewer insults accumulated on a daily basis that trigger the physiological stress process, the greater the chance that positive processes are set in motion instead. For example, a girl who is not exposed to demeaning cues in school about girls and math will perform better on her math tests, and that success can expand her future academic and professional opportunities. If she enters a STEM field, she will be in a better position to thrive and less likely to suffer the low-grade stress of stereotype threat that leads to burnout.[12] A Black college student who is not challenged by stereotype threat in his organic chemistry course, and therefore performs better, may be more likely to realize his potential and ambition to become a physician, while avoiding some of the everyday stressors that are weathering, at least at school.[13]

In general, practices that reduce stereotype threats to underrepresented group members in integrated settings such as schools lead to better life prospects for those individuals, while also paving the way for a better future for the people who follow in their footsteps. Why? Because over time those members who succeed at becoming respected professionals — teachers, doctors, lawyers, engineers, scientists, etc. — will diversify the academy and the labor force. This will naturally improve the prospects for success in the next generation of people from groups that have been marginalized in the past, because they will see their own faces and identities reflected in the world they aspire to be part of. In short, their success will contribute to dismantling negative stereotypes, and in doing so, mitigate the severity of the damage caused by identity threat across generations.

Many of the guiding principles and approaches for the creation of identity-safe environments in schools can be applied to other institutional settings, such as workplaces, health-care facilities, police-community relations, and the media.[14]

Encouraging Stigmatized People to Develop Counternarratives about Their Predicaments

Creating counternarratives that mitigate the physiological impact of toxic cues is another effective strategy for harm reduction. Having the skills to take an oppositional gaze and deploy these narratives can sometimes inoculate people against the potentially damaging health impact of negative identity cues, or at least lessen the severity of their impact. Counternarratives are alternative explanations to the dominant marginalizing narrative. They explain a situation without denigrating a person based on their social identity alone, and they can be helpful in critiquing widely shared narratives that are shaped by racist, sexist, homophobic, Islamophobic, or other-ist and other-phobic ideas. A counternarrative is more than an affirmation; it involves an analytic deconstruction of the traditionally accepted narrative and the inclusion of socially situated additional information that provides a more accurate context. In effect, a marginalized person is changing the posters in their brains themselves. For example, instead of taking personally my eleventh grade math teacher's charge that I could do well in math only by cheating, and instead of wondering what was wrong with me that provoked his distrust and hostility, and instead of seeing dropping out of his class and avoiding math for a decade as the only solution, I might have taken an oppositional gaze and said to myself, "Wait a minute. I've always excelled in math. I get better grades than most of the boys in my classes. I know I didn't cheat. I don't know why the teacher is so crabby and accusatory about it, and it will make the rest of the semester in his class uncomfortable, but there's no need to give up math altogether because he is sexist. Most of my math teachers in the past have been supportive. His sexism doesn't have to become my problem."

Institutions can help oppressed people develop these counternarratives. They can help expose and defuse the cues of stigma or entitlement attached to social identity in order to alter social dynamics and reduce related identity threat. Counternarratives, critical-consciousness raising, and protest are historically important ways for changing hearts and minds—or at least protecting stigmatized people from the most pernicious impacts of threatening cues, and offering a means of resistance.[15]

In the school setting, stereotype-threat researchers have systematically tested and found that the following strategies can neutralize marginalizing narratives:

1. Having students affirm their most valued sense of self, early in a school term, helping to inoculate them from threats. This has been accomplished as simply as by administering a one-page anonymous paper-and-pencil questionnaire that asks the student to affirm their core values.

2. Fostering intergroup exchanges that substitute familiarity and firsthand knowledge for stereotype-driven assumptions. This can be as simple as having informal diverse small group exchanges.

3. Helping students develop a narrative about the setting that explains their frustrations. This can often be accomplished through social ties, cross-group friendships, and role models. When students are facilitated in getting to know one another through social activities or study groups or peer mentorship, they have a chance to learn from others' experiences. For instance, as an eleventh grader I might have discovered that all women who were in my AP Math teacher's classes over the years were treated with derision, so he wasn't singling me out because of something that was untrustworthy about me, per se.

Longitudinal studies show that these scalable interventions improve academic performance of students of color in the short term and have continuing positive effects on their academic performance over many years.[16]

Sending New Social-Identity Cues through Storytelling Media

The media can also help create positive counternarratives—as opposed to the ubiquitous negative narratives that it has historically perpetuated. Storytelling media in all its forms—television, movies, podcasts, etc.—has become an ever more influential generator of cues about social identity. Plots, protagonists, villains, actors, and dialogue project stereotypes, reinforce them, and fill the very air we breathe. Dating back to the 1970s, the late and beloved professor and cultural critic bell hooks wrote books in which she dissected the ways media representations of Black people were inaccurate, racist, and reductive.[17] Having grown up in the 1950s, hooks was troubled both by how scarce representation of characters from adversely racialized populations were in the early days of television, and how problematic. Her parents watched TV shows with her and encouraged her to deconstruct the racist depictions on those shows.

The digital age continues to be rife with misrepresentations, some of which are obvious (for example, video game avatars that project powerfully racist or sexist images). As part of the racial socialization of their children—the process through which parents help their children understand what it means to be Black—today's parents, like hooks' parents, can help their children call out and name these surface cues to racism, thereby neutralizing them and depriving them of their power. Parents in families of color already include the so-called Talk as part of the racial socialization of their children. Through the Talk, parents are taking steps to inoculate their children from the worst reactions to threatening surroundings and interactions, as well as decreasing chances of escalation into an immediately life-threatening predicament. But these are only partial solutions, which place the burden on parents to take responsibility for decoding these messages and then teaching their children how to decode them. Instead, these threats should be excised in everyday life by the people, institutions, and systems that perpetrate and proliferate them.

Decoding and Dismantling the Negative Cues Delivered by Social and Digital Media

In today's digital world, decoding overt racist representations in the media only scratches the surface of the ways it participates in the systemic degradation and demeaning of vulnerable targets, proliferating racist, classist, and sexist ideologies.

In small and sensational doses, the public has been alerted to cues from social media that might adversely affect its teenage users. For example, much was made of the possibility that features of Instagram might negatively affect body image among teenage girls, perhaps coaxing them toward eating disorders, depression, and even suicide.[18] The scientific data on this is more nuanced than the public knows, but the idea that cues in social media could be harmful to the physical and psychological health of members of specific social identity groups — Black Americans, Native Americans, Mexican Americans, Appalachian Americans, and other historically oppressed groups — needs to be explored, and any harmful practices reined in, for example through regulation or through developing best practices for social media.[19]

Currently, for example, AI researchers are studying what D. Fox Harrell, director of the Imagination, Computation, and Expression Laboratory at MIT, calls "phantasmal media" to uncover how biases emerge in computing systems and design systems that are responsive to diverse stakeholders, enriching their user experiences and avoiding overt or subliminal stereotyping and bias.[20]

Big Data and Social Stereotyping

There is another little-known and almost invisible route through which racist narratives are promoted, sometimes to deadly effect. In her brilliant and haunting book *Weapons of Math Destruction*, the mathematician Cathy O'Neil deconstructs the ways that the ever-growing use of computer algorithms applied to or derived from Big Data and machine-learning technologies has contributed to the denigration of culturally oppressed and marginalized groups.[21] Operating quietly beneath the surface, these algorithms both encode and exacerbate prejudice, and they can have a powerful effect on every facet of our lives, from assessments of creditworthiness to decisions about where to concentrate police, whom to admit to college, whom to hire, whom to rent or sell a residence to, and more. They can be a devastating form of stealth inequity.

One area in which these algorithms have become pervasive is in medical decisions about diagnosis and treatment. Because their conclusions are seemingly objective, based on mathematical rather than personal criteria, they are believed to be neutral and fair, but in fact they are often the opposite. In a study published in *Science*, health economists found that an algorithm widely used by physicians to determine which patients require more intense, tailored, and holistic treatment regimens showed significant racial bias, leading to Black patients being vastly underserved.[22] Remedying this disparity would increase the percentage of Black patients receiving more intensive treatment from 17.7 percent to 46.5 percent, they said. That's a staggering statistic, and highly suggestive of the cost Black patients pay for being Black. The researchers concluded that the bias arises because the algorithm predicts health-care costs rather than illness, but unequal access to care means that less money is spent caring for Black patients than for white patients. Thus, despite health-care cost appearing to be an effective quantifiable proxy for health by some measures of predictive accuracy, large racial biases arise. The researchers suggest that the choice of convenient, seemingly effective proxies for ground truth can be an important source of algorithmic bias in many contexts.

Other researchers found that algorithms determining how to advertise job openings for CEO and other highly paid positions are rigged so that news of these job opportunities is less likely to be presented to qualified women.[23] Law enforcement operations are increasingly turning to facial recognition, yet the accuracy of this technology varies widely according to your race and gender. Because facial recognition software is trained on photosets containing a disproportionate number of white faces, it works best on white people, which means Black people have a higher chance of being incorrectly identified as criminals by a technology widely believed to be nearly infallible.

The widespread and growing use of computerized algorithms and machine-learning technologies is an increasing source of stealth inequity. To remedy this injustice will require a deliberate and informed attempt by both the programmers and the consumers of such algorithms. The first step, as with the resetting of so many of the cues we've been discussing, is to recognize the dangerous bias encoded in them.

Being Attentive to the Expressive Role of Law and Current Events

An increasing amount of scientific evidence is showing that laws can serve as cues to the inclusion or exclusion of social identity groups and that this "expressive role of law" can have both positive and negative health impacts.[24] Studies show that laws banning indoor smoking shifted public opinion against smoking and against smokers. Laws against gay marriage increased homophobia.[25] Some laws, such as same-sex marriage bans, miscegenation laws, and voter suppression laws, are purposefully enacted to undermine identity safety. These can exert pernicious health effects beyond the legal constraints they place on a marginalized population. However, in many other cases, the consequences of laws and policies for identity-safe contexts may be unknown and, if adverse, unintended.

Mark Hatzenbuehler and colleagues studied gay and bisexual men in Massachusetts, analyzing their health before and after same-sex marriage was legalized there in 2003. In the year following same-sex marriage legalization, both mental and physical health improved in these men as a group: They experienced an 18 percent reduction in hypertension, a 14 percent reduction in depression, and a 15 percent reduction in health-care costs, compared with the twelve months before the legalization.[26] In contrast, health-care costs during this same period increased for the general population in Massachusetts.

Similarly, a national longitudinal survey of Black Americans from 1979 to 1992 found that self-rated physical and psychological health was most positive in 1988, the year when the survey respondents were also the least likely to report experiences of racial discrimination.[27] No objective evidence to explain their greater well-being in that particular year was discerned. The researchers argued that the presidential election that year—whereby the Reagan era might come to a close (it didn't) and a Black man, Jesse Jackson, ran a serious campaign for president with early signs of success—may have encouraged them that a better day for racial equality was coming. This cue may have provided them some hope and respite from the ceaseless barrage of negative stereotypes of the urban underclass as welfare queens, crack dealers, addicts, and superpredators that pervaded the airwaves beginning in the 1980s, and perhaps reduced their chronic biopsychosocial stress. But positive developments such as these appear to persist only as long as they are actively sustained and promoted. By the 1992 wave of the survey, after the George H. W. Bush administration (1989–93) continued the Reagan-era political climate, there was no longer any such effect. Likewise, after Barack Obama was nominated for president in 2008, researchers found self-rated health increased among Black and Latinx Ohio residents—but not white residents—even net of income, education, health insurance, age, sex, marital status, Dow Jones average, and the unemployment rate.[28] Another positive "Obama effect" was found in a study showing that between the time Obama was nominated and his election, stereotype threat had a smaller adverse influence on Black students' academic performance and, in fact, Black students' academic performance improved.[29] These positive impacts were fragile. Following the 2016 presidential election, positive Obama effects on health were diminished, if not entirely eliminated. Virulent and racist backlash against Obama from some white quarters proved that Black Americans' earlier beliefs that Obama's presidency heralded a "post-racial" or deeply multicultural America were naive.

These examples demonstrate why it is important to include weathering considerations in racial impact statements, including explicit discussion of the extent to which proposed policies maximize an identity-safe culture. In conjunction with the many other insights into how to resist, mitigate, or disrupt weathering, the strategies of Jedi public health do their bit by making everyday life less automatically stressful, making the biopsychosocial playing field more level, and diminishing the power of dominant cultural ideologies to derail those whose options, resources, and lived experience it neglects.

Weathering and health inequity will not be eliminated until we neutralize the pernicious effects of the ubiquitous cues that put marginalized populations on the defensive and spontaneously activate their physiological armor. JPH initiatives acknowledge the destructive power of such cues and offer possibilities for resetting them to neutral or positive cues that individuals can adopt in any setting, even with limited time, effort, and money. Such actions will help alleviate some of the stressful challenges of everyday life for those on the margins. Given how easy it is to put these initiatives into practice, it would be a shame not to start implementing them immediately, even before more systemic and structural changes can be made. Simple as they are, their effects can be profound, setting into motion virtuous cycles that expand opportunities for many, and contributing, over time, to a more equitable landscape and life experience for all. Not utilizing them will only reinforce and extend the places and experiences where weathering occurs, including in high-stakes settings.

But let's be clear. While the strategies suggested in this chapter will indeed have an effect, they cannot alone end structural racism, classism, or sexism. Yes, the students who find questions relevant to their social identity at the end of the test they are taking are less likely to be cued to the stereotypes that brand them as deficient or limited. Likewise, the children who watch movies and television shows that depict members of their identity group in positive ways will feel better about themselves and their options, as so many of them have testified they do. Yet this will in no way end the reality of entrenched racism, classism, and sexism in our society. Systemic problems call for systemic change. The guidelines in the following chapters will lead us in that direction.

10.

Think Holistically: Transcend Departments, Compartments, and Determinants

Within the field of public health, an increasing number of stakeholders are calling for a Health in All Policies (HiAP) approach to policy making, which addresses what are known as the Social Determinants of Health (SDOH).[1] These include entrenched poverty, unsafe housing and neighborhoods, medical underservice, and unequal access to healthy food, safe exercise spaces, education, job opportunities, etc. The idea is to take health and health equity considerations into account when developing or evaluating social policies and programs, including policies that do not, at first blush, appear health related.

This is an admirable goal—as far as it goes. But making responsive and sustainable inroads toward promoting health equity takes addressing overlapping systems of oppression, not only specific "social determinants" as defined by government agencies and bureaucracies. These are limited, in the main, to concrete, measurable, and documentable inadequacies in physical and built environments, and to spatial and material barriers to routinely incorporating features of a healthy lifestyle for those living in high-poverty segregated and disinvested neighborhoods. HiAP approaches too often take on one "social determinant of health" at a time, each in isolation from the others, and construe them as influences on individuals rather than as products of racist or classist systems. Many HiAP proposals suggest policies that seem to exist in a vacuum rather than in the real world. How we define a problem will determine how we arrive at its solutions—and how effective those solutions will be.

HiAP approaches can lead to important and measurable improvements: Add grocery stores and farmers markets to food desert neighborhoods; build parks and recreational facilities in communities that lack green spaces; create bike lanes and well-lit walking paths where none exist. This approach is certainly preferable to placing the full burden of adopting healthy lifestyles on individuals and denigrating or punishing them for failing to do so. And it recognizes the geographic distribution of food deserts, namely low-income areas where high proportions of the population have little access to quality grocery stores or fresh fruits and vegetables, even as their access to liquor stores and processed foods is unimpeded.

But there are limitations to HiAP, beginning with the fact that if we restrict our understanding of the impediments to health equity to factors in the immediate physical environment, we can never truly get to the roots of the problem, such as the dominance of age-washed personal-responsibility and makers-versus-takers conceptual frameworks. And this narrow focus means there is no guarantee that these welcome additions to underinvested communities will be widespread or long-lasting. Changes in funding and the shifting winds of politics, policy, and the economy may doom them to a relatively brief existence, after which the stores and farmers markets leave, the parks fail to be maintained by the city, the lights on those paths go dark, and so forth.

For example, in the wake of the 2008 banking crisis, city governments turned to austerity urbanism, essentially the extreme tightening of their budgets.[2] This harmed the residents of many low-to-moderate-income cities with large populations of color. As noted earlier, austerity urbanism after the Great Recession led Detroit to reduce its municipal workforce by nearly half. The state's decreased commitment to funding public services in Detroit was also manifest in Detroit's renegotiated pay and pensions for the current and former public service workforce, its approximately 78,000 abandoned buildings, its scarcity of working residential streetlights, and the residential water shutoffs that were protested by the UN as a human rights violation.[3]

Alternatively, neighborhood improvement approaches can be "too successful," pricing current residents out of their homes and neighborhoods. As a matter of equity, steps must be taken to ensure that urban revitalization does not drive up the cost of living to the point where community residents are displaced after they have withstood decades of disinvestment and its weathering impacts.[4] Examples of ways to do this include community benefits requirements with teeth, rent controls, and eviction moratoria that safeguard the right of the original residents to remain in their neighborhoods.

Also, and fundamentally, limited HiAP approaches leave intact the age-washed ideologies that are informed by the personal-responsibility narrative. In short, this approach has the potential to backfire because of how it can be used against those whose health it hopes to improve. As a cautionary tale illustrating how this can happen, consider the conclusions reported by the UK Commission on Race and Ethnic Disparities as recently as March 2021.[5] One of the four major recommendations of the report is to "create agency"—in other words, to give members of marginalized groups greater ability to make "healthy" lifestyle choices. This is another way of expressing the personal-responsibility narrative. Apropos of health disparities, the report states that "individuals and communities of all ethnicities should be encouraged to take control of their own health [...] in relation to changing their own behaviours."

The report goes on to highlight top-down improvements that Britain has made over the last fifty years in "opening doors" for the marginalized but acknowledges that stark racial/ethnic disparities in outcomes persist. As for why that is, the report has this to say:

"Participation, however, is not just about opening the doors, we also speak to the need for communities to run through that open space and grasp those opportunities."

The suggestion here is that ethnic working-class populations in the UK have not sufficiently exercised their newly "granted" agency and therefore bear much responsibility for the persistence of inequity. In the US, we have seen marginalized groups going to great lengths to exert agency autonomously, but with returns on that investment in agency that are in no way commensurate with the energy, planning, coordination, and trade-offs required of them. There is reason to imagine marginalized and racialized groups in the UK are in a similar predicament. It takes a lot of hubris to turn this emphasis on agency into a vehicle for blaming those who are so profoundly disadvantaged, but this is a problem that is inherent to the personal-responsibility approach.

In short, if, having enacted some of these HiAP measures, we believe we have leveled the playing field for practicing healthy behaviors and thereby improving health, the American Creed has primed decision-makers to think it has done everything it could. And if stark inequities in health nonetheless persist, it must be the fault of those they were trying to assist. We built the level playing field; "they" did not come. We opened the door; "they" did not run through it to grasp the opportunities we offered.

Being stuck in this mind-set, the broader public may fail to see that any benefits the marginalized may have gained from taking advantage of new grocery stores and walking paths could be vastly outweighed by the chronic weathering experiences in their everyday lives. If they still start each day with hours-long commutes on standing-room-only, poorly ventilated transit systems; spend their waking time strategizing how to choose between paying for food, medications, rent, electricity, and water service as they fulfill their work obligations and force smiles for their landlords and bosses, and end each day exhausted in pest-infested, lead-paint-covered, overcrowded, poorly heated or cooled homes, engaging with media that promulgates racist ideas, weathering will continue. And all the well-intended initiatives that were supposed to offer them better opportunities for healthy living will be futile.

Some HiAP proposals are more expansive, taking into account other social sources of health inequities, for example promoting job creation and economic stability, transportation access and mobility, a strong agricultural system, environmental sustainability, and quality proximate health-care services and educational institutions. Policies informed by this more holistic understanding of the problems are more likely to have substantial positive effects than those that simply try to make a healthy lifestyle more affordable and accessible. I cannot emphasize enough what a leap forward this is when compared to the reigning individual behavioral approaches of the past forty years.

However, even these approaches can fall somewhat short of what it would take to address weathering. And because of the likelihood that influential thinkers and politicians will object to including transportation access, job creation, and other, less intuitive "social determinants of health" within policies intended to improve the overall health of oppressed populations, such an approach risks political failure or, at best, political fragility. Its architects will be attacked as exploiting the system in order to fulfill a "progressive wish list." Unfortunately, these kinds of attacks are typically effective in weakening popular support for holistic, ambitious policies, at least at the federal level. It may be politically unfeasible to expect these types of programs to gain political traction on a national level in the short term. However, in some localities, initiatives that take a more holistic and intersectional approach and pursue "high-road" development are already being implemented.[6] High-road development treats shared prosperity, environmental sustainability, and efficient democracy as necessary complements to each other, not as trade-offs.

I will describe this concept in greater detail and provide an example in chapter thirteen. These local initiatives are providing proof of concept, showing that new intersectional approaches that have larger missions and constituencies than simply improving one SDOH at a specific moment in time, such as housing, for example, and are community driven rather than top down, can succeed at multiple health-and-social-equity-promoting goals at once; realize economies of scale, breadth, and depth of buy-in; and be regenerative and sustainable within specific communities, as well as be reproducible in others.

11.

Do Not Erase Oppressed Stakeholders: Do Nothing about Us without Us

In mapping the way forward toward equitable policies, effective solutions will not come only from the mouths or minds of those who fancy themselves experts. They may be the lead dancers in today's oppressive tango, but if they expect to eliminate weathering among oppressed groups, they cannot be allowed to dictate and proscribe, center their own needs and perspectives, or rely on their own commonsense formulas for living. Without being proactive in guarding against this tendency, it will be the default.

The divisions between those with authority in the dominant culture and those they think their actions benefit are so entrenched that even the privileged who actively and open-mindedly seek to learn the truth about how people on the "other side of the tracks" live are too far removed to fathom it. I am reminded of a conversation the medical anthropologist Seth Holmes described in his book on Latinx immigrant farmworkers, *Fresh Fruit, Broken Bodies*.[1] In this passage, he is reporting on his experience as a graduate student engaged in a participant observation study focused on undocumented Mexican American farm workers. The conversation was started when a farm worker observed:

"Right now you and I are the same, we are poor. But later you will be rich and live in a luxury house."

The anthropologist explained that "he did not want a luxury house, but rather a little, simple house." The farm worker replied: "But you will have a bathroom inside, right?"

Just as the anthropologist took indoor plumbing for granted, members of dominant populations neither know nor suspect how insidious weathering can be in the lives of their racialized, working-class, or poor neighbors. The existence of weathering compels us to recognize the marginalized as the ultimate experts on their own lives.

Incorporating the voices of those in the communities who will be affected by any policies enacted, and partnering with communities to assess and develop policies, is both practical and respectful. As an example of how the failure to do so can result in an incomplete understanding of their challenges, consider the Urban Institute's attempt to evaluate the impact of school-choice programs on transportation times for high school students in Detroit.[2] Looking at only direct drive times, they concluded that on average, students lived only about a ten-minute drive from their elected schools. But the researchers must have been unaware that the ten-minute drive time was irrelevant for the majority of the students. Many of these students did not get to school by car but rather by bus. By focusing on car travel, the researchers did not anticipate the problems associated with relying on public transportation, including long and sometimes unsafe walks to bus stops, unreliable bus schedules, and buses so packed that they skip stops, forcing students to wait, sometimes for a considerable period of time, for the next bus.

Issues with public transit were not the only factor obscured by the Urban Institute's reliance on its expertise alone. Recall the qualitative study led by Linnea Evans in which we discovered that even for girls with access to a car for transportation, a commute from home to school was rarely a simple point A to point B drop.[3] More often than not, a student's drive to school had to accommodate the schedules of multiple people in the family, which lengthened commuting time. By listening to the girls themselves, we learned that their commutes were dramatically longer and more complicated than the ten-minute drive the Urban Institute researchers estimated. Grasping all the factors that make the commute to school long and complex—like the early wake-times required to accommodate bus schedules or to coordinate with others traveling to work, school, or the bus stop in the same car—could not be accomplished by the Urban Institute researchers who relied on the ostensibly objective distance between homes and schools to arrive at their estimates.

In other words, however good their intentions, the Urban Institute researchers likely extrapolated from their own experience of having a reliable car that could be driven directly from home to school to make their estimate. As a result, they vastly misapprehended the reality of the students' lives. The Urban Institute could have come up with a better and more comprehensive picture of the impact of school choice on transit time if they'd included voices of people with ground-truth knowledge of their transportation needs who would have to live with the policy.

Taking Pregnant and Birthing Women's Voices Seriously

We've seen that one prominent theme in the stories about Black mothers who had pregnancy-associated death or near-death experiences—even the wealthiest, like Serena Williams, or most highly educated, like Shalon Irving—is that their concerns were not taken seriously by their medical team, no matter how persistently they attempted to express them. Another example comes from Tressie McMillan Cottom, a sociologist, research professor at UNC–Chapel Hill, MacArthur Fellow, and writer. Cottom shared details of her own horrible birthing experience, during which her concerns about being in premature labor were dismissed by the medical professionals attending to her, who subsequently disclaimed any responsibility for the likely preventable death of her newborn daughter. Looking back on her ordeal, Cottom says:

> What I remember most [...] is how nothing about who I was in any other context mattered to the assumptions of my incompetence. I spoke in the way one might expect of someone with a lot of formal education. I had health insurance. I was married. All of my status characteristics screamed "competent," but nothing could shut down what my blackness screams when I walk into the room.[4]

We've now seen many examples of accomplished Black mothers who were disrespected by medical professionals. Had they been taken seriously, many of their own deaths and the deaths of their babies might well have been averted.

If such affluent and educated Black women can't get their voices heard, it's not surprising that the voices of poor or working-class Black mothers — the majority of Black mothers, according to national demographic statistics — are completely obliterated in the obstetrical setting, as I first saw at the clinic in Trenton. We've seen that medical personnel can contribute to maternal- and child-health inequities by allowing racist, classist, and ageist or age-washed ideas to influence how they provide care. As gatekeepers of clinical testing and treatments, clinicians need structural and cultural competency training. At the institutional level, changes need to be made in order to elevate the voices of mothers themselves as well as the nurses, midwives, and doulas who attend to them during labor, so that doctors' voices aren't the only ones that are heard in the delivery room.

All pregnant women need to feel empowered to have open and honest discussions with their health-care providers. Sascha James-Conterelli, a practicing midwife, Yale University faculty member, and recent president of the American College of Nurse Midwives, advises women that they have a right to expect providers to be willing to answer as many questions as they need to ask in order to feel comfortable and fully understand their plan of care. Women should also be entitled to bring an advocate to their visits, whether a family member, partner, or birth doula.[5]

Care providers must acknowledge that they treat women differently based on race, and that this distinction has a real effect not just on how women experience their care but on their actual risks. It is the provider's responsibility to make sure a pregnant woman knows her right to ask questions—whether they are about racism or about her birth plan—and to have her questions answered seriously and thoughtfully. But let's be clear: while entreaties like this might move the needle for individual women and care providers in the obstetrical suite, it still places the burden on individual mothers to advocate for themselves in a rigged system and will do only so much. If a member of the CDC's Epidemiology Intelligence Service, a tennis superstar with twenty-three Grand Slam titles, or a MacArthur Fellow can't get their voices heard, it's time to override clinician discretion in life-threatening circumstances to pursue equitable outcomes.

Operationalizing Equity through Mandatory Protocols in Life-Threatening Situations

In the case of maternity care, we can develop and institutionalize best-practices protocols that override clinician discretion in life-threatening situations, and, in effect, center mothers' needs over physician authority. When complications arise, these protocols can be put into action so that regardless of whatever racist beliefs clinicians may hold about the competence or character of the woman in their care, or how little they listen to her, or what their biased algorithms tell them, they can be made accountable for putting into practice the necessary actions and equipment. One example of this would be making it mandatory to use the patient safety bundles disseminated by the Alliance for Innovation on Maternal Health (AIM).[6] These bundles provide instructions for standardizing clinical response to the most common causes of preventable maternal mortality. (Each is meant to be updated as the evidence for best practices evolves.)

To date, AIM has created bundles covering the following topics:

Obstetric hemorrhage
Severe hypertension in pregnancy
Safe reduction of primary cesarean birth
Obstetric care for women with opioid use disorder
Cardiac conditions in obstetrical care
Postpartum discharge transition

As an example, consider the current bundle for obstetric hemorrhage. This protocol overrides clinician discretion by requiring, for example, that every patient be assessed for hemorrhage and that assessment not be merely impressionistic, but measured by actual quantity of blood loss. Furthermore, it mandates "readiness" in the form of having a hemorrhage cart immediately accessible, an identified response team, contingency plans for mothers with rare blood types, checklists, and unit drills to promote preparedness for when actual hemorrhages occur. To achieve greater and more diverse input from all personnel—physicians, nurses, technicians, etc.—the bundle also calls for establishing "a culture of huddles" of everyone involved with a mother who is losing blood, enabling each the opportunity and the authority to provide their observations and ideas about how best to proceed.

AIM is working with the American College of Obstetricians and Gynecologists (ACOG) and state leaders to encourage states to mandate these protocols and collect metrics on them so their impacts can be evaluated. Some states have contracted to institutionalize and evaluate these protocols, but many more states need to be compelled to do so, by legislation or accreditation requirements, if necessary.

The Fourth Trimester of Pregnancy

We must also acknowledge that the biopsychosocial impact of pregnancy and childbirth on a new mother doesn't end the moment her baby is born. Her body needs time to recover and, if she breastfeeds, to meet the new and significant physiological demands on her body. The sleep deprivation associated with having a newborn, the changing psychosocial demands of being a new mother, and the struggle to fulfill other obligations while mothering a newborn, all have adverse physiological effects. And all can compound the effects of weathering.

Currently, conventional postpartum health care in the US calls for one obstetrical visit at six weeks, during which the new mother's ob/gyn checks her blood pressure, vital signs, and physical healing. What's wrong with this picture? Our almost total lack of any other health services for women in their first months of motherhood would be considered neglect in any other high-income nation. Why? Because although about a third of maternal deaths occur during pregnancy and about a fifth on the day of delivery, the other 50 percent of maternal deaths occur after the child is born, and three quarters of those deaths occur within the first six weeks postpartum.[7] In other words, the one postpartum visit to the doctor is supposed to take place *after* the highest period of postpartum death has already passed. In contrast, the WHO recommends that a new mother have at least four health visits within the first six weeks.[8] As a culture, we do not acknowledge the holistic needs of mothers at any stage of the pregnancy experience, least of all the postpartum period.

After experiencing a very difficult twin pregnancy, including months of physician-ordered bedrest, delivering one of my sons breech and the other by emergency C-section, then getting so little sleep once they came home that I began to hallucinate, my chair refused my request to postpone a guest lecture he wanted me to give in his class when my sons were a month old. He added: "I understood when you were pregnant and experiencing complications that you couldn't be expected to take on extra assignments, but now that your babies are born, aren't you just in the same boat as the rest of us who are parents?" I was in no position—and probably too sleep-deprived—to say "Hell, no!" and, anyway, he didn't appear interested in my answer to what sounded to me like a smug rhetorical question.

Since my sons were born, the University of Michigan has made changes to allow new parents to modify the distribution of their duties, although the new policies may or may not have protected me from a Department Chair underestimating what a huge ask it was to expect me to prepare and give a guest lecture while I was still recovering from a difficult twin pregnancy and birth, not to mention the severe sleep deprivation that followed, especially as I worked with my babies to establish nursing. Still, the restrictions my job placed on me were much less severe or health harmful than those placed on less educated and poorly paid service, factory, or farm workers. I share my personal story here because it exemplifies the depth of our culture's ignorance about the needs of new mothers and babies. If this kind of thinking could prevail in such a privileged, professional space—a top-ranked school of public health, in the department that housed its Child and Family Health program, no less!—it's easy to see how deeply it's embedded in our culture and policies (or lack thereof). Our society's failure to grant parents at least a few months of paid parental leave is a disgrace, and again a departure from what just about every other affluent country does. In fact, we make virtually no institutional accommodation for the needs of new mothers.

The US also lags far behind these countries in guaranteeing postpartum visits. All other high-income countries mandate (and pay for) multiple postpartum visits. These start in the first week after hospital discharge, most within twenty-four hours of going home from the hospital. These are home visits by midwives or nurses who are mandated to spend *several hours* per visit to support mothers recovering from childbirth.

Such policies weren't always as unheard-of in this country as they are today. In 1921, Congress passed the Sheppard–Towner Act.[9] One hundred years ago, this bill provided millions of federal dollars to states to support home visits for new mothers by midwives, and to establish child and maternal health-care centers in impoverished areas across the country, all for the purpose of increasing access to prenatal care and prenatal education. The provisions of the Sheppard–Towner Act, particularly the home visits and the accessible health-care centers, were estimated to have contributed to about half of the net decrease in infant mortality rates witnessed during the eight years the act was in effect.

Unfortunately, the American Medical Association and other powerful political groups that accused the legislation of being a "communist plot" successfully opposed its reenactment when it expired in 1928. We have been stuck in some version of this specious argument against sensible measures to support new mothers, babies, and families (and many other kinds of social welfare legislation) ever since, the result being that we provide less such support than any other affluent country (and many not so affluent countries) in the world.

Another legacy of the AMA's lobbying against the act is that physicians, rather than midwives, now oversee the bulk of maternity care. This is unfortunate because midwives typically provide a more holistic form of care. They are better at listening to women who are pregnant/giving birth, and taking them seriously. But the women-centered approach midwives take to childbirth was (and is) viewed as a threat to the professional status of physicians, who assume that their expertise and status should elevate them above not only the birthing mother but also all other kinds of birth attendants in the hierarchy of authority. Doctors have been attacking midwives since the turn of the nineteenth century (and before that, too, when they were under suspicion of witchcraft).

In 1928—the same year that the Sheppard–Towner Act failed to be reauthorized—Joe P. Bowdoin, then the director of the Division of Child Hygiene at the Georgia State Board of Health, published an article in *JAMA*, the leading medical journal, entitled "The Midwife Problem," which can be seen as a landmark in its racism, classism, and its sexism. Bowdoin asserted that in the Southeast, where he practiced, the shortage of obstetricians was a compelling problem because the midwives who usurped physicians' roles in childbirth were incompetent: "Practically all midwives are negroes [*sic*] who have reached middle age or over," he observed, continuing: "They are, as a rule, ignorant and superstitious, having absorbed many things from the traditions of the race. Most of them are unable to read; consequently, teaching them is a slow process."[10]

This and other similar attacks nearly succeeded in driving midwives out of business in the US. Since then, the practice of midwifery has been revived and professionalized. Midwives today are medically trained and licensed professionals, who, depending on the state in which they practice, are allowed to perform gynecological examinations, write prescriptions, care for a woman during labor and delivery, perform fetal monitoring, and deliver babies. So what do midwives do that doctors *don't*? Plenty—and at a much lower cost. Moreover, what they don't do is in some ways as important as what they do. The MDs who currently rule the roost often objectify the birthing mother by focusing on machines monitoring her vital signs and those of her fetus, at the expense of actually listening to the woman herself and responding to her concerns. Midwives, by contrast, try to minimize the use of technological interventions, believing that birth is a natural life process rather than a medical problem—though they are also trained to know when labor is *becoming* a medical problem and to bring in a doctor when necessary. Midwives are generally more responsive to the emotional as well as the physical needs of women in labor, and they are also experienced by women as less threatening than physicians.

As discussed earlier, the International Center for Traditional Childbearing (ICTC), the nonprofit organization that trains Black women aspiring to become midwives in collaboration with Portland State University, takes an explicitly African-centered approach. In an implicit rebuke to obstetricians like Bowdoin, ICTC's method "encompasses oral traditions from Africa, the Caribbean, and the 'Deep South.' "[11]

The movement to train and incorporate more Black midwives and doulas in the birthing process is a critical step forward. But we still lag far behind other high-income countries in making use of the services of midwives, which is unfortunate, because we have a profound shortage of clinicians providing maternity care, particularly in high-poverty urban and rural areas. Relative to other high-income countries, the US has the fewest maternity-care providers per thousand live births. Among those we do have, ob/gyns are overrepresented, while midwives are in vast undersupply. In fact, the US has the lowest proportion of maternity-care providers who are midwives relative to doctors (as shown in the figure on the next page). Of only fifteen maternity-care providers per thousand live births, fewer than five are midwives. In contrast, other high-income countries have more than double the number of providers (some have four or even five times the number!), and a much larger proportion of those providers are midwives. Austria and Sweden have seventy-five and seventy-eight providers per thousand births respectively, and the vast majority are midwives: 91 percent in Austria and 75 percent in Sweden. Both of these countries boast substantially lower infant and maternal mortality rates than the US and dramatically lower per capita health-care costs.[12]

Number and Composition of Maternity-Care Providers per Thousand Live Births in the US and Other High-Income Countries

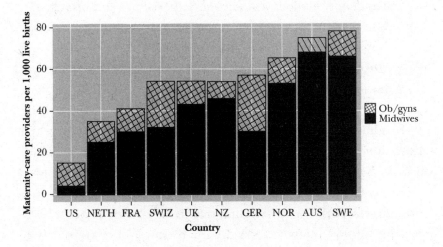

The shortage of maternity-care providers in the US, in combination with our sad excuse for postpartum care, sets weathered mothers and their babies up for the worst outcomes. The failure of the US to take pregnant, laboring, and postpartum women's voices seriously or center their needs is now a century-plus-old and epic systemic failure. However, increasing rates of maternal death over the last thirty years have gained public attention, and the steps identified previously to remediate the situation are straightforward, are already being taken in some places, and would result in lower health-care costs than business as usual if we made them matters of policy.

In 2016, the 4th Trimester Project convened a group that included mothers, health-care providers, and other stakeholders to propose the restructuring of postpartum care. Taking all stakeholders' voices seriously, they concluded standard practice should institutionalize the concept of the fourth trimester of pregnancy. As they summarized their discussion, four major areas of concern emerged:[13]

1. The intense focus on prenatal health to the near exclusion of adequate postpartum care
2. Medical practice guidelines that often do not align with women's experiences
3. Lack of validation of women as experts on their infants and failure to understand that elevating their strengths as mothers is necessary for achieving health goals
4. The need for comprehensive care, which is difficult to provide because of numerous system constraints

In addition to changes in maternity care, universal paid parental leave during the fourth trimester is the necessary minimum policy action that should be instituted in support of this model. Three months of paid maternity leave—compared to zero, which is the prevailing model!—may seem like a lot to ask. Yet every other high-income country offers at least that much; most offer considerably more—and to both parents! While the wealthy US guarantees *no* paid parental leave, the next-shortest paid leave provided by a wealthy country is fourteen weeks (Switzerland). Norway guarantees the most—ninety-one weeks!—and the UK falls in the middle at thirty-nine weeks.[14]

No Erasure: Voting Rights

In addition to speaking with words, Americans speak with their vote. In the United States, after centuries of de jure and de facto disenfranchisement of Black Americans, the Voting Rights Act of 1965 resulted in a mass enfranchisement of poor and Black Americans. Today, however, erosion of these rights is demonstrable. Several governmental decisions and practices, often at the state level, appear to be selectively and intentionally undermining the prohibition against voting rights discrimination on the basis of race and class, first set forth in the Fifteenth Amendment to the US Constitution.[15]

The trend toward shortened poll hours and more-stringent voter ID policies in several states has disproportionately negative effects on voting among the nonwhite and the poor.[16] Gerrymandering electoral boundaries that concentrate racial/ethnic groups into minority districts also reduces their political influence.[17] Felony disenfranchisement laws in many states have a significant discriminatory impact on outcomes given racial/ethnic variations in the prosecution and sentencing of drug-related crimes. All of these trends weaken the voice that Black and impoverished Americans have through voting to help shape government priorities.

Weathering further disenfranchises marginalized populations. In a study on which I collaborated—with lead investigator Javier Rodriguez, a political scientist, economist John Bound, and geographer Danny Dorling—we calculated that at least 1 million Black likely voters were lost to early death by the 2004 election cycle. That is, there would have been 1 million additional Black voters if Black and white Americans' life expectancies were equal.[18] Based on their past behavior, the largest proportion of the lost Black voters would have voted for the Democratic Party candidates. In fact, many close state-level elections would likely have had Democratic rather than Republican winners if voting-age Black Americans had the mortality profiles of voting-age white Americans.

Our calculations also show that premature deaths among Blacks are most common at the ages where Americans are most likely to exercise their right to vote. The gutting of the Voting Rights Act by the Supreme Court in 2013, along with rising levels of excess mortality among the working class, imply that voice erasure through disenfranchisement and health inequity is larger today than it was in 2004. Systematic disenfranchisement of racialized and impoverished populations undermines democracy. US voting patterns show that Black disenfranchisement reduces the odds that elected officials will have mandates to eliminate health inequities, among other ways it distorts social mandates. In other words, along with the more-recognized causes of disproportionately Black disenfranchisement, large and persistent inequities in life expectancy between Black and white Americans may have been both a cause and a consequence of partisan US politics since the political realignment of the 1960s. By weakening Black political power through the various means of disenfranchisement, governments become less inclined to invest in programs to promote health equity. And strategies to weaken the voice of Black, poor, rural, and student populations continue to be proffered and instituted.

Restoring and protecting voting rights is necessary to ensuring democracy and allowing marginalized stakeholders to elevate their political voice to equitable levels. Over the longer term, it is likely to reverse the trend toward intensified weathering we have experienced over the past thirty-plus years. There is a growing movement against gerrymandering and stringent voter ID laws, and several states have ended felony disenfranchisement once sentences have been served. Applying sustained energy to these movements is a step any concerned citizen can take. The weathering-induced loss of electoral voice, along with its implications for excess death of voting-age Black Americans, also requires sustained and systematic action.

12.

Reorient Public-Health Science and Practice to Better Address the Needs of Working- and Reproductive-Age Adults

Many public-health initiatives target or favor the health and well-being of children or the elderly over those of working-age adults. Through an age-washed lens, which assumes that young through middle-aged adults—roughly ages twenty-five to sixty-five—are able-bodied and in their prime, both the young and the old are viewed as being more at risk, and therefore more deserving of support.

However, evidence that weathering is most pronounced among working- and reproductive-age adults should give us pause. The health problems of young through middle-aged adult members of oppressed communities are vast. And if we are taking marginalized perspectives seriously—"nothing about us without us"—we'll realize that there are important needs for this age group, too. Since these are the people who are most critical to the functioning of their families and communities, it behooves us to address their needs. The benefits of doing so will also redound to their children, their elders, and society at large.

It doesn't take a lot of imagination—or even empathy—to see why this would pay off. The high level of weathering-induced disability among working-age people limits their ability to work full-time jobs and support their families economically, in addition to putting immense pressure on working-class family caretaking systems. Women who undergo difficult or life-threatening childbirth obviously require longer-than-normal recovery times and are less able to take care of their babies. Whether they are mothers or not, working- and reproductive-age women are central to the extended kin networks that sustain poor and working-class families. But having so many competing and conflicting obligations—to their family, to the larger social networks of their community, and to paid jobs—leads to early-onset stress-related disease, threatening their ability to meet all their commitments.

As we saw in the previous chapter, the US provides the least amount of maternal or family support among its peer group of nations, while having arguably the highest expectations for primary caregivers, most of whom are women. In 2019, UNICEF ranked the US last among forty-one high- and middle-income countries in "family friendliness."[1] The stressors associated with parental obligations are multiplied for working-class parents, who are least likely to be able to take any paid time off or hire help, and most likely to have stressful jobs and long commutes, live in overcrowded or dilapidated housing, and struggle with balancing their many complex and multi-generational caretaking duties.

It is in everybody's interest to invest in supportive measures that lighten the load of working- and reproductive-age adults. Instead, we expect parents to sink or swim on their own. For those who do not have the material resources to take unpaid leave or to pay for the support they need—e.g., to hire nannies and housekeepers, or to enroll their young children in quality day care and preschool—it can be an impossible ask.

Even for well-resourced parents, the lack of any kind of public safety net can send them hurtling from crisis to crisis in the face of any unexpected calamity—which is exactly what happened to parents of young children during the COVID-19 pandemic. The US is devoid of any disaster preparedness or backup plan for childcare.

Working-class and poor parents already knew this. And now, thanks to the pandemic, so do all but the most affluent and privileged parents. This is why so many women—especially women with small children—had to abandon their jobs at the start of the COVID-19 pandemic. And as late as eighteen months into the pandemic, when the Brookings Institution published a report on this issue, there was little sign of recovery in labor force participation by these women.[2]

Perhaps because the fault lines in our system were laid bare by the demands of the pandemic, federal policy proposals during the Biden administration have attempted to position parents as part of the "human infrastructure" in need of support and expansion, including family-oriented policies such as subsidized childcare, universal pre-K, family leave, child allowances, and a universal basic income or guaranteed living wage. Such policies could go a long way toward decreasing the biopsychosocial stressors faced by low-income working-age adults, at least those who are parents and also members of their support networks, as well as their material hardship. Given the impact of chronic stress on health, not to mention the impact of poor health on the productivity of the economy, implementing some or all of them should be a no-brainer. But when proposals like this come up, they often get derailed by objections to the high costs to small businesses, some imaginary slippery slope to socialism, or sudden concern about the deficit. And other priorities overtake them in government budgeting. Yet the majority of the American public thinks it's high time we joined all other affluent countries in providing some or all of these family benefits.

Human infrastructure spending would provide resources to support families. How much and whom will they support? Well, the devil is in the details. Not all approaches are equally helpful or targeted carefully enough to ensure that those most in need of the support receive it. For example, some of the family policy proposals of the last decade would have largely benefited families who were economically well-off. But other recent proposals would make meaningful improvements to our pathetic safety net, such as child tax credits that would pay low-income families a set amount per year for each child under eighteen years old. We can see the benefit of this approach by looking at the American Rescue Plan's expanded Child Tax Credit, which provided $3,600 (or $300 per month) per child per year during the pandemic, and was estimated to have cut child poverty by 30 percent or more.

Beyond this, and germane to weathering disruption, Senator Michael Bennet, who was central to developing the plan, noted, "Not only did the world not come to an end, but the families I talked to, who spent the money on everything from school clothes to a bicycle, were relieved of stress. That was the word they used with me. They were relieved of enormous, backbreaking stress."[3]

But the program expired at the end of 2021 and, although its impact underwent extensive study and its many benefits were documented—including rescuing about a third of the 9 million American households where children regularly don't have enough to eat from food insecurity—Congress declined to renew it. Republicans actively positioned themselves against it by leveraging old tropes with new coding, following the Southern Strategy playbook but replacing explicitly racist and classist language with vague or abstract language that evokes zero-sum-game moral panic.[4] In light of weathering and growing income inequality, it's well past time to call bullshit on these tired arguments against providing support to parents. Given the scope of its demonstrated benefits in only one year, one can imagine how much more could be achieved toward health equity if it were reinstated with a longer time horizon, or better yet, permanently.

Reproductive Justice: The Doulas and Don'ts

A critical way the US does not support the needs of working-class adults is its failure to promote the conditions for reproductive justice. First set forth by Loretta Ross and the collective in which she participated, SisterSong, the reproductive justice framework offers grounding for social or public health policies and clinical practices that aim to promote the health and well-being of a large set of intersectional identities.[5] In so doing, it promotes equity and it disrupts rather than exacerbates weathering. This framework can respond to the wide array of socially structured and culturally variable reproductive experiences that US women face in our diverse and inequitable society.

The three core principles of reproductive justice for all women are:

1. The right to have a child
2. The right to not have a child
3. The right to parent a child or children in safe and healthy environments

In reality, our political discourse and policy debates center on the second principle of reproductive justice alone. In line with our age-washed tendency to see reproduction in terms of individual behavior that, if enacted responsibly, will result in childbirth and parenting at the right age, in the right sequence, and under the right material conditions, we have put too many eggs (pun intended) in the basket of birth control (contraception or abstinence) as the primary means to eliminate our scandalously high level of maternal and child health inequity. As essential as having the right to regulate your fertility autonomously is, birth-control access and practice are an insufficient answer to these multidimensional problems of racialized social, economic, and health inequity.

I've found that the idea that contraception is not the full answer baffles many privileged people, including those who are genuinely concerned about the challenges of living in a racist society. So when I've presented weathering research that shows maternal mortality rates rising when Black women bear children at older ages, I find that the educated and professional people in my audiences often throw up their hands and say, sometimes sincerely, sometimes sarcastically, "What are you going to do, promote teen childbearing among poor Black women?"

To be clear, my answer to this question is a resounding "No."

The solution to misguided policy is not to turn to its binary opposite: promoting teen childbearing rather than preventing it. In any case, it is not for outsiders, no matter their apparent "expertise," to decide on a universally best age for childbearing for anyone and everyone. Yet, in April 2018, after the increasing and increasingly inequitable rates of maternal mortality of the past twenty to thirty years were placed on the front burner for redress, the American College of Obstetricians and Gynecologists (ACOG) uploaded a seemingly serious question to its Instagram account:

What's the primary way of preventing maternal mortality? ACOG18

Teasing its followers with this life-or-death question, ACOG then revealed an answer—in the form of a cartoon that appeared on both its Facebook and Instagram pages and stunned readers with its insensitivity. It pictured a weird, personified cartoon condom with a grin.[6]

So, using a condom is the answer to preventing maternal mortality? And, by logical extension, Black couples in particular should therefore more often be using condoms because their maternal mortality rates are highest? I wish I could tell you that ACOG didn't actually post this, but it did.

The post provoked swift and heartfelt rebukes. Of the more than seven hundred reactions to the post on Facebook, fewer than a hundred were likes or loves or laughter; five hundred and seventy-four registered anger; the remaining reactions included expressions of surprise or sadness. This was a typical comment:

It seems that the suggestion here is, "If you don't want to die in child-birth, don't get pregnant." I don't appreciate the flippant tone of a smiling condom when we are talking about maternal mortality. Especially knowing that the medical care field needs vast improvement in caring for women of color, who are three times more likely to die in childbirth than a white counterpart. If it's not a joke to you, don't treat it like one. Shameful.

Another commenter summarized her disgust in one pithy question: "Honestly the best you can come up with to save women is to tell them not to procreate???"

Indeed, with so much evidence in favor of straightforward ways to reduce maternal mortality, such as those I have already discussed— e.g., mandating patient safety bundles in hospitals, increased training and deployment of midwives and doulas in maternity care at all stages, and expanded, holistic postpartum care—one wonders why condom use was brought up at all.

Equitable access to birth control and abortion are of course necessary components of ensuring all people's reproductive rights. Universal access to these technologies must be protected. However, advocating birth control and abortion access is not a sensible go-to approach for addressing every health or social problem associated with childbearing among culturally oppressed people. The belief that they are central rests more on shared acceptance of the personal-responsibility narrative than on evidence-based research. Furthermore, advocating birth-control use as the front-line method for improving maternal and infant health relies on the age-washed and demonstrably wrong notion that the health problems associated with childbearing will naturally go away if women postpone childbearing to older ages. As we've seen, maternal mortality rates increase sharply with age for Black American women, beginning in their early twenties, which belies the wishful thinking that increasing the use of birth control among adolescents will solve the problem. Furthermore, US birth rates are at their lowest levels since the Great Depression, and teen birth rates are at all-time lows, which suggests that sexually active teenagers are already making effective use of contraception. Yet maternal mortality rates are still rising. Why? In part because, as explored in chapter four, of the reality that more births are taking place at older ages in fact puts more women and their babies in jeopardy.

As we reflexively turn to authorities who advocate birth control as the silver bullet answer to inequitable and rising infant and maternal mortality rates, we should instead ask ourselves: How will contraception spare Latina women from ICE raids? Or poor Appalachian Kentucky women from environmental toxins? Or working-class Black women from hours-long toxic commutes each day to perform degrading and physically taxing work for starvation wages? How would using birth control have prevented Kira Johnson and other accomplished Black mothers from having their cries for assistance ignored as they bled to death in a hospital? The driving cause of maternal mortality inequities isn't pregnancy itself; it's weathering and the racialized lived experiences that precipitate it.

When ACOG attempted to quell the outrage their cartoon condom provoked by editing the Facebook post, they doubled down on birth control's being a primary tool for reducing maternal deaths. Judging by the uniformly critical responses, ACOG's apology fell nearly as flat as the original tone-deaf joke. To many readers, it appeared half-hearted and patronizing. It also came across as defending the idea that contraception should play a significant role in reducing maternal mortality. While it is offensive to recommend, even in jest, that if women don't want to die they should just refrain from getting pregnant, that is, in essence, the extent of our official approach to the problem of maternal mortality. Yet, if we are ideologically boxed into an age-washed personal-responsibility ethos regarding the timing of childbearing, it's hard to come up with any new ideas.

The sad state of our official policy agenda for reducing preventable maternal deaths is based on the belief that using birth control is some kind of superpower. In 2020, the Department of Health and

Human Services set forth its official national public health objectives for the next decade in a report titled Healthy People 2030.[7] Acknowledging that reducing maternal and infant death rates is a high-priority goal, the department focused on three basic routes to that end, two of which—the emphasis on individual behavior, and the oversized role for birth control—have failed to result in major improvements in the past and are not likely to do so in the future. The official recommendations are concerned with changing individual behavior either before pregnancy (e.g., reduce teenage and unintended pregnancy by increasing effective use of birth control; women should avoid being overweight at conception) or during pregnancy (e.g., abstain from drug and alcohol use during pregnancy, get prenatal care, avoid contracting syphilis). None of their proposals acknowledged the vast and growing Black/white health inequities that result in those deaths, or the basic structural remedies that would be required to dismantle those inequities. When evaluated through a weathering framework, it is likely that the implementation of these specific goals would, on balance, increase rather than decrease rates of Black maternal and infant deaths, along with those of poor and working-class white women and babies.

We can do better.

To even begin to address the problem of eliminating maternal and infant health inequities we must clear our collective consciousness of its single focus on family planning—essential as it is to reproductive justice writ large—as the answer.[8] At a time when the fertility rate is decreasing with each passing year but mortality rates are rising anyway, the focus on birth control instead of more thoughtful and evidence-based approaches is simply a lazy and irrelevant response to addressing an entrenched and growing public health problem. Meanwhile, mothers and babies are dying.

There are additional and better ways to understand and address the systemic social forces that undergird increasing rates of maternal mortality and the substantial inequities in them. Achieving reproductive justice for all people requires lifting the veil on the ways our reproductive fates our linked. We need to recognize that the status quo places all mothers and babies in greater harm's way than they need be. All working families—whether professional or working class—would benefit from greater societal support.

The Exaggerated Virtues and Downplayed Costs of Postponing Childbearing

As a society, we are stuck on the imagined ideal life-course scenario of postponing parenthood until after we have attained professional security. We already know that as a consequence of this press to postpone childbearing, some Black women are paying with their lives, and even more are paying with their health. Given the high cost of housing, childcare, and college, and resultant decades of compounding student loan debts, many college-educated workers of all races or ethnicities must put in many years of work before they feel ready, according to what the dominant culture deems "readiness," to become parents. If a bow in our quiver for targeting weathering is paying better attention to the needs of working- and reproductive-age adults, the consequences of our understanding of the components of "readiness," along with the structural impediments to achieving them, must be taken seriously.

In addition to questioning the racist narratives that have been discussed throughout the book, we should also reconsider the trifecta of questionable axioms that pressure so many aspiring parents to delay childbearing:

- Respectable and responsible parenthood first requires that all one's socioeconomic ducks be in a row.
- It's impossible to train for a secure, fulfilling, prestigious, or well-renumerated career while at the same time parenting an infant or young child.

- Assisted reproduction using the latest technology will protect individuals or couples who want children from increased risk of infertility if they delay childbearing until they feel ready to become parents in their mid-to-late thirties and into their forties.

It is a law of nature that the ability to become pregnant, have a healthy pregnancy, and have a healthy baby wanes with maternal age. However, there is no such law of nature that dictates that the only way for couples who both aspire to full-time jobs or professional careers and want to raise children is to put professional security and accomplishment ahead of childbearing. If proper supports were put in place—e.g., a minimum of several months of parental leave, flexible work hours, and limits on required business travel for new parents—these two goals could both be accomplished, either in reverse order or simultaneously.

Indeed, as we have opened the doors for an increasingly diverse range of people to enter fields that require ever longer periods of education, training, and total commitment to proving oneself on the job, we have become all the more fixated on the goal of postponing parenthood, without regard to the inequitable implications across diverse groups. And people have complied. In 2016, for the first time, the CDC reported that US women in their thirties were having more children than those in their twenties.[9]

The consequences of this trend for the most educated and accomplished women were the subject of a 2022 story in the *New York Times* featuring Ariela, a thirty-four-year-old hematologist at the Mayo Clinic in Minnesota:

From the start [she] proceeded with the conviction that if she worked harder, longer and better, she would succeed. And she did: She graduated as high school valedictorian, attended an elite university and was accepted into a top medical school.

But one achievement eluded her: having a baby. She had postponed getting pregnant until she was solidly established in her career, but when she finally decided to try to have children, at thirty-four, she was surprised to find that she could not, even with fertility drugs.[10]

The article notes that Ariela's personal story is an example of a broader phenomenon. Surveys have found that female physicians who try to become pregnant face roughly double the rate of infertility of the general public.[11] Similarly, a survey of women surgeons found that 42 percent had suffered a pregnancy loss.[12] Again, this is more than twice the rate of the general population. Furthermore, they suffered a much higher rate of pregnancy complications than the general population.

Across racial groups, women who choose to become mothers are starting families at later and later ages, when the risks of infertility and poor birth outcomes are greater than they would have been for the same women at younger ages. This is certainly true for Black women, both professional and poor or working-class, as we have discussed at length. To a less severe extent, it also applies to privileged, highly educated white women, who have been both culturally and financially incentivized to put education and professional success ahead of childbearing. Complying with these cultural and social norms has led to widespread burnout and structurally induced infertility among professional women. It has also resulted in increased maternal and infant morbidity among white professional mothers and babies—which is not as shockingly high as it is for Black women, including professionals, but higher than it need be.

However, one reason for our current predicament is that professional training programs and work schedules adhere to models that were developed at a time when it was mainly men who were tasked with being breadwinners, while women were the primary caregivers. Another key reason for the apparent incompatibility of professional aspirations and a healthy family life is our economy's unregulated turn over the last forty years toward what economists call monopsony capitalism, in which huge companies, in the absence of regulation or any competition (especially once they have driven their competition into the ground) are so powerful that they can depress wages and weaken or eliminate benefit packages for their employees.[13]

Monopsony capitalism is not free-market capitalism. Monopsony concentrates power at the top and renders everyone else powerless and dependent on its goodwill—which is slim since its raison d'être is profit. But it is ascendant, as we have seen with the stunning rise of companies like Amazon, Apple, Facebook, Tesla, and Google.

Deregulation has resulted in largely unchecked monopoly and monopsony power among a very few corporate behemoths in recent decades. A monopoly is to the cost and supply of products as monopsony is to working conditions, wages, and job security. And just as monopoly is harmful to consumers, monopsony is harmful to workers. As a direct result of the absurdly outsized share of the labor market claimed by a few industry giants, and also through collusion among some of these big firms, working-class wages have dropped precipitously. Mergers and the strategic use of nondisclosure agreements, noncompete clauses, and no-poaching arrangements tie workers' hands. Less-skilled workers are provided fewer opportunities for well-paid work or benefits, or even predictable work schedules.

Monopsony capitalism affects high-salaried and professional workers, as well as the working class. It pressures salaried workers to put in longer and longer hours with no boundaries between work time and personal time. There is also pressure to travel out of town for work (less pressure of this kind during the COVID-19 pandemic, obviously), which can wreak havoc on a household with two parents who are both high-level professionals. Salaried employees also face increased job insecurity under monopsony conditions, making them less likely to rebel against pressures to work early, late, or on weekends. To the extent their problems are acknowledged at all, workers are encouraged to cope with stress, loss of control over their time, and even burnout by meditating and exercising and eating more healthfully. But their biggest coping mechanism, without which none of this would be possible, is to rely on outside help to keep their households and families afloat. And that, in turn, has a huge impact on weathering—that is, *on the weathering of people from less affluent, marginalized communities.*

In a society that offers almost no institutional or financial support for families, privileged parents have been able to enjoy the benefits of being successful working couples only because they have also been able to outsource most of their domestic labor.[14] They depend more and more on the working class to watch their children, clean their houses, deliver their groceries, cook their meals, walk their dogs, and even serve as their gestational surrogates—even while these workers must struggle, often to the point of total exhaustion, to perform such duties for their own families. Thus, in yet another instance of how we are all part of the same ecosystem no matter how its effects on us may differ, the pressure on professional workers to delay childbearing and work longer and longer hours likely contributes to the further weathering of marginalized workers.

Rather than be guided by the dominant culture's "ideal life course" or "success sequence" for major life events and accomplishments, we must remember that as we press working-class and poor young women to postpone childbearing beyond their late teens and early twenties, and discourage more affluent or socioeconomically mobile women of color who want to become mothers from bearing children before they have completed their educations and are ensconced in their intense professional careers, we are also promoting their weathering. If, as a society, we want to promote childbearing at a later age, we must think about what we must do to reduce the weathering that makes it unsafe. And we must find ways to protect pregnant women from the everyday biopsychosocial stressors that are so commonly faced by members of poor and marginalized communities. These are matters of reproductive justice.

To achieve full reproductive justice, including reproductive health equity, the ability of the more privileged to enjoy the pleasures of family life cannot be predicated on the exploitation and weathering of working-class people. If our abhorrent rates of maternal and infant morbidity and mortality are to be reduced, and inequity in these rates eliminated, we must push for explicit regulation to limit the powers of monopsony capitalism as well as offer family supports.

Some of the greatest beneficiaries of monopsony capitalism are the industry giants of Silicon Valley. They are also major protagonists in the press for highly successful professional women to delay childbearing—even if they may have fooled us and themselves into thinking the opposite is true. Silicon Valley companies have a history of offering what appear to be generous perks—company bus rides to work, free food, massages, a gym, yoga classes, and even dry-cleaning services at the office—but the flip-side of all these perks is that they encourage employees to spend ever longer hours at their jobs. These companies offer several months' maternity or paternity leave (generous by US standards), which was modeled by the Facebook CEO when each of his two daughters was born. This is of course commendable. But what consideration do these companies give to making day-to-day job expectations and responsibilities compatible with being pregnant or raising a family for the years it will take after parental leave has ended? True, salaries are high for professionals at these companies, providing them the financial means to pay for private household help. But the overall culture at these companies is not nearly as family-friendly as they'd have us believe.

In recent years, companies including Apple, Google, and Facebook began offering a new kind of perk, advertised as a compassionate response to the (very rare) employee who might experience premature menopause, such as a woman whose ability to ovulate is ended by undergoing cancer treatment. While this could have been offered as an option only for women employees who face this tragic circumstance, instead they offer all of their young female professional employees (but notably not their warehouse or other lower-paid employees) this rather unusual fringe benefit: coverage for having their eggs frozen as insurance against future infertility.[15]

Egg freezing might seem like the ultimate perk for professional employees, especially those who have become structurally induced workaholics. Little consideration is given to the number of potential health consequences connected to this process that have not been sufficiently explored, researched, debated, or regulated. To freeze her eggs, a woman must undergo two weeks of hormone injections per cycle and egg extraction under general anesthesia. Many who have undergone this procedure report experiencing an additional two-week recovery time before they feel "back to normal." Furthermore, women often undergo these procedures over multiple cycles, either because viable eggs are not harvested the first time or to help ensure that enough frozen eggs are harvested to supply multiple IVF cycles once a woman decides to use them.

There's an additional dark side to this perk: it's a bit of a bait-and-switch. The success rate of having a live birth at a later age using frozen eggs is less than 15 percent (about 1 in 7). Companies are presenting the appearance of being family-friendly while in reality undermining the chances that women who take advantage of egg freezing will actually become pregnant. In doing so, these companies help ensure they can get the most out of their female employees before burnout takes too strong a toll. Whether or not this perk gives female employees greater options for and control of their fertility and careers, it certainly offers substantial benefits to the companies themselves: keeping their employees focused on their jobs. And it is easier for companies to offer a technological perk like egg freezing than to find ways to fundamentally change a toxic or exploitative work culture.

What it means for companies is that female employees who delay childbearing with the expectation of using those frozen eggs when they decide to have a child won't, for the time being, be distracted by the competing obligations of family life. Young tech-firm employees often work sixteen-hour days and are expected to travel all over the world for days or weeks at a time at the drop of a hat. Women and men who have delayed childbearing can work these crazy schedules without their bosses having to make allowances for children's illnesses, school holidays, after-school activities, or any of the other issues that arise among employees with children. Culturally, such an approach also serves to stigmatize those workers who choose to bear children in their twenties or early thirties, setting them up to be viewed as insufficiently committed to their careers at a cultural moment where the highest-ranking female Facebook executive advises that the recipe for female professional success is to "lean in."

Bad as these working environments are for the tech professionals employed in them who are or hope to become parents, consider the domino effect exerted by the pressure that is placed on them. If they must work long hours and hectic schedules as their corporate employers try to squeeze ever more value out of them, they in turn will expect the "help"—mostly women, and disproportionately women of color—to work longer hours, too. Weathering among domestic and other family service workers will be exacerbated in turn, which will increase their already shockingly high risk of maternal and infant morbidity and mortality.

There is a saying, "When a white person gets a cold, a Black person gets pneumonia." One reason for this is that weathered Black working-class and poor people who already have "pneumonia" are called upon to nurse affluent white people through their "colds." And this applies exponentially in the realm of maternal and child health. If the danger to professional women who delay childbearing because of societal expectations is unnecessarily high, it is all the higher for the working class, the poor, and women of color.

If we are sincere in our intention to minimize weathering and its intergenerational impact, and are committed to achieving true reproductive justice and social equity, those with resources cannot simply advocate for themselves while failing to recognize that the way they cope burdens others. Nor should well-compensated workers settle for piecemeal perks of ambiguous value like egg freezing rather than a real, society-wide commitment to supporting the needs of all working-age adults and their families.

13.

Recognize All Our Fates Are Linked

Failing to grapple with the physical, social, and economic costs of weathering is simply not sustainable in the long run — not for those who most immediately bear its impact, nor for society at large. We cannot afford to think in binaries, whether winners versus losers, deserving versus undeserving, or makers versus takers. Inequities of the magnitude we see in the United States today, in income, health, and political inclusion, threaten the fabric of our society. Whether we admit it or not, all our fates are linked. Everyone can benefit from a new social vision.

As Heather McGhee eloquently argues in her book, *The Sum of Us*, American political and policy logic often holds us hostage to the belief that each of us — whether as individuals or as members of social identity groups — must advocate for our own interests in a zero-sum game.[1] That there need always be "winners" and "losers" is as much an illusion as its corollary that winners earned their status and losers deserve theirs. The fallacy of this logic becomes clear when we look concretely at important public-policy issues, such as health-care costs and climate change, as I will do on the pages that follow. With these and many other issues, we are all stakeholders, and we are all implicated. Taking weathering into account as we address these social issues is imperative for success and will benefit all of us.

Health-Care Spending

Weathering has a profound impact on US health-care spending, and how it affects us all is straightforward. Even the wealthiest among us need health services, yet the US health-care system is financially unsustainable. It gorges on a huge share of GDP without producing a commensurately healthy population.[2] Meanwhile, it places an exorbitant burden on the budgets of both our families and the nation.[3] Health-care spending is a primary contributor to ballooning US debt, crowding out other budget priorities. Anxiety about how to pay medical bills keeps many Americans—especially but not only those most subject to weathering—one health crisis away from being able to pay their utility bills, their rent, or worse. To reduce the demand for health care, we need to invest in people and places in ways that disrupt the inequities that cause weathering and improve the overall health of the population. Happily, some interventions in the medical care system that disrupt weathering themselves are also less costly than current medical practice—as I noted in the context of maternity care. In other cases, such as regionalizing tertiary care for rural residents, making the necessary investments may be costly in the short term; but in the long term, failure to make these changes will cost a lot more.

It's simple: Our health-care system will not be viable for any of us unless growing demand for health care is slowed. Ignoring weathering takes us in the opposite direction, affecting us all.

Climate Change

It's easy to see how weathering increases health-care costs; how these costs impact all of us, even those who aren't weathering themselves; and how addressing weathering will thus benefit all of us. Climate-change policy may seem like a less obvious example. What could it have to do with weathering?

Many people believe that addressing climate change is largely a matter of technological and political innovation. But in reality our capacities to address climate change and weathering are linked. We will not be able to address climate change if we do not take into account the ways that racism has sustained it through race-conscious suburbanization, the proliferation of cars, and the subsequent urban disinvestment and decay that fueled white flight. These trends have in turn exacerbated both weathering and climate change. Nor will we be able to address climate change if we do not consider equity and weathering in our attempts to revitalize urban centers, build a green economy, and increase public transit. I will address all of this in more detail later in this chapter, including examples where weathering and equity were not considered, to everyone's detriment, as well as a promising example where these factors are being considered. But first, let's clarify the ways our fates are linked as we face the existential threat climate change poses to the habitability of our planet.

While the worst ravages of climate change are felt by the least privileged (and exacerbate their weathering), no one can fully escape the destruction of climate change. Scorched-earth heat waves and the raging fires that accompany them destroy the hugely expensive homes on Malibu Beach just as readily as they do the much more modest homes and trailer parks of Paradise, California. No matter how much fun the richest men on earth have floating weightless for three or four minutes at the edge of space in an obscenely expensive phallic capsule, even they need to come back to earth. No one will escape the threats posed by reduced biodiversity and the impact on our food supply, dwindling supplies of fresh water, and the increase in pestilence and disease. Not to mention the social unrest that will result as climate refugees seek new places to live, and as wars are waged over dwindling resources.

The fact that none of us is safe, even now, became personal to me when I was skimming the *Detroit News* one morning in the summer of 2021. I was horror-struck to read: "Rebecca Copeland, a twenty-nine-year-old University of Michigan graduate, was found dead in frigid water Thursday after an overnight flash flood at the Grand Canyon washed away her campsite."[4]

I knew Rebecca, who had graduated a month or so before her death, with joint master's degrees in public health and public policy. She was on vacation in Arizona, rafting the Colorado River, prior to beginning her dream job with the Center for Medicare and Medicaid Innovation. Now her body had been found lifeless, ice cold, and bludgeoned by debris.

Rebecca's rafting group had set up its overnight camp at an established site about a quarter of a mile from the slot canyon where her dead body was discovered. Like so many parts of the country, Arizona experienced torrential rains that summer, often provoking flash floods like the one that ripped Rebecca from her base camp and killed her. Climate change is thought to be—at least, in part—responsible for this flooding.

Contemporaneous with such flooding, parts of the country in the American West are suffering from a megadrought, the worst since 800 CE, according to the UCLA hydroclimatologist Park Williams, who links this state of affairs to climate change as well. He noted that "the last twenty-two years actually rank as the driest twenty-two-year period in at least 1,200 years, based on tree ring records."[5] This scorching drought is quickly draining reservoirs and fueling deadly heat waves and raging wildfires in the western states. It is devastating agricultural workers' livelihoods and making a healthy diet less economically attainable for a broad swath of people: scarcity of water and arable land, plus increasing irrigation costs, contribute to ever-rising fruit, vegetable, and grain prices.

Climate change also threatens job and broader economic security and opportunities for upward socioeconomic mobility. A TV news report featured Joe Del Bosque's melon farm in the Central Valley of California that is plagued by drought; he is hemorrhaging farm workers as the threat of lost profits looms. He has also had to downsize his plantings due to water scarcity. Mr. Del Bosque is unsure whether his farm and the livelihoods it provides will survive this megadrought at all. When asked by a reporter, "if you were starting all over, knowing what you know about this climate now, would you do this?" Del Bosque replied:

> I don't know. It was like a dream for me to be able to do this. Because I was the son of farm workers. I have a lot of people that depend on me. There's hundreds of people working in the fields, picking melons, that are people just like my ancestors that came here, worked hard to try to make a living for their kids, so their kids could go to college like I did. And this is gonna end their dream, too.[6]

Addressing climate change is imperative despite the resistance of powerful groups. And an effective solution must take into consideration the ways that systemically applied racist and classist ideologies have brought us to the brink of climate chaos and catastrophe while extracting a consistently large toll from the health of marginalized groups via environmental racism and the biopsychocial stressors associated with the coping required by day-to-day life.

Suburbanization and Reurbanization: The Links between Climate Change and Weathering, Historically and Now

One fundamental reason we have reached such a level of climate disaster is suburbanization and urban sprawl, which was made possible by twentieth-century decisions to invest in roads and cars rather than public transit.[7] Sprawl accounts for much of the greenhouse gas emissions in the US, and the US is a world leader in greenhouse gas emissions. Driving-related emissions have increased sharply as sprawl has held steady or intensified in most US metropolitan areas

over recent decades, despite the fact that everybody hates traffic congestion and long commutes, and polls show that the majority of
Americans want a greener future.

Why is this happening?

At its root is racial residential segregation and the racist ideology
that sustains it, even now that it is illegal. Living in the suburbs versus staying in the cities was not and is not simply a choice anyone can
make. Twentieth-century redlining practices undermined housing
values and investment in urban neighborhoods of color, and disqual-
ified residents of these neighborhoods from the mortgages needed
to buy new suburban homes.[8] As suburban developers built more
and more housing, it came with the development of land use restrictions (zoning) that, for example, prohibited building multifamily
dwellings in suburbs, whether duplex houses or apartment buildings, which would have been affordable to the working class and
would have facilitated the maintenance of multigenerational kin
networks. Zoning laws in many suburbs require that each single-
family home be built on a large lot, which puts the price of homeownership even further out of the working class's reach. Restrictive
covenants on individual home deeds legally precluded selling suburban homes to Black people (and, in some cases, to Asian or Jewish
families).

These laws and practices encouraged white movement to the suburbs, facilitated by new highway construction in the mid-twentieth
century that linked suburban whites to metropolitan cultural centers. Continuing white flight from the city in response to the growth
and decay of disinvested and stigmatized "inner-city neighborhoods," followed by middle-class Black, Latinx, and Asian flight once
restrictive covenants were outlawed, has been the driving force of
continued urban sprawl, maintaining grave inequities in the quality
and conditions of life between the largely white suburbs and the predominantly minoritized poor and working-class populations in
major cities.

Urban sprawl continues to be the staging ground for racial segregation and inequities in housing, education, toxic environmental exposure, and employment. This process contributes to the pervasiveness of biopsychosocial stressors that fuel weathering in people of color who are ghettoized into increasingly disinvested urban neighborhoods, many of which were cut off from cultural centers, employment, members of their families, and kin networks by the highway construction in the mid-twentieth century.[9]

For white people, early entrée into suburban housing has been the gift that keeps on giving. Many are aware that my generation—the children of the original white suburban homeowners in the 1950s and 1960s—and, by extension, our children have continued to benefit from the vast appreciation in suburban housing values since that time. The median home price in 1940 (six years after the New Deal created federally backed low-interest mortgages) was just $2,938 ($30,600 in today's dollars). By 2000, the median home price was $119,600.

Today, thanks in part to this appreciation, homeownership is the number one source of wealth for most Americans. Decades-long discrimination and outright exclusion from the housing market means minority families have been denied this anchor of financial security across generations that for some, particularly in the most expensive metropolitan areas, are massive windfalls of wealth. The structured creation of this race-based boondoggle alone undermines any conventional sense of who is or is not "deserving" of their current economic station.

In recent decades, pressure to revitalize urban areas has increased. Certainly, reducing urban sprawl is an important component of meaningful climate-change policy to reduce greenhouse gas emissions. However, if efforts to revitalize cities do not include an equity component or affordable housing, our good intentions will exacerbate weathering *and* do little to mitigate climate change. Let's break this down.

So far, the actions taken to reverse sprawl and reclaim urban areas for the socioeconomically advantaged have had disastrous results for poor and working-class city residents, who have been dispersed and displaced—helped along by demolition of public housing and naive theories about the social importance of "deconcentrating poverty." The increasingly affluent populations that have moved back to city centers in the past decades have fueled gentrification, leading to higher real estate prices that make it impossible for the longtime, low-income, low-wealth, and disproportionately Black and immigrant residents to remain in their homes. As a result, the fate of the urban poor and working class has fallen into three categories of housing apartheid, each with weathering consequences:

1. Those long-term working-class residents who continue to live in the city have been stuck with higher housing costs that eat into their meager budgets, leave them insufficient resources to stay financially afloat, incentivize apartment overcrowding and overuse of decaying electrical systems, and stoke social and environmental stressors in their homes and neighborhoods, while increasing fire risk, infectious disease spread, and the anxiety of looming eviction.
2. Others have been displaced to the more distant suburbs for cheaper housing, resulting in long, stressful commutes to their jobs in the city, either by public transit or, if they can afford it, by car—which of course only adds to traffic congestion and carbon emissions. Ironically, rather than reducing sprawl, we have simply played musical chairs on a regional scale.
3. Still others join the ranks of the unhoused and inadequately housed or live in informal settlements within cities—in essence, American shantytowns.

All of these housing and commuting options for people priced out of the local housing market expose the poor and working class to weathering. None of this is good for public health *or* the environment.

To address climate change, we will need to undo sprawl, which means we will need to live in more concentrated communities, thereby bringing us into closer proximity to other racial groups and economic classes. We cannot simultaneously eliminate sprawl *and* remain racially or class segregated. Although urban gentrification of the most recent decades has brought affluent white people back to urban centers, they have tended to live in racially and economically segregated areas, even gated communities. This form of reurbanization merely changes the character of sprawl rather than eliminating it, as the working class move out to the fringes of the city and far-flung suburbs in search of affordable housing. The question has become, how can we encourage and incentivize integration effectively so that people across class and race live in proximity to each other with no one gated out or gated in? And how do we neutralize the potential for othering of marginalized groups and achieve integration in ways that *ameliorate* rather than *exacerbate* weathering among the poor, exploited, or oppressed?

It is hard to exaggerate what a major challenge true equitable urbanization will be for US public policy, politics, and society. Neither people of color nor suburban white people are likely to welcome such a mandate. Historically, Black Americans have viewed the environmental movement with suspicion and, for good reason, felt that it focused on changes that only the well-off can afford to make: drive a Tesla, buy from clean-energy companies, install solar panels, etc. However, now indigenous American, Black, and Latinx people are on the front lines of community organizing for environmental justice, as they understand that structural changes are needed that go well beyond making expensive personal green lifestyle choices.

If we are to become integrated into dense urban and equitable communities, it will require more than providing economic incentives or mandates that individuals make green lifestyle choices.

An Equitable Green Economy

Many herald the push to green cities as a way to open up new working- and middle-class job opportunities in the wake of deindustrialization, as untold numbers of workers will be required to retrofit old, energy-inefficient buildings and build new, more environmentally friendly ones; build new transit systems, wind farms, and ecologically sound water management systems; and fulfill the countless other aims of the new green economy. With transportation costs rising, many manufacturers will find it cost-effective to produce locally, so there will be new manufacturing jobs as well. But nothing about this process is automatic. There is nothing intrinsic to green construction jobs that will make them good jobs. Construction jobs were good jobs historically because they were unionized and paid well.

Furthermore, for this green economy to fulfill its potential of providing good job opportunities for a large and inclusive workforce, the problems wrought over decades of disinvestment in high-poverty, racially segregated urban centers—in particular, profound educational and health inequities—must be addressed. J. Phillip Thompson, a former deputy mayor of New York City and now a professor of urban planning at MIT, observes:

> The big questions for the green workforce if it is to be an inclusive one are: Will these workers be well-trained and well-paid for this work? How will the training take place, at scale? Who will pay for it? What about the fact that training for electricians and plumbers requires a twelfth grade reading and math level, while many young underemployed people have a fourth grade functional reading and math level? How is the remedial training going to take place? How will wage standards get set? It will take new public policies to ensure that the jobs created through greening our cities lift people out of poverty, and don't just create handfuls of new millionaires.[10]

Successful greening of cities cannot sidestep the issues Thompson describes, nor can it ignore the reality of weathering. We have seen that weathering robs the working class of their lives and, before that, their physical abilities. Those who are not disabled face competing obligations between work opportunities and caring for dependents—whether their children, chronically ill or disabled adults, or the frail elderly. All of this further fuels their weathering and robs families *and the workforce* of critically needed workers. We will not be able to create a green economy if those seeking jobs do not have the requisite education or health for the newly available jobs. What might seem to be merely a technological fix will require attention toward promoting equity and eliminating weathering.

Improving Public Transit

Many Americans who prioritize moving toward a green economy share a consensus that energy-efficient, expanded, and upgraded public transportation is key. Approached equitably, improving public transportation will reduce weathering stressors among its largely poor and working-class ridership, while also increasing ridership across class, and reducing greenhouse gas emissions. However, many approaches that have been taken so far are neither equitable nor effective. Unfortunately, this is a story I could tell many times over with examples from Long Island, New York, to Portland, Oregon.[11] Portland is a good place to start.

A self-identified climate-friendly city, Portland has failed to meet its ambitious goals to reduce greenhouse gas emissions specifically because it failed to consider equity in its original calculations. In selected white and affluent parts of Portland, efforts to add bike-share stations, bike lanes, and dependable streetcars, and improve the walkability of neighborhoods, have succeeded in allowing those who can afford to live there to do so car-free. Yet, the low-income and racially diverse neighborhoods of East Portland saw no such improvements.

As housing prices in the walkable neighborhoods have continued to skyrocket, low-income residents have been pushed out to places like East Portland, where a car is a necessity. Now, to ease growing traffic congestion, many Portland citizens are advocating for expanding the number of lanes in existing highways, which will increase greenhouse gas emissions, particularly in predominantly minoritized neighborhoods. Traffic congestion has become so severe that students at Harriet Tubman Middle School, located on the I-5 freeway, are expected to limit their time outside in order to reduce their exposure to toxic fumes.[12] To preserve student and teacher health given highway pollution, a multimillion-dollar air filtering system was recently installed in the school, draining money that could otherwise have been spent on educational needs. No equity here.

The ultimate consequence of these selective and hoarded greening efforts is that greenhouse gas emissions in Portland continue to increase overall, despite the new highly walkable neighborhoods. Of little reassurance about the future, although perhaps some poetic justice, is that during the heatwave of summer 2021, the unprecedented scorching temperatures melted streetcar cables in the greenest neighborhoods in Portland.[13]

More hopefully, and perhaps with a nod to necessity as the mother of invention, community groups in greater Portland have turned to the principles of the energy democracy movement to promote equity in greening Portland. In 2018, Black, Indigenous, and other communities of color organized a ballot initiative to require corporations with gross revenue of at least $500,000 in Portland-based sales to contribute 1 percent of their annual gross income to a locally managed Portland Clean Energy Fund. Thanks to the painstaking community-building, educational and canvassing efforts, and get-out-the-vote activities led by communities of color, the measure passed in a landslide two-thirds majority. A critical part of their educational efforts was their work to bring local businesses and labor leaders on board. As a result, the Portland Clean Energy Fund is now in the position to distribute about $40 million to $60 million annually to support home retrofits and upgrades, living-wage job training to residents, renewable energy projects, and urban gardens and green space for the poorest communities and families of color in the greater Portland area.

Los Angeles, another city with ambitious goals for a greener future, is at a crossroads and could take note of Portland's initial mistakes.

In 2006, when I drove my then-teenage daughter into LA for the first time, she gasped at the sight of gray skies on a sunny day. Anyone who has seen the smog in LA (even now that it has been reduced from its highest levels), or has been caught in LA traffic, has experienced the results of the twentieth-century choice to invest in highways for affluent, suburban commuters rather than equitable, livable city centers for all.

In recent years, Los Angeles has created broad sustainability goals, including an announcement of the city's own Green New Deal in 2019, which places it ahead of the curve compared to most places in America.[14] Its achievement would have huge benefits for a city that is currently heavily polluted, spectacularly sprawling, and reliant on congested freeways. To provide additional resources toward greening transit in LA, the Measure M sales tax was passed with the goal of raising $860 million yearly for LA transit.[15] In addition, more than $2 billion from the LA County budget in the 2020 fiscal year was earmarked for expanding the county's Metro rail system, which links some of the far-flung neighborhoods of the county to the city.[16]

All of this sounds very promising. In addition to reducing greenhouse gases, improving public transit could, in theory, decrease weathering stressors. Due to a long history of underinvesting in transit, and because LA has seen its working class move farther and farther away from their jobs, long daily commutes to work for domestic and essential workers are exhausting and dispiriting—and potentially toxic. For example, Maria, a domestic worker in her fifties, rides the bus more than three hours each day to get to work at her job cleaning homes in an affluent neighborhood. She and her family have been forced to move to inner-ring suburbs farther and farther away from her work, because rent and housing prices have skyrocketed while working-class wages have stagnated or declined in real value—the same kind of housing crisis afflicting people in many other cities across the country.[17]

Yurithza, a young student, spends five hours a day commuting thirty miles to and from California State College, Northridge, in LA, a trip that requires her to be at the bus stop by 6 a.m. to start her three-bus, one-train commute. She cannot afford to live closer to school or to buy a car. Her frustration is palpable as she states, "On the bus, I just can't get from Point A to Point B whenever I need to. I hate it."[18]

Because of the extraordinary toll exacted by long daily commutes—disrupted or curtailed sleep, exposure to diesel and car exhaust fumes, extended discomfort while enduring prolonged wait times at bus stops, including in inclement weather, and sheer frustration—riders face transportation-specific weathering stressors daily. When such aspects of the long commuting experience activate physiological stress processes, as they inevitably do, the resulting elevated heart rates can persist for hours or throughout the day (and night) as they accumulate with other stressors faced. These additional stressors can include exposure to indignities, trying physical labor, and toxic chemicals in cleaning products for domestic workers like Maria, or the vigilance to stereotype threat and code-switching that provide students like Yurithza with the armor they need to survive in a college setting that was not designed for them.

Thus, improving public transit could have an immediate material impact on the health of the people most subject to weathering stressors in their daily lives. Unfortunately, whether LA's new initiatives will help residents like Maria and Yurithza is still up for debate. For now, LA is dangerously close to following Portland's missteps. While the poorest residents rely on buses, not trains, a wildly disproportionate share of the new public transportation funding in LA has been earmarked for tunnel and rail projects that cater to the affluent and to tourists. The cost of building these new rail lines often ends up much higher than what residents were initially promised, leaving the county scrambling to find money to shore up the project.[19] Predictably, this affords the system even less money for badly needed improvements in bus service, at a time when budget cuts have led to reduced service hours and routes.

In the words of Channing Martinez, director of organizing at the Labor Community Strategy Center in Los Angeles, LA Metro is "stealing money from the buses [...] in order to build their rail system."[20] This is a pattern with a long history in Los Angeles and, in past decades, it has taken creative, grassroots collective action to halt it. In 1996, for example, the Los Angeles Bus Riders Union (BRU) sued the city and successfully proved in court that LA was violating bus-dependent riders' civil rights and creating separate and unequal systems.[21] This was an enormous victory and forced Metro to invest $2 billion in the bus system over the next ten years. Sadly, when the consent decree expired in 2006, Metro returned to cutting much-needed bus services.

While the prioritization of rail poses an immediate inequity, it also creates long-term tension with the stated goals of increasing public transit ridership. The investments in bus services won by the BRU translated to a 20 percent increase in ridership. This kind of transformation has positive impacts not only for those who depend on the bus, but also for the environment and for other commuters, for whom better bus service means less traffic congestion. Furthermore, it is hard to imagine a reality where LA commuters are able to take advantage of rail systems without the support of a robust bus system to supplement it. As Eric Mann, the director of the Los Angeles Bus Riders Union and Strategy Center, argues: "Rail has no flexibility, it's a straight shot. If you're going from Point A to Point B, that's great. But if you're not, and you get off the train, where are you going? You need a bus."[22]

Unfortunately, the successes of campaigns like that of the BRU are temporary reprieves in what is otherwise a predictable pattern — recent years have seen a *decrease* in transit ridership even as Metro makes enormous investments. Other cities have experienced something similar, but not at such scale. In the twenty-first century, about 90 percent of major metropolitan areas have lost public transportation ridership, with LA Metro suffering the steepest decline among major transit systems in the country. Thus, contrary to the stated goals, traffic congestion has increased, and any major reduction in greenhouse gas emissions by the target date of 2030 will happen only if the city makes serious midcourse corrections. Some are being made; others may not be. Observers have noted, for example, that LA's Green New Deal did not include any mention of increased investment in the current bus system.[23]

In hopes of attracting greater ridership, there is a plan for a $250 million pilot program, funded by the Measure M sales tax, which would make LA bus ridership free for twenty-three months.[24] This is certainly a positive step for the low-income riders who will be the main beneficiaries. However, it's only a pilot program, and, in any case, it does not address the many other deep systemic problems with bus service. Grassroots organizations like Alliance for Community Transit and Strategic Actions for a Just Economy have called for a permanently fare-free system, using the agency's own data and reports to point out that going fareless would be the single most effective thing the agency could do to increase ridership and decrease traffic congestion.[25] Progress toward institutionalizing the pilot fareless system permanently is bogged down in makers versus takers logic.

In addition to adopting a fareless system, there are ways to spend funds allocated to rail projects more equitably, including: switching to a new, electric bus fleet; adding bus routes; increasing the frequency and hours of bus service; creating dedicated rapid-transit lanes for buses; and improving the lighting and general safety, comfort, and attractiveness of bus stops. Paying attention to equity and making the bus a more efficient and appealing option would reduce weathering stressors, increase ridership, and decrease both the number of cars on the road and greenhouse gas emissions. With the new LA Metro funding, most or all of these improvements could be paid for, if there were the political will to do so. However, at this writing, the future of these improvements is still being debated.

A positive development in the LA case is the proactive attempt to prevent gentrification near new LA Metro train lines by using a method known as land-banking. History tells us that, without land-banking, a likely consequence of building light rail systems is that it opens up opportunities for developers to build high-priced real estate along the rail lines. What happens then? At best, low-income essential workers will be displaced even farther away, leading them to face commutes that are more, not less, weathering. New highway expansion will also be a likely, though unintended, consequence if affluent inhabitants of new developments want highway expansion to their communities in addition to the high-speed rail. If this anticipatable cascade occurs, we would be back to square 1950s again!

LA has seen this happen in the past: LA Metro builds a new train line, nearby land and property values explode; small businesses and low-income renters, often people of color, are displaced in favor of luxury development. In June 2022, the LA Metro board of directors set in motion a means of preventing this default scenario through land-banking. The plan is for LA Metro itself to buy and "bank" land near future train lines, enforce protections for current low-income residents to remain in place, and also facilitate affordable housing development by requiring low rents and prohibiting land speculation.[26] This should increase affordable housing opportunities in LA, allow renters to benefit from new rail lines, and preserve existing and diverse low-income communities. This approach is equitable and will disrupt weathering in multiple ways, including by keeping support networks and communities together, shortening commute times, providing greater accessibility to other parts of the city, and helping local small family businesses to thrive.

The importance of practices like land-banking highlights the reality that simply budgeting large sums for public transportation, or supporting a vague goal of going green, does not ensure that any of the overarching goals of equity, weathering-prevention, and pollution-reduction will be fulfilled. In fact, a green energy goal is only as good as its attention to equity, and thus weathering.

Vital Brooklyn: Centering Equity through Holistic and Community-Based Urban Planning

Other groups across the country are promoting economic and health equity as they take on the challenge of moving to a renewable energy society. An example is Vital Brooklyn, a New York City program that is taking an explicitly anti-weathering approach it calls wellness-based development as it promotes an intersectional, high-road approach to economic equity and city greening. Before we look more closely at the specifics of Vital Brooklyn's approach, let me briefly discuss what it means to take an intersectional, high-road approach toward greening.

High-road development is an approach that sees beyond binaries and trade-offs such as makers versus takers, jobs versus the climate, or competitive and compartmentalized action versus democratic and intersectional action. Instead, through process and goal, high-road development strives for shared benefits and prosperity, environmental sustainability, democracy, and local control.[27] This is the approach of the environmental democracy movement.

Such an approach requires community organizing and collaboration among multiple stakeholders. In the case of greening disinvested city neighborhoods, rural communities, and tribal lands, environmental democracy requires turning to smaller public, locally owned, worker-owned, or collectively owned energy grids and away from aging and sprawling grids controlled by major corporations. This shift facilitates accountability, preparedness for swift disaster response (as opposed to, for example, rolling blackouts or prolonged loss of power, particularly in remote and high-poverty communities), lower energy bills, more disposable income to apply to additional bundled hardships (such as the "heat-or-eat" dilemma), local jobs, and job training.[28]

Applying a bottom-up approach and an equity lens means bringing more voices to the table, which, as we have discussed, makes a community more likely to arrive at the most meaningful and equitable solutions. And local ownership and buy-in are likely to yield stronger commitments to energy conservation and best practices. While this may seem too slow an approach, the investment will pay off and be regenerative and sustainable in the longer run compared to top-down and private free-market approaches that have less stakeholder participation, buy-in, or accountability. Here, I elaborate on one example, Vital Brooklyn. (For those with greater interest in energy democracy, turn to the work of the Emerald City Collaborative ECC, a national nonprofit network of organizations that have been working together since 2009 to advance a sustainable environment while creating just and inclusive economies that ensure an equity stake for low-income communities of color and disadvantaged local businesses of color as we transition to a green economy.[29])

We've seen time and time again that when equity isn't centered, well-intentioned policy often *increases* weathering stressors, and can even be counterproductive to the policy's stated goals. But what happens when policy makers *do* center equity? Vital Brooklyn, which was launched in 2021, is one example of a plan that centers equity in its approach to addressing health, economic development, education, and housing issues in a coordinated and intersectional vision and plan.

Vital Brooklyn is a $1.4 billion program funded through the New York State government and serving Central Brooklyn neighborhoods including Bedford-Stuyvesant, Brownsville, Bushwick, Canarsie, Crown Heights, Cypress Hills / Ocean Hill, East Flatbush, East New York, Prospect Heights, and Prospect Lefferts Gardens.[30] The original Vital Brooklyn proposal was built on the premise that "the social ills of society accumulate in our bodies." If that sounds to you like an acknowledgment of weathering, you're correct. I collaborated with an architect of the program in its formative stages, and the plan incorporates ways to promote health equity refracted through a weathering lens.[31]

Vital Brooklyn aims to reverse the effects of mid-twentieth-century policies that resulted in gross inequities in health, opportunities, and living and working conditions in Central Brooklyn. Those policies, which included the withdrawal of municipal services from racially segregated neighborhoods as part of the public disinvestment in the inner city, led to predominantly Black and working-class neighborhoods' becoming burned-out, blighted, high-poverty areas.[32] Meanwhile, macroeconomic restructuring and globalization robbed these neighborhoods of decent local employment opportunities.

To remediate these problems, Vital Brooklyn takes an approach that is diametrically opposed to the policies of the 1990s, which focused on "deconcentrating poverty" by displacing and scattering public housing residents to outlying areas. By contrast, Vital Brooklyn operates on the assumption that poor and working-class neighborhoods with high concentrations of people of color need and deserve social and economic investment as a matter of equity and restorative justice, and also as a way of maximizing the already existing and abundant positive qualities and strong networks of those people and places.

To achieve its goals, Vital Brooklyn embraces many of the guide-lines for equitable and weathering-informed social policy:

Think holistically and ecologically
Do not erase oppressed stakeholders: "do nothing about us with-out us"
Pay attention to the needs of working- and reproductive-age adults
Recognize all our fates are linked

Rather than assuming that they are the experts, the architects of Vital Brooklyn took "nothing about us without us" seriously. The initiative began in 2016 by surveying Brooklyn residents themselves about the problems in their community. The results of these interviews, which were used to frame the initiative's priorities and approaches in Central Brooklyn, were found to be: "open space and recreation; healthy food; education; economic empowerment; community-based violence prevention; community-based health care; affordable housing; and (environmental) resiliency." Vital Brooklyn understands that these issues are interconnected and aims to address them holistically, rather than compartmentalizing them. Recognizing that all our fates are linked, Vital Brooklyn also partners with and fosters collaborations between government, local businesses, nonprofits, labor unions, local universities, hospitals, and community organizations in an integrated and intersectional way. And by mandating local procurement opportunities; providing educational, employment, and affordable housing opportunities; keeping local hospitals afloat that serve as anchor institutions, yet were headed for bankruptcy; and making buildings healthier, Vital Brooklyn is clearly paying attention to the needs of working- and reproductive-age adults.

Some examples of Vital Brooklyn initiatives include: creating green spaces within a ten-minute walk of every member of a community; planning thousands of new affordable housing units with input from the community; offering retrofitting loans to landlords for solar-energy adoption, lead-paint abatement, and pest control; and providing employment and training for residents of all ages, including in the areas of STEM, health care, and local habitat restoration.

Vital Brooklyn excels by maximizing local resources, keeping community dollars within local businesses, generating healthy opportunities within arm's reach of community members, and using a community-oriented economic development approach. For example, Vital Brooklyn works to increase urban farming and create a local, sustainable food system that will make fresh produce more accessible. It creates social connection and community around physical exercise, develops more locally owned and cooperatively run gyms, rehabilitates parks and increases walkability between them, and rehabilitates housing to make it healthier and more energy-efficient. By reducing energy insecurity, ambulance wait times, and distances traveled to green space, gyms, and nutritious produce, and by providing income through local procurement opportunities—e.g., facilitating and obtaining personnel, services, supplies, and equipment from residents and local businesses—as well as jobs, job training, and local pre-apprentice programs to prepare youth to participate in the emerging green economy, Vital Brooklyn addresses the everyday stresses of weathered communities and provides local residents with realistic, community-based solutions for a sustainable, healthier life.

This initiative is underway and has forged the collaborations, stakeholder buy-in, and funding needed to fulfill its promises. Once it's been fully implemented, it will need to be evaluated. Surely there will be lessons to be learned. But in concept and direction, the Vital Brooklyn approach is a strong model for how equity-centered initiatives can and should be holistically formulated and community-driven. And it offers a template that can spread and adapt to other disinvested urban or rural areas and populations across the country.

From a weathering point of view, Vital Brooklyn takes some steps toward Jedi public health practices that mitigate biopsychosocially induced weathering and may improve school and work performance. By maintaining the density of long-term residents as a matter of equity, and by providing local educational and economic opportunities, residents will be subjected to fewer microaggressions, indignities, or anxieties on a day-to-day basis. This will likely decrease the biopsychosocial stressors of ubiquitous othering, chronic vigilance, and code-switching experiences. One might see in this approach some analogies to the health benefits of attending a historically Black college compared to a predominantly white institution for a Black student.

However, local communities that undergo such transformation do not exist in a vacuum. Their residents remain subject to marginalizing and unresponsive dominant cultural values, commonsense judgments, algorithms, national and state laws, and media representations that wreak weathering havoc. The Vital Brooklyn model leaves open for now the question of how we might achieve its same identity-safety benefits in integrated settings, including at the national level.

Going Forward

One hope is that local model plans in the mold of Vital Brooklyn across the country will denaturalize some of our most embedded racist and classist stereotypes as diverse residents of these areas are enabled to become better-educated, economically self-sufficient, and healthier—not only because of their greater access to healthy diets and exercise, but also because other critical contributors to human health and wholeness are enhanced: living in a nontoxic physical environment, having access to local educational and job opportunities, participating in activities that provide purpose and meaning, and being close to strong networks of kin.

As we learn from ambitious, holistic, community-driven intersectional approaches like Vital Brooklyn, we will find answers to questions about how to make green, equitable, and more densely inhabited cities where Americans will want to live. Although there remain powerful political and economic barriers to scaling up such projects nationally, there are also unprecedented opportunities to expand them. Many cities are increasingly developing coalitions of young residents who are deeply concerned about their own futures, as well as the future of the planet and of democracy. Neither they nor their rural counterparts facing poverty, long-term joblessness, and increasing job loss are ready to see weathering, poverty, oppression, and death as options anymore.

In addition, HR 3684, the Infrastructure and Investment Jobs Act, signed into law by President Biden on November 15, 2021, offers funding to update US physical infrastructure.[33] It has massive transformational potential, but it is essential for those who understand the benefits of high-road, equitable, and intersectional approaches to act aggressively and in a coordinated fashion to shape the projects that will be funded through this law. If addressing equity, which will also disrupt weathering, is not a focal part of the planning process, and is not reinforced by guidelines that have teeth to keep stakeholders accountable, then the plans are doomed to failure. Furthermore, without a focus on equity, we are likely to spend large sums of money on infrastructure that will serve only the most affluent, and that, therefore, will have a negligible impact on greenhouse gas emissions (or perhaps the opposite impact from what we want!).

But there is also hope. The intensity of feeling, commitment, and drive to focus on equity is seen in cases such as the Portland Clean Energy Fund and other local ballot initiatives across the country, as well as pending national legislation such as HR 448, the Energy Resilient Communities Act.[34] The establishment in 2022 of a new federal office of environmental justice was informed by the idea that all people have an equal right to protection from environmental and health hazards and integrates EPA and Department of Justice actions and missions toward this end.[35]

Certainly, we are at a critical juncture with regard to democracy, the environment, and population health, and those of us who endorse equity and democracy have lost important battles. But the country's extreme political polarization can be a double-edged sword. While the corporatized and centralized fossil fuel economy remains powerful, and the sharply rightward tilt of the Supreme Court has by edict already eviscerated the power of the EPA to regulate industry and drastically undermined access to critical health services for populations most subject to weathering, at least half the country is infuriated by these decisions and ready to organize and fight for a more progressive vision. This is the broader social vision into which policies and social change to disrupt and eliminate weathering must fit.

The time is past ripe to act. There's much we know how to do and there are steps we can take today as well as tomorrow. Lives depend on taking action toward eliminating weathering and promoting health equity. The clock is ticking. All our fates are linked.

Acknowledgments

I have been encouraged by many and have considered writing a book about weathering on and off for thirty years. Until recently, I demurred. Book writing is not my medium. But I was stopped cold in my tracks when I saw that US maternal mortality rates, in particular preventable deaths of Black, Indigenous, Latinx, and rural white mothers, rose dramatically over these same thirty years. I wondered if weathering belonged in the public conversation.

I am grateful to journalists Linda Villarosa, Nina Totenberg, Renee Montagne, Mara Gay, Kai Wright, Gene Denby, and David Harewood, who interviewed me and, through their reporting, showed me that it did. Linda Villarosa, in particular, continued to nudge me from time to time, providing encouragement and holding me accountable for my claim that I was really writing a book.

I owe a huge debt to Kari Hong, an immigration attorney who requested my expert testimony in support of habeas (early release) petitions for pro bono cases she represented of detained immigrant asylum-seekers. Each faced daunting risks of acquiring and dying from COVID-19 that grew exponentially with each hour they languished in detention centers where COVID-19 spread like wildfire. Based on weathering, Kari sought to make the case that these clients—none of whom had been convicted of any crime—were biologically older than their chronological age and deserved release just as senior citizen detainees had been released during the pandemic. Under Kari Hong's watch, many were released, suggesting that adding weathering science to the broader conversation could be consequential.

I am profoundly grateful to those whose stories I invoke in hopes of helping new insights to penetrate a worldview defined by the same venomous race fiction that had a hand in their early demise or that of their loved ones. At the same time, I am aware that including their stories may trigger or re-traumatize readers from racialized groups. My deepest hope is that I did not misjudge how to strike the balance.

There would be no book without the perfectly paced and proffered advice and encouragement of my agent, Nate Muscato of Aevitas Creative Management. Nate is a writer-whisperer of extraordinary insight, skill, and compassion. He knew just when to encourage my foot back onto the gas pedal when I was having doubts. Equally important, he knew just when and how to encourage me to pump the brakes on my championship tendency to digress in my writing. Nate also knew just when to take the steering wheel for a brief spell. He always steered it in the right direction for just the right amount of time until I was ready to take back the wheel.

I am deeply grateful to my editor at Little, Brown Spark, Tracy Behar, who saw the spark in my book proposal. Tracy has been an exceptional guide to realizing its promise ever since, including providing essential ideas on how best to structure it. I am very grateful for the support of her outstanding team, in particular Ian Straus, Karina Leon, and Liz Garriga. I am beholden to other consultants who enhanced the book's readability: Beth Rashbaum for her insightful edits, Renee Harleston for her keen discernment of how others might perceive my words differently than I intended, Matt Hutson for his highly informed help with the citations, and Albert LaFarge for thoughtful, thorough, and meticulous copyediting.

Throughout my educational and professional history, I have had the good luck to encounter guiding lights whose fingerprints continue to be visible on my written pages. Some provided enduring building blocks of my intellectual worldview, others provided just the right advice or puzzle piece at just the right moment. Among them, I am indebted to Sheldon Wolin and Steve Esquith, who opened my eyes to the importance of structure and power to forging and maintaining dominance, marginalization, and exploitation; to Bob LeVine, who provided me the conceptual anthropological tools to think systematically about the innumerable combinations and permutations of the facts and values of everyday life that inform our personal or collective actions that give life purpose and meaning; Jane Lancaster, who helped me consider how these coalesce into varying population-level stakes and tradeoffs; to Carol Stack and Linda Burton, who illuminated ground truths and nuance through the concrete examples of weathering portrayed in their ethnographies; to Sherman James and Claude Steele, without whose work, mentorship, and collaboration I might have missed the crucial importance of social psychological dynamics to weathering; to Phil Thompson, whose incomparable melding of deep analytic vision and activism is consistently inspiring, as is his refusal to identify whether the cup is half full or half empty in favor of simply working to fill it up; to Bruce McEwen, whose concept of allostatic load provided a vivid and fitting biological mechanism for how entrenched structural racism could get scored into the bodies of the oppressed, marginalized, and exploited. For more than twenty years, Bruce was an energetic cheerleader for weathering theory and was eager to read and comment on the manuscript. I know this would have been a better book if he had lived to critique it.

This book gains its evidentiary base from almost four decades of research, much of it with collaborators. The debt I owe to these colleagues is enormous, in particular to John Bound, Phil Thompson, Jay Pearson, Tim Waidmann, Sherman James, Marianne Hillemeier,

Sandy Korenman, Cindy Colen, Rachel Snow, Brenda Henry-Sanchez, Danya Keene, Linnea Evans, Erin Linnenbringer, Louis Graham, Mark Hatzenbeuhler, Mary Murphy, Sylvia Tesh, Aresha Martinez-Cardoso, Nicole Novak, Carmen Stokes, Angela Reyes, Amy Schulz, Cleo Caldwell, Annie Ro, Kristefer Stojanovski, Landon Hughes and Alexa Eisenberg. Early on, Charlie Westoff, Steve Gortmaker, and Adolph Reed, Jr. provided training, opportunities, and welcome moral support that helped my emerging weathering research take off. Though far too many to name, all of my students over four decades of teaching occupy a special and motivational place in my heart. I love that now, through your careers, I get to learn from you!

Most of my research would not have been possible without generous funding of specific projects by the Eunice Kennedy Shriver National Institute of Child Health and Human Development, the National Institute on Aging, the National Institute on Minority Health and Health Disparities, the Centers for Disease Control and Prevention, the William T. Grant Foundation, the Russell Sage Foundation, and the Robert Wood Johnson Foundation.

Residencies as a Visiting Fellow at the Center for Advanced Study in the Behavioral Sciences at Stanford and as a Visiting Scholar at the Russell Sage Foundation provided me space and time to clarify weathering-related ideas at various stages of their development. These residencies fulfilled their promise of facilitating intellectual synergies with co-resident Fellows across disciplines. In addition to some already mentioned, key among them are Larry Bobo, Sterling Stuckey, Skip Gates, Anne Petersen, Harry Holzer, Joan Fujimura, D. Fox Harrell, Katherine Isbister, Fred Turner, Alice O'Connor, Sam Myers, Steven Othello Roberts, Diana Hernandez, and Kirsten Swinth.

In the historical dimension, I owe everything to my parents, grandparents, and shtetl ancestors who persevered in the face of genocide in Eastern Europe, and later xenophobic and working-class oppression in the United States—all while living large parts of their lives in exile from the loved ones, home places, and traditions they held dear. I thank my cousins, Sharon Greene and Joyce Tichnell, and my sisters, Edie Walsh and Susan Geronimus, for adding their collective memories of our parents and grandparents to mine, helping me reconstruct their histories.

In the contemporary dimension, I owe everything to my husband and frequent research collaborator, John Bound, and my children Miriam, Aidan, and Charlie Geronimus. All four spent time they did not have reading, editing, and commenting on parts of the draft manuscript, leading to tangible improvements in the book. More than once they got me over humps that threatened to derail me, whether through their concrete suggestions or the boundless inspiration they provided. Working with my children revealed that each has grown up to neither tolerate erasure of any group nor hoard their accident-of-birth privileges. Getting to know each of them better as adults, especially during a pandemic when in-person visits were off the table, turned out to be the most serendipitous gift I received from taking on book writing. As always, John, Miriam, Aidan, and Charlie reminded me what makes everything in life worthwhile.

Notes

INTRODUCTION

1. M. Heckler, "Report of the Secretary's Task Force on Black and Minority Health" (Washington, DC: US Department of Health and Human Services), 1985.
2. Infoplease Staff, "Life Expectancy at Birth by Race and Sex, 1930–2010," *Infoplease,* February 28, 2017, https://www.infoplease.com/us/population/life-expectancy-birth-race-and-sex-1930-2010.
3. National Center for Health Statistics, "Healthy People," CDC, n.d., https://www.cdc.gov/nchs/healthy_people/index.htm.
4. Heckler, "Report of the Secretary's Task Force."
5. T. A. LaVeist and J. M. Wallace Jr., "Health Risk and Inequitable Distribution of Liquor Stores in African American Neighborhood," *Social Science and Medicine* 51, no. 4 (2000): 613–617; T. A. LaVeist and L. A. Isaac, ed., *Race, Ethnicity, and Health: A Public Health Reader,* vol. 26 (San Francisco: John Wiley, 2012); A. T. Geronimus, L. J. Neidert, and J. Bound, "Age Patterns of Smoking in US Black and White Women of Childbearing Age," *American Journal of Public Health* 83, no. 9 (1993): 1258–1264.
6. B. C. Booske, S. A. Robert, and A. M. Rohan, "Awareness of Racial and Socioeconomic Health Disparities in the United States: The National Opinion Survey on Health and Health Disparities, 2008–2009," *Preventing Chronic Disease* 8, no. 4 (July 2011).
7. Author's calculations using Cohort Birth Files for the years 1989–2019 from Centers for Disease Control and Prevention Vital Statistics Data, 1968–2019.
8. Ibid.
9. Author's calculations using Cohort Birth Files for the years 1989–2019 and Period/Cohort Linked Birth-Infant Death Data Files for the years 1989–2020, from Centers for Disease Control and Prevention Vital Statistics Data.
10. A. T. Geronimus et al., "Excess Mortality Among Blacks and Whites in the United States," *New England Journal of Medicine* 335, no. 21 (1996): 1552–1558; A. T. Geronimus et al., "Inequality in Life Expectancy, Functional Status, and Active Life Expectancy Across Selected Black and White Populations in the United States," *Demography* 38, no. 2 (2001): 227–251.
11. For a review, see: D. R. Williams, "Miles to Go Before We Sleep: Racial Inequities in Health," *Journal of Health and Social Behavior* 53, no. 3 (2012): 279–295.
12. B. Jordan, "Authoritative Knowledge and Its Construction," in *Childbirth and Authoritative Knowledge: Cross-Cultural Perspectives,* ed. Davis-Floyd and C. Sargent (Berkeley: University of California Press, 1997), 55–79.

13. K. W. Crenshaw, *On Intersectionality: Essential Writings* (New York: New Press, 2023).
14. C. Cheng, "Are Asian American Employees a Model Minority or Just a Minority?," *Journal of Applied Behavioral Science* 33, no. 3 (1997): 277–290.
15. T. C. Masters-Waage, N. Jha, and J. Reb, "COVID-19, Coronavirus, Wuhan Virus, or China Virus? Understanding How to 'Do No Harm' When Naming an Infectious Disease," *Frontiers in Psychology* 11 (December 2020): 561270.
16. I. Disha, J. C. Cavendish, and R. D. King, "Historical Events and Spaces of Hate: Hate Crimes Against Arabs and Muslims in Post-9/11 America," *Social Problems* 58, no. 1 (2011): 21–46.
17. A. L. Reed Jr., *The South: Jim Crow and Its Afterlives* (New York: Verso, 2022).
18. L. D. Hughes et al., "U.S. Black-White Differences in Mortality Risk Among Transgender and Cisgender People in Private Insurance, 2011–2019," *American Journal of Public Health,* 112 (10): 1507–1514.

PART I

1. *Fannie Lou Hamer's America*, February 22, 2022, PBS, directed by J. Davenport.

CHAPTER 1

1. M. Levenson, "11 Days After Fuming About Coughing Passenger, a Bus Driver Died from the Coronavirus," *New York Times,* April 4, 2020, https://www.nytimes.com/2020/04/04/us/detroit-bus-driver-coronavirus.html.
2. J. Hargrove, Facebook, March 22, 2020, https://www.facebook.com/photo/?fbid=10222511706481725.
3. J. Hargrove, Facebook, March 21, 2020, https://www.facebook.com/Dj.Infiniti/videos/10222496193013898.
4. G. Russonello, "Why Most Americans Support the Protests," *New York Times,* June 5, 2020, https://www.nytimes.com/2020/06/05/us/politics/polling-george-floyd-protests-racism.html.
5. HRC Foundation, *Violence Against the Transgender and Gender Non-Conforming Community in 2020,* n.d., https://www.hrc.org/resources/violence-against-the-trans-and-gender-non-conforming-community-in-2020.
6. M. Alsan, A. Chandra, and K. Simon, "The Great U: Initial Health Effects of COVID-19 in the United States," *Journal of Economic Perspectives* 35, no. 3 (2021): 25–46.
7. A. T. Forde et al., "The Weathering Hypothesis as an Explanation for Racial Disparities in Health: A Systematic Review," *Annals of Epidemiology* 33 (May 2019): 1–18.
8. CDC, "Risk for COVID-19 Infection, Hospitalization, and Death by Race/Ethnicity," June 2, 2022, https://www.cdc.gov/coronavirus/2019-ncov/covid-data/investigations-discovery/hospitalization-death-by-race-ethnicity.html.
9. D. L. Hoyert, "Maternal Mortality Rates in the United States, 2020," CDC, February 2022, https://www.cdc.gov/nchs/data/hestat/maternal-mortality/2020/maternal-mortality-rates-2020.htm.
10. Author's calculations based on data from Centers for Disease Control and Prevention, Pregnancy Mortality Surveillance System, https://www.cdc.gov/reproductivehealth/maternal-mortality/pregnancy-mortality-surveillance-system.htm.
11. J. Vaupel, "Setting the Stage: A Generation of Centenarians?," *Washington Quarterly* 23, no. 3 (2000): 195–200.
12. *Time,* February 23, 2015.
13. Age of Happiness, "These 60-and-Older Seniors Will Destroy Your Age Stereotypes," *Bored Panda,* 2015, https://www.boredpanda.com/senior-citizen-ageing-stereotypes-age-of-happiness-vladimir-yakovlev.
14. B. Kantrowitz, P. King, and S. Downey, "The Road Ahead: A Boomer's Guide to Happiness," *Newsweek,* April 3, 2000, 56–59.

15. G. Cowley & A. Underwood, "How to Get to Your Golden Years," *Newsweek*, April 4, 2000, 72–74.

16. J. Kluger, "How Your Mindset Can Change How You Age," *Time*, February 23, 2015, 82–86.

17. J. A. Pearson, "Can't Buy Me Whiteness: New Lessons from the Titanic on Race, Ethnicity, and Health," *Du Bois Review: Social Science Research on Race* 5, no. 1 (2008): 27–47; J. A. Pearson and A. T. Geronimus, "Race/Ethnicity, Socioeconomic Characteristics, Coethnic Social Ties, and Health: Evidence from the National Jewish Population Survey," *American Journal of Public Health* 101, no. 7 (2011): 1314–1321.

18. *Statista*, "Life Expectancy (from Birth) in the United States, from 1860 to 2020," August 2019, https://www.statista.com/statistics/1040079/life-expectancy-united-states-all-time//.

19. A. Gopnik, "Can We Live Longer But Stay Younger?," *New Yorker*, May 13, 2019, https://www.newyorker.com/magazine/2019/05/20/can-we-live-longer-but-stay-younger.

20. J. Bound et al., "Measuring Recent Apparent Declines in Longevity: The Role of Increasing Educational Attainment," *Health Affairs* 34, no. 12 (2015): 2167–2173; A. T. Geronimus et al., "Inequality in Life Expectancy, Functional Status, and Active Life Expectancy Across Selected Black and White Populations in the United States," *Demography* 38, no. 2 (2001): 227–251; A. T. Geronimus et al., "Weathering, Drugs, and Whack-A-Mole: Fundamental and Proximate Causes of Widening Educational Inequity in US Life Expectancy by Sex and Race, 1990–2015," *Journal of Health and Social Behavior* 60, no. 2 (2019): 222–239; and author's calculations based on the 1990, 2000, and 2010 decennial census of the United States.

21. A. T. Geronimus et al., "Excess Black Mortality in the United States and in Selected Black and White High-Poverty Areas, 1980–2000," *American Journal of Public Health* 101, no. 4 (2011): 720–729.

22. Ibid.; A. T. Geronimus et al., " 'Weathering' and Age Patterns of Allostatic Load Scores Among Blacks and Whites in the United States," *American Journal of Public Health* 96, no. 5 (2006): 826–833; A. T. Geronimus et al., (2007), "Black-White Differences in Age Trajectories of Hypertension Prevalence Among Adult Women and Men, 1999–2002," *Ethnicity and Disease* 17, no 1 (2007): 40–49.

23. J. DeMuth, "Fannie Lou Hamer: Tired of Being Sick and Tired," *Nation*, June 1, 1964, https://www.thenation.com/article/archive/fannie-lou-hamer-tired-being-sick-and-tired//.

24. V. Wang, "Erica Garner, Activist and Daughter of Eric Garner, Dies at 27," *New York Times*, December 30, 2017, https://www.nytimes.com/2017/12/30/nyregion/erica-garner-dead.html.

25. *Politics Nation*, January 7, 2018, "Transcript 1/7/18 Politics Nation," https://www.msnbc.com/transcripts/politicsnation/2018-01-07-msna1058631.

26. Wang, "Erica Garner."

27. DeMuth, "Fannie Lou Hamer."

28. J. M. Burns, *The Crosswinds of Freedom, 1932–1988* (New York: Open Road Media, 2012).

29. W. J. Barber, "America, Accepting Death Is Not an Option Anymore!," sermon, June 14, 2020, *Repairers of the Breach*, https://www.breachrepairers.org/blogs/accepting-death-is-not-an-option-anymore.

30. *Morning Joe*, January 2020, MSNBC, Reverend Barber interview.

CHAPTER 2

1. J. Salah, "All-Women's Alzheimer's Report: Stress, Midlife Crisis and Other Demons," *Guardian Liberty Voice*, October 1, 2013, https://guardianlv.com/2013/10/all-womens-alzheimers-report-stress-midlife-crisis-and-other-demons//.

2. J. Kluger, "How Your Mindset Can Change How You Age," *Time*, February 23, 2015, 82–86.

3. H. Epstein, "Ghetto Miasma: Enough to Make You Sick," *New York Times Magazine*, October 12, 2003, 10–16.

4. A. T. Geronimus et al., "'Weathering' and Age Patterns of Allostatic Load Scores Among Blacks and Whites in the United States," *American Journal of Public Health* 96, no. 5 (2006): 826–833.
5. L. M. Burton and L. Bromell, "Childhood Illness, Family Comorbidity, and Cumulative Disadvantage," *Annual Review of Gerontology and Geriatrics* 30, no. 1 (2010): 233–265.
6. A. T. Geronimus et al., "Excess Mortality Among Blacks and Whites in the United States," *New England Journal of Medicine* 335, no. 21 (1996): 1552–1558; A. T. Geronimus, J. Bound, and T. A. Waidmann, "Poverty, Time, and Place: Variation in Excess Mortality Across Selected US Populations, 1980–1990," *Journal of Epidemiology and Community Health* 63, no. 6 (1999): 325–334; A. T. Geronimus, "Economic Inequality and Social Differentials in Mortality," *Economic Policy Review* 5 (September 1999): 23–36; A. T. Geronimus et al., "Inequality in Life Expectancy, Functional Status, and Active Life Expectancy Across Selected Black and White Populations in the United States," *Demography* 38, no. 2 (2001): 227–251; A. T. Geronimus et al., "Urban-Rural Differences in Excess Mortality Among High-Poverty Populations: Evidence from the Harlem Household Survey and the Pitt County, North Carolina, Study of African American Health," *Journal of Health Care for the Poor and Underserved* 17, no. 3 (2006): 532–558; A. T. Geronimus, J. Bound, and C. G. Colen, "Excess Black Mortality in the United States and in Selected Black and White High-Poverty Areas, 1980–2000," *American Journal of Public Health* 101, no. 4 (2011): 720–729.
7. Geronimus, Bound, and Colen, "Excess Black Mortality."
8. Geronimus et al., "Inequality in Life Expectancy."
9. A. T. Geronimus et al., "Weathering, Drugs, and Whack-A-Mole: Fundamental and Proximate Causes of Widening Educational Inequity in US Life Expectancy by Sex and Race, 1990–2015," *Journal of Health and Social Behavior* 60, no. 2 (2019): 222–239.
10. Ibid.
11. B. S. McEwen, "Stress, Adaptation, and Disease: Allostasis and Allostatic Load," *Annals of the New York Academy of Sciences* 840, no. 1 (1998): 33–44.
12. Greater Good Science Center, "Robert Sapolsky: The Psychology of Stress," March 20, 2012, YouTube, https://www.youtube.com/watch?v=bEcdGK4DQSg.
13. R. M. Sapolsky, *Why Zebras Don't Get Ulcers: The Acclaimed Guide to Stress, Stress-Related Diseases, and Coping*, 3rd ed. (New York: Henry Holt, 2004); B. S. McEwen and R. M. Sapolsky, "Stress and Cognitive Function," *Current Opinion in Neurobiology* 5, no. 2 (1995): 205–216.
14. B. J. Ellis et al., "Hidden Talents in Harsh Environments," *Development and Psychopathology* 34, no. 1 (2022): 95–113.
15. D. Young, "I Pray for Murder Sometimes," *New York Times*, September 28, 2019, https://www.nytimes.com/2019/09/28/opinion/sunday/black-men-murder-death.html.
16. E. J. Kim, B. Pellman, and J. J. Kim, "Stress Effects on the Hippocampus: A Critical Review," *Learning and Memory* 22, no. 9 (2015): 411–416.
17. R. S. Duman and L. M. Monteggia, "A Neurotrophic Model for Stress-Related Mood Disorders," *Biological Psychiatry* 59, no. 12 (2006): 1116–1127.
18. K. M. Roy, C. Y. Tubbs, and L. M. Burton, "Don't Have No Time: Daily Rhythms and the Organization of Time for Low-Income Families," *Family Relations* 53, no. 2 (2004): 168–178.
19. L. M. Burton and K. E. Whitfield, "'Weathering' Towards Poorer Health in Later Life: Co-morbidity in Urban Low-Income Families," *Public Policy and Aging Report* 13, no. 3 (2003): 13–18.
20. D. Sontag, "For Poor, Life 'Trapped in a Cage,'" *New York Times*, October 6, 1996, https://www.nytimes.com /1996/10/06 /us/for-poor-life-trapped-in-a-cage.html.
21. M. Desmond, *Evicted: Poverty and Profit in the American City* (New York: Crown, 2016).
22. A. Elliott, *Invisible Child: Poverty, Survival and Hope in an American City* (New York: Random House, 2021).

23. A. Eisenberg et al., "Toxic Structures: Speculation and Lead Exposure in Detroit's Single-Family Rental Market," *Health and Place* 64 (July 2020): 102390.
24. Ibid.
25. J. McKenzie, "Detroit's Foreclosure Crisis and the Need for 'Information Justice,'" *Bloomberg*, March 8, 2017, https://www.bloomberg.com/news/articles/2017-03-08/detroit-s-foreclosure-crisis-and-the-need-for-information-justice.
26. J. Gallagher, "In Detroit, More People Rent Homes Than Own Them," March 19, 2017, *Detroit Free Press*, https://www.freep.com/story/money/business/john-gallagher/2017/03/19/detroit-poverty-mortgages-economy-homeownership/98957798/.
27. J. Akers and E. Seymour, "The Eviction Machine: Neighborhood Instability and Blight in Detroit's Neighborhoods," *Poverty Solutions*, University of Michigan, June 2019.
28. J. Kurth and M. Wilkinson, "Detroit Demo Blitz Linked to Rising Lead Levels in Children," *Bridge Michigan*, November 13, 2017, https://www.bridgemi.com/children-families/detroit-demo-blitz-linked-rising-lead-levels-children.
29. H. A. Washington, *A Terrible Thing to Waste: Environmental Racism and Its Assault on the American Mind* (New York: Little, Brown Spark, 2019); K. Chandramouli et al., "Effects of Early Childhood Lead Exposure on Academic Performance and Behaviour of School Age Children," *Archives of Disease in Childhood* 94, no. 11 (2009): 844–848; S. A. Mayfield, "Language and Speech Behaviors of Children with Undue Lead Absorption: A Review of the Literature," *Journal of Speech, Language, and Hearing Research* 26, no. 3 (1983): 362–368.
30. D. J. Vagins and J. McCurdy, "Cracks in the System: Twenty Years of the Unjust Federal Crack Cocaine Law," American Civil Liberties Union, October 2006.
31. D. Wallace and R. Wallace, "Urban Systems During Disasters: Factors for Resilience," *Ecology and Society* 13, no. 1 (2008); D. Wallace and R. Wallace, *A Plague on Your Houses: How New York Was Burned Down and Public Health Crumbled* (London and New York: Verso, 1998).
32. C. Tsigos and G. P. Chrousos, "Hypothalamic–Pituitary–Adrenal Axis, Neuroendocrine Factors and Stress," *Journal of Psychosomatic Research* 53, no. 4 (2002): 865–871.
33. B. S. McEwen and P. J. Gianaros, "Central Role of the Brain in Stress and Adaptation: Links to Socioeconomic Status, Health, and Disease," *Annals of the New York Academy of Sciences* 1186, no. 1 (2010): 190–222.
34. M. H. Schernthaner-Reiter et al., "The Interaction of Insulin and Pituitary Hormone Syndromes," *Frontiers in Endocrinology* 12 (2021): 626427.
35. Mary F. Dallman, Norman C. Pecoraro, Susanne E. la Fleur, Chronic stress and comfort foods: self-medication and abdominal obesity, Brain, Behavior, and Immunity, Volume 19, Issue 4, 2005, Pages 275-280.
36. Author's calculations using Centers for Disease Control and Prevention, Pregnancy Mortality Surveillance System, https://www.cdc.gov/reproductivehealth/maternal-mortality/pregnancy-mortality-surveillance-system.htm.
37. J. Gonnerman, "Kalief Browder, 1993–2015," *New Yorker*, June 7, 2015, https://www.newyorker.com/news/news-desk/kalief-browder-1993-2015.
38. B. McEwen, "Neurobiological and Systemic Effects of Chronic Stress," *Chronic Stress* 1 (January-December 2017): 2470547017692328; D. Pagliaccio et al., "Stress-System Genes and Life Stress Predict Cortisol Levels and Amygdala and Hippocampal Volumes in Children," *Neuropsychopharmacology* 39, no. 5 (2014): 1245–1253.
39. M. Nolan et al., "Hippocampal and Amygdalar Volume Changes in Major Depressive Disorder: A Targeted Review and Focus on Stress," *Chronic Stress* 4 (September 2020): 2470547020944553.
40. K. Hughes et al., "The Effect of Multiple Adverse Childhood Experiences on Health: A Systematic Review and Meta-Analysis," *Lancet Public Health* 2, no. 8 (2017): e356–e366.
41. S. Jacobs and J. Annese, "Mom Dies of 'Broken Heart' After Son Kalief Browder Killed Himself Last Year," *New York Daily News*, October 16, 2016, https://www.nydailynews.com/new-york/bronx/exclusive-mom-late-kalief-browder-dies-broken-heart-article-1.2833023.

CHAPTER 3

1. A. M. Tuchman, *Diabetes: A History of Race and Disease* (New Haven, CT: Yale University Press, 2020).

2. A. L. Beaudet and L. Meng, "Gene-Targeting Pharmaceuticals for Single-Gene Disorders," *Human Molecular Genetics* 25, no. R1 (2016): R18–R26.

3. M. F. Fraga et al., "Epigenetic Differences Arise During the Lifetime of Monozygotic Twins," *Proceedings of the National Academy of Sciences* 102, no. 30 (2005): 10604–10609.

4. L. L. Simpson and Society for Maternal-Fetal Medicine (SMFM), "Twin-Twin Transfusion Syndrome," *American Journal of Obstetrics and Gynecology* 208, no. 1 (2013): 3–18.

5. J. O. Hill and J. C. Peters, "Environmental Contributions to the Obesity Epidemic," *Science* 280, no. 5368 (1998): 1371–1374.

6. C. Bouchard, "Genetics of Obesity: Overview and Research Directions," in *The Genetics of Obesity*, ed. C. Bouchard (Boca Raton, FL: CRC Press, 2020), 223–233.

7. 23andMe, "23andMe Releases First-of-Its-Kind Genetic Weight Report," 23andMe Blog, March 2, 2017, https://blog.23andme.com/health-traits/23andme-releases-first-of-its-kind-genetic-weight-report/.

8. L. O. Schulz and L. S. Chaudhari, "High-Risk Populations: The Pimas of Arizona and Mexico," *Current Obesity Reports* 4, no. 1 (2015): 92–98.

9. R. A. Kittles and K. M. Weiss, "Race, Ancestry, and Genes: Implications for Defining Disease Risk," *Annual Review of Genomics and Human Genetics* 4, no. 1 (2003): 33–67.

10. R. S. Cooper, "Race and Genomics," *New England Journal of Medicine* 348, no. 12 (2003): 1166.

11. E. Evangelou et al., "Genetic Analysis of Over 1 Million People Identifies 535 New Loci Associated with Blood Pressure Traits," *Nature Genetics* 50, no. 10 (2018): 1412–1425.

12. R. S. Cooper et al., "An International Comparative Study of Blood Pressure in Populations of European vs. African Descent," *BMC Medicine* 3, no. 1 (2005): 1–8.

13. J. S. Kaufman and S. A. Hall, "The Slavery Hypertension Hypothesis: Dissemination and Appeal of a Modern Race Theory," *Epidemiology* 14, no. 1 (2003): 111–118.

14. K. Esoh and A. Wonkam, "Evolutionary History of Sickle-Cell Mutation: Implications for Global Genetic Medicine," *Human Molecular Genetics* 30, no. R1 (2021): R119–R128.

15. J. Diamond, "Race Without Color," *Discover*, November 1, 1994, https://www.discovermagazine.com/mind/race-without-color.

16. E. S. Epel et al., "Accelerated Telomere Shortening in Response to Life Stress," *Proceedings of the National Academy of Sciences* 101, no. 49 (2004): 17312–17315.

17. S. R. Chan and E. H. Blackburn, "Telomeres and Telomerase," *Philosophical Transactions of the Royal Society of London, Series B: Biological Sciences* 359, no. 1441 (2004): 109–122.

18. K. de Punder et al., "Stress and Immunosenescence: The Role of Telomerase," *Psychoneuroendocrinology* 101 (2019): 87–100.

19. J. Yang et al., "The Paradoxical Role of Cellular Senescence in Cancer," *Frontiers in Cell and Developmental Biology* 12 (August 2021): 2200.

20. J. Zhang et al., "Ageing and the Telomere Connection: An Intimate Relationship with Inflammation," *Ageing Research Reviews* 25 (2016): 55–69.

21. S. Tsalamandris et al., "The Role of Inflammation in Diabetes: Current Concepts and Future Perspectives," *European Cardiology Review* 14, no. 1 (2019): 50–59.

22. L. Duan, X. Rao, and K. R. Sigdel, "Regulation of Inflammation in Autoimmune Disease," *Journal of Immunology Research* 2019 (February 28, 2019): 7403796–7403796.

23. G. Multhoff, M. Molls, and J. Radons, "Chronic Inflammation in Cancer Development," *Frontiers in Immunology* 2 (2012): 98.

24. G. K. Hansson, "Inflammation, Atherosclerosis, and Coronary Artery Disease," *New England Journal of Medicine* 352, no. 16 (2005): 1685–1695.

25. J. F. Bentzon et al., "Mechanisms of Plaque Formation and Rupture," *Circulation Research* 114, no. 12 (2014): 1852–1866.

26. E. Linnenbringer, S. Gehlert, and A. T. Geronimus, "Black-White Disparities in Breast Cancer Subtype: The Intersection of Socially Patterned Stress and Genetic Expression," *AIMS Public Health* 4, no. 5 (2017): 526.
27. P. P. Souza and U. H. Lerner, "The Role of Cytokines in Inflammatory Bone Loss," *Immunological Investigations* 42, no. 7 (2013): 555–622.
28. Z. Wang et al., "Potential Role of Cellular Senescence in Asthma," *Frontiers in Cell and Developmental Biology* 8 (2020): 59.
29. C. C. Walton et al., "Senescence as an Amyloid Cascade: The Amyloid Senescence Hypothesis," *Frontiers in Cellular Neuroscience* 14 (2020): 129.
30. C. Franceschi et al., "Inflamm-aging: An Evolutionary Perspective on Immunosenescence," *Annals of the New York Academy of Sciences* 908, no. 1 (2000): 244–254.

CHAPTER 4

1. L. M. Burton and L. Bromell, "Childhood Illness, Family Comorbidity, and Cumulative Disadvantage: An Ethnographic Treatise on Low-Income Mothers' Health in Later Life," *Annual Review of Gerontology and Geriatrics* (2010): 231–265.
2. C. Nathanson, *Dangerous Passage: The Social Control of Sexuality in Women's Adolescence* (Philadelphia: Temple University Press, 1991).
3. C. Jencks, "What Is the Underclass—and Is It Growing?," *Focus* 12, no. 1 (1989): 14–26.
4. J. R. Anderson et al., "Revisiting the Jezebel Stereotype: The Impact of Target Race on Sexual Objectification," *Psychology of Women Quarterly* 42, no. 4 (2018): 461–476.
5. United Health Foundation, "America's Health Rankings Annual Report," 2021, https://assets.americashealthrankings.org/app/uploads/americashealthrankings-2021annual report.pdf.
6. D. M. Ely and A. K. Driscoll, "Infant Mortality in the United States, 2019: Data from the Period Linked Birth/Infant Death File," *National Vital Statistics Reports* 70, no. 14 (2021): 1–18.
7. G. K. Singh and M. Y. Stella, "Infant Mortality in the United States, 1915–2017: Large Social Inequalities Have Persisted for Over a Century," *International Journal of Maternal and Child Health and AIDS* 8, no. 1 (2019): 19–31.
8. D. L. Hoyert, "Maternal Mortality Rates in the United States, 2020," CDC, February 2022, https://www.cdc.gov/nchs/data/hestat/maternal-mortality/2020/maternal-mor tality-rates-2020.htm.
9. N. J. Kassebaum et al., "Global, Regional, and National Levels of Maternal Mortality, 1990– 2015: A Systematic Analysis for the Global Burden of Disease Study 2015," *Lancet* 388, no. 10053 (2016): 1775–1812.
10. Author's calculations based on Centers for Disease Control and Prevention, Pregnancy Mortality Surveillance System, https://www.cdc.gov/reproductivehealth/maternal-mor tality/pregnancy-mortality-surveillance-system.htm.
11. Hoyert, "Maternal Mortality Rates."
12. R. Montagne, "For Every US Mother Who Dies for Pregnancy-Associated Reasons, Another 70 Mothers Come Close to Dying," NPR, May 10, 2018, https://www.npr.org /2018/05/10/607782992/for-every-woman-who-dies-in-childbirth-in-the-u-s-70-more -come-close.
13. N. J. Kassebaum et al., "Global, Regional, and National Levels."
14. **For 1990–2015** Centers for Disease Control and Prevention, "Births: Final Data for 2015," *National Vital Statistics Reports* 66, no. 1 (2017), https://www.cdc.gov/nchs/data /nvsr/nvsr66/nvsr66_01.pdf.
15. Personal communication with the author.
16. Author's calculations using Cohort Birth Certificate Files for babies born from 1989 through 2019 provided by Centers for Disease Control and Prevention.

17. K. Mikkola et al., "Neurodevelopmental Outcome at 5 Years of Age of a National Cohort of Extremely Low Birth Weight Infants Who Were Born in 1996–1997," *Pediatrics* 116, no. 6 (2005): 1391–1400.

18. A. L. Beam et al., "Estimates of Healthcare Spending for Preterm and Low-Birthweight Infants in a Commercially Insured Population: 2008–2016," *Journal of Perinatology* 40, no. 7 (2020): 1091–1099, https://www.nature.com/articles/s41372-020-0635-z.

19. Author's calculations using Cohort Birth and Death Certificate Files.

20. A. T. Geronimus, "What Teen Mothers Know," *Human Nature* 7, no. 4 (1996): 323–352.

21. Author's calculations using Cohort Birth Certificate Files.

22. CDC, "High Blood Pressure During Pregnancy," May 6, 2021, https://www.cdc.gov/bloodpressure/pregnancy.htm.

23. T. Shih et al., "The Rising Burden of Preeclampsia in the United States Impacts Both Maternal and Child Health," *American Journal of Perinatology* 33, no. 4 (2016): 329–338; J. Winter, "Why a Life-Threatening Pregnancy Complication Is on the Rise," *New Yorker,* August 12, 2022, https://www.newyorker.com science annals-of-medicine/why-a-life-threatening-pregnancy-complication-is-on-the-rise.

24. T. Field and M. Diego, "Cortisol: The Culprit Prenatal Stress Variable," *International Journal of Neuroscience* 118, no. 8 (2008): 1181–1205.

25. M. D. Esteban-Vasallo et al., "Mercury, Cadmium, and Lead Levels in Human Placenta: A Systematic Review," *Environmental Health Perspectives* 120, no. 10 (2012): 1369–1377; H. Bové et al., "Ambient Black Carbon Particles Reach the Fetal Side of Human Placenta," *Nature Communications* 10, no. 1 (2019): 1–7.

26. M. A. Kioumourtzoglou et al., "Traffic-Related Air Pollution and Pregnancy Loss," *Epidemiology* 30, no. 1 (2019): 4.

27. C. Winder, "Lead, Reproduction and Development," *Neurotoxicology* 14, no. 2–3 (1993): 303–317; H. Hu et al., "Fetal Lead Exposure at Each Stage of Pregnancy as a Predictor of Infant Mental Development," *Environmental Health Perspectives* 114, no. 11 (2006): 1730–1735; H. A. Washington, *A Terrible Thing to Waste: Environmental Racism and Its Assault on the American Mind* (New York: Little, Brown Spark, 2019).

28. A Eisenberg, et al., "Toxic Structures: Speculation and Lead Exposure in Detroit's Single-Family Rental Market," *Health and Place* 64 (July 2020): 102390.

29. L. D. Klein et al., "Concentrations of Trace Elements in Human Milk: Comparisons Among Women in Argentina, Namibia, Poland, and the United States," *PloS One* 12, no. 8 (2017): e0183367.

30. M. Jaishankar et al., "Toxicity, Mechanism and Health Effects of Some Heavy Metals," *Interdisciplinary Toxicology* 7, no. 2 (2014): 60–72.

31. A. T. Geronimus et al., "Black-White Differences in Age Trajectories of Hypertension Prevalence Among Adult Women and Men, 1999–2002," *Ethnicity and Disease* 17, no. 1 (2007): 40–49.

32. A. A. Creanga et al., "Pregnancy-Related Mortality in the United States, 2006–2010," *Obstetrics and Gynecology* 125, no. 1 (2012): 5–12.

33. Author's calculations using data from Centers for Disease Control and Prevention, Pregnancy Mortality Surveillance System, https://www.cdc.gov/reproductivehealth/maternal-mortality/pregnancy-mortality-surveillance-system.htm.

34. N. Martin and R. Montagne, "Black Mothers Keep Dying After Giving Birth. Shalon Irving's Story Explains Why," NPR, December 7, 2017, https://www.npr.org/2017/12/07/568948782/black-mothers-keep-dying-after-giving-birth-shalon-irvings-story-explains-why.

35. C. Jackson, "East Orange Police Sgt. Tahmesha Dickey Dies During Childbirth," East Orange (NJ) Public Information, January 14, 2018, https://www.tapinto.net/towns/paterson/articles/east-orange-police-sgt-tahmesha-dickey-dies-duri-4.; E. Brady et al., "Dying to Deliver: The Race to Prevent Sudden Death of New Mothers," ABC News, May 16, 2018, https://abcnews.go.com/Health/dying-deliver-race-prevent-sudden-death-mothers/story?id=55015361.

36. S. Alisobhani, "A Call to Action: Responding to the Crisis of Maternal Mortality," *Ms.*, February 17, 1011, https://msmagazine.com/2022/02/07/maternal-mortality-kira-john son-black-women-health/; Associated Press, "Lawsuit Says a Black Patient Bled to Death Because of a Hospital's Culture of Racism," NPR, May 5, 2022, https://www.npr.org /2022/05/05/1096833756/racism-lawsuit-cedars-sinai-medical-center-wife-death; A. Helm, "Kira Johnson Spoke 5 Languages, Raced Cars, Was Daughter in Law of Judge Glenda Hatchett. She Still Died in Childbirth," *The Root*, October 19, 2018, https://www.theroot .com/kira-johnson-spoke-5-languages-raced-cars-was-daughte-1829862323; S. Young, "Confronting Racial Bias in Maternal Deaths," *Grow by WebMD*, January 17, 2020, https://www.webmd.com/baby/news/20200117/confronting-racial-bias-in-maternal -deaths.

37. J. Burton, "Serena Williams Called 'Crazy' by Nurse Amid Pregnancy Blood Clot Scare," *Newsweek*, April 7, 2022, https://www.newsweek.com/serena-williams-nurse-called-crazy -pregnancy-blood-clot-ordeal-1695869; R. Haskell, "Serena Williams on Motherhood, Marriage, and Making Her Comeback," *Vogue*, January 10, 2018, https://www.vogue.com /article/serena-williams-vogue-cover-interview-february-2018; A. Macon, "Serena Wil liams's New HBO Documentary Sparks the Breastfeeding Conversation We Should All Be Having," *Vogue*, May 16, 2018, https://www.vogue.com/article/serena-williams -breastfeeding-motherhood-wedding-hbo-documentary-being-serena.

38. H. Southwick, "Talk About a Grand Slam! Inside Serena Williams' Net Worth and How She Made It," *Parade*, July 1, 2022, https://parade.com/1400745/hannah-southwick /serena-willliams-net-worth/.

39. I. Kendi, *Stamped from the Beginning:* The Definitive History of Racist Ideas in America (New York: Nation Books, 2016); L. Villarosa, *Under the Skin:* The Hidden Toll of Racism on American Lives and on the Health of Our Nation (New York: Doubleday, 2022).

40. N. Natale, "Venus Williams Opens Up About Rare Autoimmune Disease as She Prepares for the U.S. Open," *Prevention*, July 30, 2019, https://www.prevention.com/health /a28446557/venus-williams-sjogren-syndrome/.

41. Shine My Crown Staff, "Serena Williams: 'I Know Firsthand the Sexism and Racism the Media Use to Vilify Women of Color,' " *Shine My Crown*, March 8, 2021, https://shinemy crown.com/serena-williams-i-know-firsthand-the-sexism-and-racism-the-media -use-to-vilify-people-of-color//.

42. Villarosa, *Under the Skin*.

43. S. Cruickshank, "The Death of a Young Black Mother Brings Attention to the Issue of Racial Health Disparities," *Hub*, February 26, 2019, https://hub.jhu.edu/2019/02/26/ shalon-irving-maternal-mortality-symposium//.

44. Burton, "Serena Williams Called 'Crazy.' "

45. Haskell, "Serena Williams on Motherhood."

46. M. Osterman et al., "Births: Final Data for 2020," *National Vital Statistics Reports* 70, no, 17 (2021): 1–50.

47. S. J. Ventura, B. E. Hamilton, and T. J. Matthews, "National and State Patterns of Teen Births in the United States, 1940–2013," *National Vital Statistics Reports* 63, no. 4 (2014): 1–34, https://www.cdc.gov/nchs/data/nvsr/nvsr63/nvsr63_04.pdf.

CHAPTER 5

1. R. A. LeVine et al., *Child Care and Culture: Lessons from Africa* (Cambridge: Cambridge University Press, 1994).

2. R. Blythe, *The View in Winter: Reflections on Old Age* (London: Allen Lane/Penguin, 1979).

3. A. T. Geronimus et al., "Inequality in Life Expectancy, Functional Status, and Active Life Expectancy Across Selected Black and White Populations in the United States," *Demography* 38, no. 2 (2001): 227–251, and additional author's calculations to update to more recent years.

4. M. Gilens, *Why Americans Hate Welfare* (Chicago: University of Chicago Press, 1999).

5. L. M. Burton, "Teenage Childbearing as an Alternative Life-Course Strategy in Multi-generation Black Families," *Human Nature* 1, no. 2 (1990): 123–143.

6. K. L. Brown, *Gone Home: Race and Roots Through Appalachia* (Chapel Hill: University of North Carolina Press, 2018).

7. C. Stack, *All Our Kin: Strategies for Survival in a Black Community* (New York: Basic Books, 1974).

8. In this regard, it is critical to distinguish shared responsibilities across generations that include more fluid expectations of the capacities and responsibilities of older youth in the face of deep collective need from "adultification bias" in institutions like schools and the juvenile justice system. Adultification bias is when people in authority view Black youth as less innocent or needing of comfort or gentle guidance than white youth. Such dominant cultural bias can result in devastating outcomes for Black youth, for example, when a Black juvenile offender is tried and punished as an adult, while his white counterpart is treated leniently, his offense brushed off as "boys will be boys." Instances of adultification bias among the powerful must be called out and eradicated. The fact that my uncle Henry was expected to shoulder responsibility to maintain his family's livelihood when my grandfather became ill does not imply that he should be viewed as less innocent or deserving of empathy than the children his age who were able to continue their schooling.

9. D. Brooks, "The Nuclear Family Was a Mistake," *Atlantic*, March 2020, https://www.the atlantic.com/magazine/archive/2020/03/the-nuclear-family-was-a-mistake/605536/.

10. D. Cohn et al., "The Demographics of Multigenerational Households," Pew Research Center, March 24, 2022, https://www.pewresearch.org/social-trends/2022/03/24/the -demographics-of-multigenerational-households//.

11. J. V. Ward, *The Skin We're In: Teaching Our Children to Be Emotionally Strong, Socially Smart, Spiritually Connected* (New York: Simon and Schuster, 2000).

12. C. B. Stack and L. M. Burton, "Kinscripts," *Journal of Comparative Family Studies* 24, no. 2 (1993): 157–170.

13. A. T. Geronimus, S. Korenman, and M. M. Hillemeier, "Does Young Maternal Age Adversely Affect Child Development? Evidence from Cousin Comparisons," *Population and Development Review* 20, no. 3 (1994): 585–609; A. T. Geronimus, "On Teenage Child-bearing and Neonatal Mortality in the United States," *Population and Development Review* 13, no. 2 (1987): 245–279.

14. L. Mullings, "The Sojourner Syndrome: Race, Class, and Gender in Health and Illness," *Voices* 6, no. 1 (2002): 32–36.

15. D. Young, *What Doesn't Kill You Makes You Blacker: A Memoir in Essays* (New York: Ecco, 2019).

16. C. Chambers, *Hill Women: Finding Family and a Way Forward in the Appalachian Mountains* (New York: Ballantine Books, 2021).

17. S. Hicks-Bartlett, "Between a Rock and a Hard Place: The Labyrinth of Working and Parenting in a Poor Community," in *Coping With Poverty: The Social Contexts of Neighborhood, Work, and Family in the African-American Community,* ed. S. Danziger and A. C. Lin (Ann Arbor: University of Michigan Press, 2000), 27–51.

CHAPTER 6

1. *abUSed: The Postville Raid,* film produced and directed by L. Argueta (United States: New Day Films, 2011).

2. J. Friesen, "Hardening the Line on Illegal Workers," *Globe and Mail (Toronto),* May 24, 2008.

3. J. M. Krogstad, "In Postville, Shock But No Surprise," *Waterloo–Cedar Falls (IA) Courier,* May 13, 2008, https://wcfcourier.com/news/metro/in-postville-shock-but-no-surprise /article_205edba8-a0e1-59be-a16b-13ceae6628d6.html.

4. E. Camayd-Freixas, "Interpreting After the Largest ICE Raid in US History: A Personal Account," in *Behind Bars: Latinos/as and Prison in the United States*, ed. S. Oboler (New York: Palgrave Macmillan, 2009), 159–173.

5. Krogstad, "In Postville, Shock."

6. Camayd-Freixas, "Interpreting After the Largest ICE Raid."

7. M. Hemingway and B. Weingarten, "Op-Ed: Feds Ignore Illegal Alien ID Theft Plaguing Americans as U.S. Coffers Fill," *The Center Square*, June 30, 2022, https://www.thecen tersquare.com/national/op-ed-feds-ignore-illegal-alien-id-theft-plaguing-americans -as-u-s-coffers-fill/article_28cf76dc-f8be-11ec-92ec-b3950c9a0650.html.

8. C. C. García Hernández, "Naturalizing Immigration Imprisonment," *California Law Review* (2015): 1449–1514.

9. R. Brito, "Europe Welcomes Ukrainian Refugees—Others, Less So," AP News, February 28, 2022, https://apnews.com/article/Russia-ukraine-war-refugees-diversity-230b0cc 790820b9bf8883f918fc8e313.

10. García Hernández, "Naturalizing Immigration Imprisonment."

11. N. L. Novak, A. T. Geronimus, and A. M. Martinez-Cardoso, "Change in Birth Outcomes Among Infants Born to Latina Mothers After a Major Immigration Raid," *International Journal of Epidemiology* 46, no. 3 (2017): 839–849.

12. T. Saul, "Eastern Iowa Hispanic Community Fears More Raids," *Sioux City Journal*, May 22, 2008, https://siouxcityjournal.com/news/eastern-iowa-hispanic-community-fears-more -raids/article_20a51fb3-24e0-55be-b65b-98b82089b5ae.html.

13. E. Christensen, "Area Hispanics Scurry to Get Paperwork in Line," *Courier (Waterloo, IA)*, May 12, 2008, https://postvilleproject.org/stories/items/show/28.

14. J. Jacobs and J. Perkins, "Immigration Raid: Workers, Take Care, Take Cover," *Des Moines Register*, May 13, 2008, https://www.fosterglobal.com/news/ImmigrationRaidWorkers TakeCareTakeCover.pdf; "90 Miles Away, Postville Raid's Impact Is Still Being Felt," *Globe Gazette (Mason City, IA)*, May 25, 2008, https://globegazette.com/news/local/90 -miles-away-postville-raids-impact-is-still-being-felt/article_ed576161-6c5c-5543-8d9b -ac0857480bd3.html.

15. Camayd-Freixas, "Interpreting After the Largest ICE Raid."

16. D. S. Lauderdale, "Birth Outcomes for Arabic-Named Women in California Before and After September 11," *Demography* 43, no. 1 (2006): 185–201.

17. D. S. Curtis et al., "Highly Public Anti-Black Violence and Preterm Birth Odds for Black and White Mothers," *SSM—Population Health* 18 (June 2022): 101112.

18. D. S. Curtis et al., "Highly Public Anti-Black Violence Is Associated with Poor Mental Health Days for Black Americans," *Proceedings of the National Academy of Sciences* 118, no. 17 (2021): e2019624118.

19. C. M. Steele, *Whistling Vivaldi: How Stereotypes Affect Us and What We Can Do* (New York: W. W. Norton, 2011).

20. L. Feinberg, *Stone Butch Blues* (Sydney, Australia: ReadHowYouWant.com, 2010).

21. A. Ashe and A. Rampersad, *Days of Grace: A Memoir* (New York: Ballantine Books, 1994).

22. J. H. Davis, S. G. Stolberg, and T. Kaplan, "Trump Alarms Lawmakers with Disparaging Words for Haiti and Africa," *New York Times*, January 11, 2018.

23. J. A. Pearson, "Can't Buy Me Whiteness: New Lessons from the Titanic on Race, Ethnicity, and Health," *Du Bois Review: Social Science Research on Race* 5, no.1 (2008): 27–47.

24. *Seinfeld* (season 6, episode 24), "The Understudy," directed by A. Ackerman, written by L. David, J. Seinfeld, M. Gross, and C. Leifer, Sony Pictures Entertainment.

25. V. Bashi and A. McDaniel, "A Theory of Immigration and Racial Stratification," *Journal of Black Studies* 27, no. 5 (1997): 668–682; D. W. Carbado, "Racial Naturalization," *American Quarterly* 57, no. 3 (2005): 633–658; Pearson, "Can't Buy Me Whiteness."

26. R. Kaestner et al., "Stress, Allostatic Load, and Health of Mexican Immigrants," *Social Science Quarterly* 90, no. 5 (2009): 1089–1111.

27. K. Kozlowski, "Detroit's 70-Year Population Decline Continues; Duggan Says City Was Undercounted," *Detroit News*, August 12, 2021, https://www.detroitnews.com/story/news

/local/detroit-city/2021/08/12/census-detroit-population-decline-u-s-census-bureau /5567639001//.

28. C. Gibson and K. Jung, "Historical Census Statistics on Population Totals by Race, 1790 to 1990, and by Hispanic Origin, 1970 to 1990, for Large Cities and Other Urban Places in the United States" (Washington, DC: Population Division, US Census Bureau, 2002).

29. For a poignant and devastating example, see the op-ed on thegrio.com written by another former doctoral student I taught, Dr. Rahwa Haile, now an associate professor in the State University of New York College system: R. Haile, "The Attacks on Black Maternal Health Go Far Beyond Roe," June 8, 2022, https://thegrio.com/2022/06/08 /the-attacks-on-black-maternal-health-go-far-beyond-roe/.

30. T. J. Sugrue, "The Rise and Fall of Detroit's Middle Class," *New Yorker,* July 23, 2013, https://www.newyorker.com/news/news-desk/the-rise-and-fall-of-detroits-middle -class.

31. L. Deng et al., "Saving Strong Neighborhoods from the Destruction of Mortgage Fore-closures: The Impact of Community-Based Efforts in Detroit, Michigan," *Housing Policy Debate* 28, no. 2 (2018): 153–179.

32. Annie E. Casey Foundation, *The 2014 KIDS COUNT Data Book,* July 22, 2014, https:// www.aecf.org/resources/the-2014-kids-count-data-book//.

33. UN Office of the High Commissioner for Human Rights, "Detroit: Disconnecting Water from People Who Cannot Pay—An Affront to Human Rights, Say UN Experts," June 25, 2014, https://www.ohchr.org/en/press-releases/2014/06/detroit-disconnecting-water -people-who-cannot-pay-affront-human-rights-say.

34. A. T. Geronimus et al., "Weathering in Detroit: Place, Race, Ethnicity, and Poverty as Conceptually Fluctuating Social Constructs Shaping Variation in Allostatic Load," *Milbank Quarterly* 98, no. 4 (2020): 1171–1218; A. T. Geronimus et al., "Race-Ethnicity, Poverty, Urban Stressors, and Telomere Length in a Detroit Community-Based Sample," *Journal of Health and Social Behavior* 56, no. 2 (2015): 199–224.

35. E. A. Viruell-Fuentes, "Beyond Acculturation: Immigration, Discrimination, and Health Research Among Mexicans in the United States," *Social Sciences and Medicine* 65, no. 7 (2007): 1524–1535.

CHAPTER 7

1. K. Brodkin, *How Jews Became White Folks and What That Says About Race in America* (New Brunswick, NJ: Rutgers University Press, 1998); M. F. Jacobson, *Whiteness of a Different Color* (Cambridge, MA: Harvard University Press, 1999).

2. A. T. Abernethy, *The Jew a Negro: Being a Study of the Jewish Ancestry from an Impartial Standpoint* (Moravian Falls, NC: Dixie Publishing, 1910).

3. A. M. Tuchman, *Diabetes: A History of Race and Disease* (New Haven, CT: Yale University Press, 2020).

4. J. Karabel, *The Chosen: The Hidden History of Admission and Exclusion at Harvard, Yale, and Princeton* (Boston: Houghton Mifflin, 2005).

5. M. Boullier and M. Blair, "Adverse Childhood Experiences," *Paediatrics and Child Health* 28, no. 3 (2018): 132–137.

6. B. S. McEwen, "The Brain on Stress: Toward an Integrative Approach to Brain, Body, and Behavior," *Perspectives on Psychological Science* 8, no. 6 (2013): 673–675.

7. M. Lepeles, "Conservative Alumni Act to Alter Princeton Image," *New York Times,* March 3, 1974.

8. M. Devall et al., "Racial Disparities in Epigenetic Aging of the Right vs Left Colon," *Journal of the National Cancer Institute* 113, no. 12 (2021): 1779–1782.

9. L. J. Costa et al., "Recent Trends in Multiple Myeloma Incidence and Survival by Age, Race, and Ethnicity in the United States," *Blood Advances* 1, no. 4 (2017): 282–287.

10. R. Howell, "Before Their Time," *Yale Alumni Magazine,* May 2011, https:// yalealumn imagazine.org /articles /3193-before-their-time.

11. "Stanley H. Reeves '78," *Princeton Alumni Weekly,* November 13, 2019, https:// paw.princeton .edu/memorial/stanley-h-reeves-78.

12. C. G. Colen, N. Pinchak, and K. S. Barnett, "Racial Disparities in Health Among College-Educated African Americans: Can HBCU Attendance Reduce the Risk of Metabolic Syndrome in Midlife?," *American Journal of Epidemiology* 190, no. 4 (2020): 553–561.

13. Z. N. Hurston, "How It Feels to Be Colored Me," in *Worlds of Difference: Inequality in the Aging Experience,* 3rd ed., ed. Eleanor Palo Stoller and Rose Campbell Gibson (Thousand Oaks, CA: Pine Forge Press, 2000).

14. C. M. Steele, *Whistling Vivaldi: How Stereotypes Affect Us and What We Can Do* (New York: W. W. Norton, 2011).

15. C. M. Steele and J. Aronson, "Stereotype Threat and the Intellectual Test Performance of African Americans," *Journal of Personality and Social Psychology* 69, no. 5 (1995): 797–811.

16. M. C. Murphy, C. M. Steele, and J. J. Gross, "Signaling Threat: How Situational Cues Affect Women in Math, Science, and Engineering Settings," *Psychological Science* 18, no. 10 (2007): 879–885; S. J. Spencer, C. M. Steele, and D. M. Quinn, "Stereotype Threat and Women's Math Performance," *Journal of Experimental Social Psychology* 35, no. 1 (1999): 4–28.

17. N. Ambady et al., "Stereotype Susceptibility in Children: Effects of Identity Activation on Quantitative Performance," *Psychological Science* 12, no. 5 (2001): 385–390; M. Shih, T. L. Pittinsky, and N. Ambady, "Stereotype Susceptibility: Identity Salience and Shifts in Quantitative Performance," *Psychological Science* 10, no. 1 (1999): 80–83.

18. J. Stone et al., "Stereotype Threat Effects on Black and White Athletic Performance," *Journal of Personality and Social Psychology* 77, no. 6 (1999): 1213–1227.

19. S. J. Barber and M. Mather, "Stereotype Threat Can Both Enhance and Impair Older Adults' Memory," *Psychological Science* 24, no. 12 (2013): 2522–2529.

20. M. C. Murphy and V. J. Taylor, "The Role of Situational Cues in Signaling and Maintaining Stereotype Threat," in *Stereotype Threat: Theory, Process, and Application,* ed. M. Inzlicht and T. Schmader (Oxford: Oxford University Press, 2012), 17–33; C. M. Steele, S. J. Spencer, and J. Aronson, "Contending With Group Image: The Psychology of Stereotype and Social Identity Threat," in *Advances in Experimental Social Psychology,* ed. M. P. Zanna, vol. 34 (PUB LOCATION??: Academic Press, 2002): 379–440.

21. S. Cheryan et al., "Ambient Belonging: How Stereotypical Cues Impact Gender Participation in Computer Science," *Journal of Personality and Social Psychology* 97, no. 6 (2009): 1045–1060.

22. M. Inzlicht and T. Ben-Zeev, "A Threatening Intellectual Environment: Why Females Are Susceptible to Experiencing Problem-Solving Deficits in the Presence of Males," *Psychological Science* 11, no. 5 (2000): 365–371.

23. J. Blascovich et al., "African Americans and High Blood Pressure: The Role of Stereotype Threat," *Psychological Science* 12, no. 3 (2001): 225–229.

24. Murphy, Steele, and Gross, "Signaling Threat."

25. W. Mischel, *The Marshmallow Test: Understanding Self-Control and How to Master It* (New York: Random House, 2014).

26. T. W. Watts, G. J. Duncan, and H. Quan, "Revisiting the Marshmallow Test: A Conceptual Replication Investigating Links Between Early Delay of Gratification and Later Outcomes," *Psychological Science* 29, no. 7 (2018): 1159–1177.

27. C. Kidd, H. Palmeri, and R. N. Aslin, "Rational Snacking: Young Children's Decision-Making on the Marshmallow Task Is Moderated by Beliefs About Environmental Reliability," *Cognition* 126, no. 1 (2013): 109–114.

28. S. A. James, "The Narrative of John Henry Martin," *Southern Cultures* 1, no. 1 (1993), 83–106.

29. S. A. James, "John Henryism, Structural Racism, and Cardiovascular Health Risks in African Americans," in *Racism: Scientific Tools for the Public Health Professional,* ed. C. Ford et al. (Washington, DC: American Public Health Association, 2019), 56–76.

30. S. A. James, "John Henryism and the Health of African Americans,"*Culture, Medicine and Psychiatry* 18, no. 2 (1994): 163–182.

31. J. M. Booth and C. R. Jonassaint, "The Role of Disadvantaged Neighborhood Environments in the Association of John Henryism with Hypertension and Obesity," *Psychosomatic Medicine* 78, no. 5 (2016): 552–561; J. P. Godbout and R. Glaser, "Stress-Induced Immune Dysregulation: Implications for Wound Healing, Infectious Disease and Cancer," *Journal of Neuroimmune Pharmacology* 1, no. 4 (2006): 421–427; S. A. James et al., "Life-Course Socioeconomic Position and Obesity in African American Women: The Pitt County Study," *American Journal of Public Health* 96, no. 3 (2006): 554–560; N. Khansari, Y. Shakiba, and M. Mahmoudi, "Chronic Inflammation and Oxidative Stress as a Major Cause of Age-Related Diseases and Cancer," *Recent Patents on Inflammation and Allergy Drug Discovery* 3, no. 1 (2009): 73–80; V. Parente, L. Hale, and T. Palermo, "Association Between Breast Cancer and Allostatic Load by Race: National Health and Nutrition Examination Survey 1999–2008," *Psycho-Oncology* 22, no. 3 (2013): 621–628; T. Seeman et al., "Socio-Economic Differentials in Peripheral Biology: Cumulative Allostatic Load," *Annals of the New York Academy of Sciences* 1186, no. 1 (2010): 223–239; T. Seeman et al., "The Great Recession Worsened Blood Pressure and Blood Glucose Levels in American Adults," *Proceedings of the National Academy of Sciences* 115, no. 13 (2018): 3296–3301; A. Steptoe and M. Kivimäki, "Stress and Cardiovascular Disease: An Update on Current Knowledge," *Annual Review of Public Health* 34 (2013): 337–354.

32. G. E. Miller et al., "Self-Control Forecasts Better Psychosocial Outcomes But Faster Epigenetic Aging in Low-SES Youth," *Proceedings of the National Academy of Sciences* 112, no. 33 (2015): 10325–10330.

33. G. H. Brody et al., "Persistence of Skin-Deep Resilience in African American Adults," *Health Psychology* 39, no. 10 (2020): 921–926.

34. Miller et al., "Self-Control Forecasts."

35. E. Chen et al., "The Costs of High Self-Control in Black and LatinoYouth with Asthma: Divergence of Mental Health and Inflammatory Profiles," *Brain, Behavior, and Immunity* 80 (2019): 120–128.

36. G. E. Miller et al., "Youth Who Achieve Upward Socioeconomic Mobility Display Lower Psychological Distress But Higher Metabolic Syndrome Rates as Adults: Prospective Evidence from Add Health and MIDUS," *Journal of the American Heart Association* 9, no. 9 (2020): e015698.

37. L. Gaydosh et al., "College Completion Predicts Lower Depression But Higher Metabolic Syndrome Among Disadvantaged Minorities in Young Adulthood," *Proceedings of the National Academy of Sciences* 115, no. 1 (2018): 109–114.

38. G. H. Brody et al., "Resilience in Adolescence, Health, and Psychosocial Outcomes," *Pediatrics* 138, no. 6 (2016): e20161042.

39. G. H. Graf et al., "Testing Black-White Disparities in Biological Aging Among Older Adults in the United States: Analysis of DNA-Methylation and Blood-Chemistry Methods," *American Journal of Epidemiology* 191, no. 4 (2022): 613–625.

40. L. E. Davis, "Have We Gone Too Far with Resiliency?," *Social Work Research* 38, no. 1 (2014): 5–6.

CHAPTER 8

1. A. T. Geronimus et al., "Black-White Differences in Age Trajectories of Hypertension Prevalence Among Adult Women and Men, 1999–2002," *Ethnicity and Disease* 17, no. 1 (2007): 40–49; A. T. Geronimus, J. Bound, and C. G. Colen, "Excess Black Mortality in the United States and in Selected Black and White High-Poverty Areas, 1980–2000," *American Journal of Public Health* 101, no. 4 (2011): 720–729; A. T. Geronimus et al., "Weathering, Drugs, and Whack-A-Mole: Fundamental and Proximate Causes of

Widening Educational Inequity in US Life Expectancy by Sex and Race, 1990–2015," *Journal of Health and Social Behavior* 60, no. 2 (2019): 222–239.

2. A. T. Geronimus, "To Mitigate, Resist, or Undo: Addressing Structural Influences on the Health of Urban Populations," *American Journal of Public Health* 90, no. 8 (2000): 867–872.

3. Personal Responsibility and Work Opportunity Reconciliation Act of 1996, H.R. 3734, 104th Congress, https://www.congress.gov/bill/104th-congress/house-bill/3734.

4. K. Edin and H. L. Shaefer, *$2.00 a Day: Living on Almost Nothing in America* (Boston: Houghton Mifflin Harcourt, 2015).

5. R.D.G. Kelley, "Playing for Keeps: African-American Youth in the Postindustrial City," in *The House That Race Built: Black Americans/U.S. Terrain*, ed. W. Lubiano (New York: Random House, 1997), 195–231.

6. D. P. Moynihan, US Department of Labor, Office of Policy Planning and Research, *The Negro Family: The Case for National Action* (Washington, DC: US Government Printing Office, 1965). *African American Male Research*, (pp. 1–35). The full passage from Moynihan appears in chapter 4, "The Tangle of Pathology": "Nonetheless, at the center of the tangle of pathology is the weakness of the family structure. Once or twice removed, it will be found to be the principal source of most of the aberrant, inadequate, or antisocial behavior that did not establish, but now serves to perpetuate the cycle of poverty and deprivation."

7. For example, see: V. J. Hotz et al., "The Costs and Consequences of Teenage Childbearing for Mothers," in *Kids Having Kids: Economic Costs and Social Consequences of Teen Pregnancy,* ed. R. A. Maynard (Washington, DC: Urban Institute Press, 1997), 55–94. Hotz and his colleagues review studies that use various approaches to account for unobserved background factors that may confound the relationship between teenage childbearing and long-term economic outcomes. They conclude that selection bias "vastly" overstates the negative consequences of teenage childbearing estimated in cross-sectional studies and find that the reviewed studies "provide no support that there are large, negative consequences." They further conclude that the range of uncertainty is over whether the effects of teenage childbearing are "slightly negative," "negligible," or "positive." See also: A. T. Geronimus and S. Korenman, "The Socioeconomic Costs of Teenage Childbearing: Evidence and Interpretation," *Demography* 30, no. 2 (1993): 281–296, and C. A. Bachrach and K. Carver, "Outcomes of Early Childbearing: An Appraisal of Recent Evidence," Summary of a Conference Convened by the National Institute of Child Health and Human Development, Bethesda, MD, 1992.

8. J. Forman and K. Vinson, "The Superpredator Myth Did a Lot of Damage. Courts Are Beginning to See the Light," *New York Times,* April 20, 2022, https://www.nytimes.com/2022/04/20/opinion/sunday/prison-sentencing-parole-justice.html.

9. Editorial Board, "Slandering the Unborn," *New York Times,* December 28, 2018, https://www.nytimes.com/interactive/2018/12/28/opinion/crack-babies-racism.html.

10. 4President Corporation, "Bill Clinton 1996, on the Issues: Preventing Teen Pregnancy," *4President.Org.,* n.d., http://www.4president.org/issues/clinton1996/clinton1996teen.htm.

11. The prohibitions and requirements for block grant assistance include that no assistance can be given to an unmarried minor with children over twelve weeks old who is not a high school graduate and is not participating in activities leading to a high school diploma or equivalent or an alternative educational program approved by the state; nor can assistance be given to such individuals (whatever their children's age) if they do not reside in a residence maintained by a parent, legal guardian, or other adult relative, or some other form of adult-supervised living arrangement. A teen head of household who maintains satisfactory school attendance is deemed to be meeting workfare requirements. While not limited to teens, teens will be disproportionately affected by requirements that individuals cooperate with paternity establishment, with the minimum penalty for noncooperation a 25 percent reduction in the family's grant.

12. See: Personal Responsibility and Work Opportunity Reconciliation Act of 1996, and the charge of "The National Campaign to Prevent Teen Pregnancy," 2100 M Street, N.W., Suite 500, Washington, DC 20037.

13. A. T. Geronimus, "Teenage Childbearing and Personal Responsibility: An Alternative View," *Political Science Quarterly* 112, no. 3 (1997): 405–430.

14. Recent publicity given to the finding that according to some poverty measures, children's poverty rates have decreased since the early 1990s may be definitional, but is superficial and misleading. (See J. DeParle, "Expanded Safety Net Drives Sharp Drop in Child Poverty," *New York Times*, September 11, 2022, https://www.nytimes.com /2022/09/11/us /politics/child-poverty-analysis-safety-net.html.) All proposed official poverty measures are widely understood to be too low, to fail adequately to take the skyrocketing cost of living since the 1980s and 1990s into account, and to deeply draw on the lived experience and socially situated knowledge of impoverished families themselves and are pegged to nuclear families, not kin networks. Maybe a few more families technically have resources slightly above the [much too low] official poverty level, but that doesn't mean they avoid food or housing insecurity, other forms of deep, even life-threatening, material hardship, can afford needed medical care, or are able to avoid financial stressors that contribute to their continued weathering. And some related statistical findings that imply no increase in child poverty during the Great Recession are simply implausible.

15. Edin and Shaefer, *$2.00 a Day.*

16. Ibid.

17. L. M. Burton and K. E. Whitfield, " 'Weathering' Towards Poorer Health in Later Life: Co-morbidity in Urban Low-Income Families," *Public Policy and Aging Report* 13, no. 3 (2003): 13–18.

18. S. Hicks-Bartlett, "Between a Rock and a Hard Place: The Labyrinth of Working and Parenting in a Poor Community," in *Coping With Poverty: The Social Contexts of Neighborhood, Work, and Family in the African-American Community*, ed. S. Danziger and A. C. Lin (Ann Arbor: University of Michigan Press, 2000), 27–51.

19. J. Guillen, "City Inspections of Detroit Schools Find Rodents, Mold," *Detroit Free Press*, January 25, 2016, https://www.freep.com/story/news/2016/01/25/city-inspections-detroit -schools-find-rodents-mold/79311004//.

20. E. Brown, "Rats, Roaches, Mold—Poor Conditions Lead to Teacher Sickout, Closure of Most Detroit Schools," *Washington Post*, January 20, 2016, https://www.washingtonpost .com/news/education/wp/2016/01/20/rats-roaches-mold-poor-conditions-leads -to-teacher-sickout-closure-of-most-detroit-schools//.

21. L. J. Dill, O. Morrison, and M. Dunn, "The Enduring Atlanta Compromise: Black Youth Contending with Home Foreclosures and School Closures in the 'New South,' " *Du Bois Review: Social Science Research on Race* 13, no. 2 (2016): 365–377; M. F. Gordon et al., "School Closings in Chicago: Staff and Student Experiences and Academic Outcomes," University of Chicago Consortium on School Research, 2018. T. L. Green, " 'We Felt They Took the Heart out of the Community': Examining a Community-Based Response to Urban School Closure," *Education Policy Analysis Archives/ Archivos Analíticos de Políticas Educativas* 25 (2017): 1–30; B. Kirshner, M. Gaertner, and K. Pozzoboni, "Tracing Transitions: The Effect of High School Closure on Displaced Students," *Educational Evaluation and Policy Analysis* 32, no. 3 (2010): 407–429.

22. L. A. Evans, A. T. Geronimus, and C. C. Caldwell, "Systematically Shortchanged: Black Adolescent Girls in the Detroit-Metro School Reform Environment," *Du Bois Review: Social Science Research on Race* 16, no. 2 (2020): 357–383.

23. M. Pattillo, "Everyday Politics of School Choice in the Black Community," *Du Bois Review: Social Science Research on Race* 12, no. 1 (2015): 41–71.

24. D. Keene, M. Padilla, and A. T. Geronimus, "Leaving Chicago for Iowa's 'Fields of Opportunity': Community Dispossession, Rootlessness and the Quest for Somewhere to 'Be OK,' " *Human Organization: Journal of the Society for Applied Anthropology* 69, no. 3 (2010): 275–284.

25. S. Clampet-Lundquist, "'Everyone Had Your Back': Social Ties, Perceived Safety, and Public Housing Relocation," *City and Community* 91, no. 1 (2010): 87–108.
26. D. Ranney and P. Wright, "Race, Class and the Abuse of State Power: The Case of Public Housing in Chicago," *SAGE Race Relations Abstracts* 25, no. 2 (2000): 3.
27. G. T. Kingsley, J. Johnson, and K. L. Pettit, "Patterns of Section 8 Relocation in the HOPE VI Program," *Journal of Urban Affairs* 25, no. 4 (2003): 427–447.
28. S. Greenbaum et al., "Deconcentration and Social Capital: Contradictions of a Poverty Alleviation Policy," *Journal of Poverty* 12, no. 2 (2008): 201–228.
29. L. Bennett and A. Reed, "The New Face of Urban Renewal: The Near North Redevelopment Initiative and the Cabrini-Green Neighborhood," in *Without Justice for All: The New Liberalism and Our Retreat from Racial Equality,* ed. A. Reed (Boulder, CO: Westview Press, 1999), 176–192.
30. D. Keene and A. T. Geronimus, "'Weathering' HOPE VI: The Importance of Evaluating the Population Health Impact of Public Housing Demolition and Displacement," *Journal of Urban Health* 88, no. 3 (2011): 417–435.
31. E. Linnenbringer et al., "Associations Between Breast Cancer Subtype and Neighborhood Socioeconomic and Racial Composition Among Black and White Women," *Breast Cancer Research and Treatment* 180, no. 2 (2020): 437–447.
32. A. T. Geronimus et al., "Race-Ethnicity, Poverty, Urban Stressors, and Telomere Length in a Detroit Community-Based Sample," *Journal of Health and Social Behavior* 56, no. 2 (2015): 199–224.
33. M. Schmidt, "Glenn Grothman Criticized for Saying Black Lives Matter Dislikes 'Old-Fashioned Family,'" *Wisconsin State Journal,* March 12, 2021, https://madison.com/news/local/govt-and-politics/glenn-grothman-criticized-for-saying-black-lives-matter-dislikes-old-fashioned-family/article_02b5de1e-2fb6-5a06-9666-c90a9caf5d06.html.
34. R. Scott, "Washington Elites Oppose My Plan to Rescue America: Here's What's in It," *Washington Examiner,* March 14, 2022, https://www.washingtonexaminer.com/restoring-america/equality-not-elitism/washington-elites-oppose-my-plan-to-rescue-america-heres-whats-in-it.

PART II

1. https://www.bringyourownchair.org/about-shirley-chisholm/.
2. For key lessons drawn from movement experiences, and successful strategies of social movement activists as guides for those of us who want to join or emulate them, see both classic books on movement organizing and recent books including, G. Jobin-Leeds and AgitArte, *When We Fight We Win: Twenty-First-Century Social Movements and the Activists That Are Transforming Our World* (New York: New Press, 2016); P. Khan-Cullors and A. Bandele, *When They Call You a Terrorist: A Black Lives Matter Memoir* (New York: St. Martin's, 2018); S. Schulman, *Let the Record Show: A Political History of ACT UP New York, 1987–1993* (New York: Farrar, Straus and Giroux, 2021).
3. R. R. Hardeman, E. M. Medina, and K. B. Kozhimannil, "Structural Racism and Supporting Black Lives—The Role of Health Professionals," *New England Journal of Medicine,* 375, no. 22 (2016): 2113–2115.

CHAPTER 9

1. A. T. Geronimus, "Jedi Public Health: Leveraging Contingencies of Social Identity to Grasp and Eliminate Racial Health Inequality" in *Mapping "Race": Critical Approaches to Health Disparities Research (Critical Issues in Health and Medicine),* ed. L. Gómez and N. López (New Brunswick, NJ: Rutgers University Press, 2013).
2. A. T. Geronimus et al., "Jedi Public Health: Co-Creating an Identity-Safe Culture to Promote Health Equity," *SSM—Population Health* 2 (December 2016): 105–116.

3. L. Graham et al., "Critical Race Theory as Theoretical Framework and Analysis Tool for Population Health Research," *Critical Public Health* 21, no. 1 (2011): 81–93; S. A. James, "John Henryism and the Health of African Americans," *Culture, Medicine, and Psychiatry* 18, no. 2 (1994): 163–182; J. A. Pearson, J."Can't Buy Me Whiteness: New Lessons from the Titanic on Race, Ethnicity, and Health," *Du Bois Review: Social Science Research on Race* 5, no.1 (2008): 27–47.

4. A. T. Geronimus et al., "'Weathering' and Age Patterns of Allostatic Load Scores Among Blacks and Whites in the United States," *American Journal of Public Health* 96, no. 5 (2006): 826–833; S. A. James, "Racial and Ethnic Differences in Infant Mortality and Low Birth Weight: A Psychosocial Critique," *Annals of Epidemiology* 3, no. 2 (1993): 130–136; Pearson, "Can't Buy Me Whiteness"; E. Viruell-Fuentes, "Beyond Acculturation: Immigration, Discrimination, and Health Research Among Mexicans in the United States," *Social Science and Medicine* 65, no. 7 (2007): 1524–1535; E. Viruell-Fuentes, P. Y. Miranda, and S. Abdulrahim, "More Than Culture: Structural Racism, Intersectionality Theory, and Immigrant Health," *Social Science and Medicine* 75, no. 12 (2012): 2099–2106.

5. L. Villarosa, "Why America's Black Mothers and Babies Are in a Life-or-Death Crisis," *New York Times Magazine*, April 11, 2018.

6. S. K. McGrath and J. H. Kennell, "A Randomized Controlled Trial of Continuous Labor Support for Middle-Class Couples: Effect on Cesarean Delivery Rates," *Birth* 35, no. 2 (2008): 92–97.

7. ICTC, now a training program affiliated with Portland State University in Oregon. Note: I am providing this as an example, not to recommend any services.

8. J. P. Jamieson, W. B. Mendes, and M. K. Nock, "Improving Acute Stress Responses: The Power of Reappraisal," *Current Directions in Psychological Science* 22, no. 1 (2013): 51–56; A. Martens et al., "Combating Stereotype Threat: The Effect of Self-Affirmation on Women's Intellectual Performance," *Journal of Experimental Social Psychology* 42, no. 2 (2006): 236–243; T. Schmader, "Stereotype Threat Deconstructed," *Current Directions in Psychological Science* 19, no. 1 (2010): 14–18; D. Sekaquaptewa, A. Waldman, and M. Thompson, "Solo Status and Self-Construal: Being Distinctive Influences Racial Self-Construal And Performance Apprehension in African American Women," *Cultural Diversity and Ethnic Minority Psychology* 13, no. 4 (2007): 321–327; C. M. Steele, *Whistling Vivaldi: How Stereotypes Affect Us and What We Can Do* (New York: W. W. Norton, 2011); C. M. Steele and J. Aronson, "Stereotype Threat and the Intellectual Test Performance of African Americans," *Journal of Personality and Social Psychology* 69, no. 5 (1995): 797–811; C. M. Steele, S. J. Spencer, and J. Aronson, "Contending With Group Image: The Psychology of Stereotype and Social Identity Threat," in *Advances in Experimental Social Psychology*, ed. M. P. Zanna, vol. 34 (PUB LOCATION??: Academic Press, 2002): 379–440; G. M. Walton and G. L. Cohen, "A Brief Social Belonging Intervention Improves Academic and Health Outcomes of Minority Students," *Science* 331, no. 6023 (2011): 1447–1451.

9. C. S. Dweck, *Self-Theories: Their Role in Motivation, Personality, and Development* (New York: Psychology Press, 2000); C. S. Dweck and E. L. Leggett, "A Social-Cognitive Approach to Motivation and Personality," *Psychological Review* 95, no. 2 (1988): 256–273.

10. M. C. Murphy and C. S. Dweck, "A Culture of Genius: How an Organization's Lay Theory Shapes People's Cognition, Affect, and Behavior," *Personality and Social Psychology Bulletin* 36, no. 3 (2010): 283–296.

11. C. Dweck, "The Power of Believing That You Can Improve," TED Talk, 2014, https://www.ted.com/talks/carol_dweck_the_power_of_believing_that_you_can_improve.

12. M. Deziel et al., "Analyzing the Mental Health of Engineering Students Using Classification and Regression," July 2013, in *Educational Data Mining 2013*; I. H. Settles, "When Multiple Identities Interfere: The Role of Identity Centrality," *Personality and Social Psychology Bulletin* 30, no. 4 (2004): 487–500; I. H. Settles et al., "The Climate for Women in Academic Science: The Good, the Bad, and the Changeable," *Psychology of Women Quarterly* 30, no.1 (2006): 47–58; US Department of Health and Human Services. (1992).

Substance Abuse and Mental Health Services Administration, Office of Applied Studies, *Treatment Episode Data Set, 2005*; Substance Abuse and Mental Health Services Administration, Office of Applied Studies, *The NSDUH Report*, "Depression Among Adults Employed Full-Time, by Occupational Category," 2007; C. J. Taylor, " 'Relational by Nature'? Men and Women Do Not Differ in Physiological Response to Social Stressors Faced by Token Women," *American Journal of Sociology* 122, no. 1 (2016): 49–89; W. M. Hall, T. Schmader, and E. Croft, "Engineering Exchanges: Daily Social Identity Threat Predicts Burnout Among Female Engineers," *Social Psychological and Personality Science* 6, no. 5 (2015): 528–534.

13. Steele, "Whistling Vivaldi."

14. Geronimus et al., "Jedi Public Health"; A. T. et al.,"Public Health Creating Identity-Safe Culture to Promote Health Equity,"—2 (2016):

15. A. T. Geronimus and J. P. Thompson, "To Denigrate, Ignore, or Disrupt: Racial Inequality in Health and the Impact of a Policy-Induced Breakdown of African American Communities," *Du Bois Review: Social Science Research on Race* 1, no. 2 (2004): 247–279.

16. D. Kenthirarajah and G. Walton, "How Brief Social-Psychological Interventions Can Cause Enduring Effects," in *Emerging Trends in the Social and Behavioral Sciences*, ed. R. Scott and S. Kosslyn (Hoboken, NJ: John Wiley, 2015).

17. b. hooks, *Black R Looks: Race and Representation* (Boston: South End Press, 1992); b. hooks, *Reel to Real: Race, Sex and Class at the Movies* (New York: Routledge, 1996).

18. S. Lai, "How Do We Solve Social Media's Eating Disorder Problem?," *TechTank*, February 24, 2022, https://www.brookings.edu/blog/techtank/2022/02/24/how-do-we-solve-social-medias-eating-disorder-problem//.

19. R. Benjamin, *Race After Technology: Abolitionist Tools for the New Jim Code* (Cambridge and New York: Polity, 2019).

20. D. F. Harrell, *Phantasmal Media: An Approach to Imagination, Computation, and Expression* (Cambridge, MA: MIT Press, 2013).

21. C. O'Neil, *Weapons of Math Destruction: How Big Data Increases Inequality and Threatens Democracy* (New York: Crown, 2016).

22. Z. Obermeyer et al., "Dissecting Racial Bias in an Algorithm Used to Manage the Health of Populations," *Science* 366, no. 6464 (2019): 447–453.

23. I. Ajunwa, "The Paradox of Automation as Anti-Bias Intervention," *Cardozo Law Review* 16741, no. 5 (2016): 1672–1742.

24. S. Burris, "Stigma and the Law," *Lancet*, 367, no. 9509 (2006), 529–531.

25. Geronimus et al., "Jedi Public Health."

26. M. L. Hatzenbuehler et al., "Effect of Same-Sex Marriage Laws on Health Care Use and Expenditures in Sexual Minority Men: A Quasi-Natural Experiment," *American Journal of Public Health* 102, no. 2 (2012): 285–291.

27. J. S. Jackson et al., "Racism and the Physical and Mental Health Status of African Americans: A Thirteen Year National Panel Study," *Ethnicity and Disease* 61, no. 1–2 (1996): 132–147.

28. J. Malat, J. M. Timberlake, and D. R. Williams, "The Effects of Obama's Political Success on the Self-Rated Health of Blacks, Hispanics, and Whites," *Ethnicity and Disease* 21, no. 3 (2011): 349–355.

29. D. M. Marx, S. J. Ko, and R. A. Friedman, "The 'Obama Effect': How a Salient Role Model Reduces Race-Based Performance Differences," *Journal of Experimental Social Psychology* 45, no. 4 (2009): 953–956.

CHAPTER 10

1. CDC, Office of the Associate Director for Policy and Strategy, "Health in All Policies," June 9, 2016, https://www.cdc.gov/policy/hiap/index.html.

2. J. Peck, "Austerity Urbanism: American Cities Under Extreme Economy," *City* 16, no. 6 (2012), 626–655.

3. J. Lichterman and B. Woodall, "In Detroit Bankruptcy Trial, Union Says City Had Pensions in Sight," Reuters, October 23, 2013, https://www.reuters.com/article/us-usa-detroit-bankruptcy/in-detroit-bankruptcy-trial-union-says-city-had-pensions-in-sight-idUSBRE99M0U320131023; UN Office of the High Commissioner for Human Rights, "Detroit: Disconnecting Water from People Who Cannot Pay—An Affront to Human Rights, Say UN Experts," June 25, 2014, https://www.ohchr.org/en/press-releases/2014/06/detroit-disconnecting-water-people-who-cannot-pay-affront-human-rights-say.
4. M. T. Fullilove, *Urban Alchemy: Restoring Joy in America's Sorted-Out Cities* (New York: New Village Press, 2013).
5. Commission on Race and Ethnic Disparities, "The Report of the Commission on Race and Ethnic Disparities," March 31, 2021, *Gov.uk*, https://www.gov.uk/government/publications/the-report-of-the-commission-on-race-and-ethnic-disparities.
6. J. Rogers, "What Does 'High Road' Mean?," University of Wisconsin–Madison, Center on Wisconsin Strategy, 1990, https://www.cows.org/_data/documents/1776.pdf.

CHAPTER 11

1. S. Holmes, *Fresh Fruit, Broken Bodies: Migrant Farmworkers in the United States* (Berkeley: University of California Press, 2013).
2. J. Cowen et al., "Motor City Miles: Student Travel to Schools in and Around Detroit," *Urban Institute*, October 11, 2018, https://www.urban.org/research/publication/motor-city-miles-student-travel-schools-and-around-detroit.
3. L. A. Evans, A. T. Geronimus, and C. H. Caldwell, "Systematically Shortchanged, Yet Carrying On: Black Adolescent Girls in the Detroit Metropolitan School Reform Environment," *Du Bois Review: Social Science Research on Race* 16, no. 2 (2019): 357–383.
4. T. M. Cottom, *Thick: And Other Essays* (New York: New Press, 2018).
5. Sascha James-Conterelli, personal communication.
6. AIM Patient Safety Bundles, safehealthcareforeverywoman.org.
7. R. Tikkanen et al., "Maternal Mortality and Maternity Care in the United States Compared to 10 Other Developed Countries," *Commonwealth Fund*, November 18, 2020, https://www.commonwealthfund.org/publications/issue-briefs/2020/nov/maternal-mortality-maternity-care-us-compared-10-countries.
8. World Health Organization, "WHO Urges Quality Care for Women and Newborns in Critical First Weeks After Childbirth," March 30, 2022, https://www.who.int/news/item/30-03-2022-who-urges-quality-care-for-women-and-newborns-in-critical-first-weeks-after-childbirth.
9. K. Madgett, "Sheppard-Towner Maternity and Infancy Protection Act (1921)," *Embryo Project Encyclopedia*, May 18, 2017, https://embryo.asu.edu/pages/sheppard-towner-maternity-and-infancy-protection-act-1921.
10. J. P. Bowdoin, "The Midwife Problem," *Journal of the American Medical Association* 9, no. 7 (1928): 460–462.
11. ICTC, Portland State University, Oregon, 2022, https://capstone.unst.pdx.edu/partners/international-center-for-traditional-childbearing-ictc.
12. Tikkanen et al., "Maternal Mortality and Maternity Care."
13. K. P. Tully, A. M. Stuebe, and S. B. Verbiest, "The Fourth Trimester: A Critical Transition Period with Unmet Maternal Health Needs," *American Journal of Obstetrics and Gynecology* 217, no. 1 (2017): 37–41.
14. Y. Chzhen, A. Gromada, and G. Rees, "Are the World's Richest Countries Family Friendly?: Policy in the OECD and EU," UNICEF Office of Research, Florence, Italy, 2019.
15. J. Manza and C. Uggen, *Locked Out: Felon Disenfranchisement and American Democracy* (Oxford: Oxford University Press, 2006); C. Uggen and J. Manza, "Democratic Contraction? Political Consequences of Felon Disenfranchisement in the United States," *American*

Sociological Review 67, no. 6 (2002): 777–803; C. Uggen, S. Shannon, and J. Manza, "State-Level Estimates of Felon Disenfranchisement in the United States, 2010," Sentencing Project, July 12, 2012.

16. M. A. Barreto, S. A. Nuno, and G. R. Sanchez, "The Disproportionate Impact of Voter-ID Requirements on the Electorate: New Evidence from Indiana," *PS: Political Science and Politics* 42, no. 1 (2009): 111–116.

17. D. Epstein and S. O'Halloran, "Measuring the Electoral and Policy Impact of Majority-Minority Voting Districts," *American Journal of Political Science* 43, no. 2 (1999): 367–395; F. Trebbi, P. Aghion, and A. Alesina, "Electoral Rules and Minority Representation in US Cities," *Quarterly Journal of Economics* 123, no. 1 (2008): 325–357.

18. J. M. Rodriguez et al., "Black Lives Matter: Differential Mortality and the Racial Composition of the U.S. Electorate, 1970–2004," *Social Science and Medicine* 136–137 (July 2015): 193–199.

CHAPTER 12

1. Y. Chzhen, A. Gromada, and G. Rees, "Are the World's Richest Countries Family Friendly?: Policy in the OECD and EU," UNICEF Office of Research, Florence, Italy, 2019.

2. S. Aaronson and F. Alba, "The Relationship Between School Closures and Female Labor Force Participation During the Pandemic," *Brookings,* November 3, 2021, https://www.brookings.edu/research/the-relationship-between-school-closures-and-female-labor-force-participation-during-the-pandemic//.

3. E. Klein, "America Has Turned Its Back on Its Poorest Families," *New York Times,* April 17, 2022, https://www.nytimes.com/2022/04/17/opinion/biden-child-tax-credit.html.

4. For example, to derail Build Back Better or other human infrastructure plans, Senator Rick Scott's "12-point plan to rescue America" attempts to use family structure as a wedge makers-versus-takers issue. In extolling the alleged virtues of the nuclear family—and implying the failures of multigenerational and extended Black families—he never refers explicitly to race or class. Scott argues: "The fanatical left seeks to devalue and redefine the traditional family, as they undermine parents and attempt to replace them with government programs. We will not allow Socialism to place the needs of the state ahead of the family" (https://rescueamerica.com/12-point-plan). How much traction this political strategy of blaming the struggles of the working class on the allegedly powerful and threatening "fanatical left" will gain remains to be seen.

5. L. Ross and R. Solinger, *Reproductive Justice: An Introduction* (Oakland: University of California Press, 2017).

6. American College of Obstetricians and Gynecologists, Facebook, April 27, 2018, https://m.facebook.com/ACOGNational/photos/edited-post-we-hear-you-and-we-sincerely-apologize-for-the-misrepresentation-of-/1683943528326841//.

7. US Department of Health and Human Services, Healthy People 2030, *Health.gov,* n.d., https://health.gov/healthypeople.

8. Of course, this reasoning should not lead us to accept state abortion bans that have no exceptions for the health or life of the mother, which, by definition, are likely to increase pregnancy-associated mortality.

9. M. Stobbe, "Women in Their 30s Having More Babies Than Younger Moms in United States," AP News, May 21, 2017, https://apnews.com/article/053d0884bc514c2eafa-43d25a66969e6.

10. J. Mroz, "A Medical Career, at a Cost: Infertility," *New York Times,* September 13, 2021, https://www.nytimes.com/2021/09/13health/women-doctors-infertility.html.

11. N. C. Stentz et al., "Fertility and Childbearing Among American Female Physicians," *Journal of Women's Health* 25, no. 10 (2016): 1059–1065.

12. E. L. Rangel et al., "Incidence of Infertility and Pregnancy Complications in US Female Surgeons," *JAMA Surgery* 156, no. 10 (2021): 905–915.

13. E. L. Groshen and H. J. Holzer, "Labor Market Trends and Outcomes: What Has Changed Since the Great Recession?," *ANNALS of the American Academy of Political and Social Science* 695, no. 1 (2021): 49–69.

14. A. R. Hochschild, *The Outsourced Self: Intimate Life In Market Times* (New York: Metropolitan Books, 2012).

15. C. Weller, "What You Need to Know About Egg-Freezing, the Hot New Perk at Google, Apple, and Facebook," *BusinessInsider.com*, September 17, 2017, https://www.businessin sider.com/egg-freezing-at-facebook-apple-google-hot-new-perk-2017-9.

CHAPTER 13

1. H. McGhee, *The Sum of Us: What Racism Costs Everyone and How We Can Prosper Together* (New York: One World, 2022).

2. R. Nunn, J. Parsons, and J. Shambaugh, "A Dozen Facts about the Economics of the U.S. Health-Care System," *Brookings*, March 10, 2020, https://www.brookings.edu/research /a-dozen-facts-about-the-economics-of-the-u-s-health-care-system/.

3. L. Lopes et al., "Health Care Debt in the U.S.: The Broad Consequences of Medical and Dental Bills," June 16, 2022, *KFF*, https://www.kff.org/health-costs/report/kff-health -care-debt-survey//.

4. "'A Bright Light': Ann Arbor Woman Dies in Grand Canyon Flash Flood," *Detroit News*, July 16, 2021, https://www.detroitnews.com/story/news/local/michigan/2021/07/16/ann -arbor-michigan-woman-dies-in-grand-canyon-flash-flood/7990485002.

5. *Sunday Morning*, "What the Megadrought Means to the American West," July 18, 2021, CBS News, https://www.cbsnews.com/news/what-the-megadrought-means-to-the-ameri can-west//.

6. Ibid.

7. M. L. Oliver and T. M. Shapiro, *Black Wealth/White Wealth: A New Perspective on Racial Inequality* (New York and London: Routledge, 1995); R. Ewing and S. Hamidi, "Compactness Versus Sprawl: A Review of Recent Evidence from the United States," *Journal of Planning Literature* 3, no. 4 (2015): 413–432.

8. L. C. Winling and T. M. Michney, "The Roots of Redlining: Academic, Governmental, and Professional Networks in the Making of the New Deal Lending Regime," *Journal of American History* 108, no. 1 (2021): 42–69.

9. M. T. Fullilove, *Root Shock: How Tearing Up City Neighborhoods Hurts America, and What We Can Do About It* (New York: Ballantine Books, 2004).

10. J. Phillip Thompson, personal communication.

11. Editorial Board, "Is This Railroad for the Rich?," *New York Times*, June 26, 2021, https:// www.nytimes.com/2021/06/26/opinion/lirr-long-island-affordable-housing.html; N. Popo-vich and B. Plumer, "Can Portland Be a Climate Leader Without Reducing Driving?," *New York Times*, April 21, 2022, https://www.nytimes.com/interactive/2022/04/21/climate /portland-emissions-infrastructure-environment.html.

12. Popovich and Plumer, "Can Portland Be a Climate Leader."

13. Ibid.

14. S. Roth, "L.A. Mayor Garcetti's 'Green New Deal' Would Phase Out Gas-Fueled Cars," *Los Angeles Times*, https://www.latimes.com/business/la-fi-garcetti-green-new-deal-los -angeles-20190429-story.html.

15. A. Walker, "Measure M: Angelenos Vote to Tax Themselves for Better Public Transit," *Curbed Los Angeles*, November 9, 2016, https://la.curbed.com/2016/11/9/13573924 /measure-m-los-angeles-public-transit-results.

16. J. Linton, "Metro Board Approves FY2020 Budget, Locking In Rail Service Cuts," *Streets Blog Los Angeles*, May 29, 2019, https://la.streetsblog.org/2019/05/29/metro-board -approves-fy2020-budget-locking-in-transit-service-cuts//.

17. L. J. Nelson, "LA Is Hemorrhaging Bus Riders—Worsening Traffic and Hurting Climate Goals," *Los Angeles Times,* June 27, 2019, https://www.latimes.com/local/lanow/la-me-ln-bus-ridership-falling-los-angeles-la-metro-20190627-story.html.
18. Ibid.
19. L. J. Nelson, "How L.A. Metro Plans to Close Billion-Dollar Funding Gaps on Major Rail Projects," *Los Angeles Times,* https://www.latimes.com/california/story/, December 25, 2019-12-25/los-angeles-metro-rail-projects-budget-problems-2028-olympics, https://www.latimes.com/california/story/2019-12-25/los-angeles-metro-rail-projects-budget-problems-2028-olympics.
20. K. Kaufmann, "Garcetti Prioritizes Rails for the Rich Over Accessible Public Transportation," *Knock LA,* January 27, 2021, https://knock-la.com/metro-is-talking-about-more-bus-service-cuts-6927eef438cf//.
21. R. García and T. A. Rubin, "Crossroad Blues: The MTA Consent Decree and Just Transportation," in *Running on Empty: Transport, Social Exclusion and Environmental Justice,* ed. K. Lucas (Bristol, England: Policy Press), 221–256.
22. Kaufmann, "Garcetti Prioritizes Rails."
23. D. Newton, "Garcetti's Green New Deal for Los Angeles Under Attack for Being Too Car-Centric," *Streetsblog Los Angeles,* April 30, 2019, https://la.streetsblog.org/2019/04/30/garcettis-green-new-deal-for-los-angeles-under-attack-for-being-too-car-centric//.
24. P. Vega, "L.A. Metro Votes to Create Financial Plan for Offering Free Rides to Students, Low-Income Riders," *Los Angeles Times,* May 27, 2021, https://www.latimes.com/california/story/2021-05-27/l-a-metro-votes-to-create-financial-plan-to-launch-program-offering-free-rides-to-students-low-income-riders.
25. A. Walker, "L.A. Just Ran (and Ended) the Biggest Free-Transit Experiment in the U.S.," *Curbed,* January 19, 2022, https://www.curbed.com/2022/01/los-angeles-metro-free-transit-buses.html.
26. S. Scauzillo, "LA Metro Will Try to Prevent Gentrification Near Its Future Rail Lines by 'Land Banking,'" *Los Angeles Daily News,* June 27, 2022, https://www.dailynews.com/2022/06/27/la-metro-will-try-to-prevent-gentrification-near-its-future-rail-lines-by-land-banking//.
27. J. Rogers, "What Does 'High Road' Mean?," University of Wisconsin–Madison, Center on Wisconsin Strategy, 1990, https://www.cows.org/_data/documents/1776.pdf.
28. D. Hernández, "Understanding 'Energy Insecurity' and Why It Matters to Health," *Social Science and Medicine* 167 (October 2016): 1–10.
29. Emerald Cities, https://emeraldcities.org/.
30. Vital Brooklyn Initiative, https://www.ny.gov/vital-brooklyn-initiative/vital-brooklyn-initiative.
31. A. T. Geronimus and J. P. Thompson, "To Denigrate, Ignore, or Disrupt: Racial Inequality in Health and the Impact of a Policy-Induced Breakdown of African American Communities," *Du Bois Review: Social Science Research on Race* 1, no. 2 (2004): 247–279.
32. A. T. Geronimus, "To Mitigate, Resist, or Undo: Addressing Structural Influences on the Health of Urban Populations," *American Journal of Public Health* 90, no. 8 (2000): 867–872.
33. Infrastructure Investment and Jobs Act, H.R. 3684, 117th Congress,
34. Energy Resilient Communities Act, H.R. 448, 117th Congress, www.GovTrack.us.2021, July 23, 2022, https://www.govtrack.us/congress/bills/117/hr448.
35. C. Davenport, "E.P.A. Will Make Racial Equality a Bigger Factor in Environmental Rules," *New York Times,* September 24, 2022, https:// www.nytimes.com /2022 /09 /24 / climate /environmental- justice- epa.html.

Index

Page numbers followed by *f* or *t* refer to figures and tables, respectively.

About the Author

Arline T. Geronimus is a professor in the School of Public Health and a research professor in the Institute for Social Research at the University of Michigan, where she also is affiliated with the Center for Research on Ethnicity, Culture, and Health. An elected member of the National Academy of Medicine, part of the National Academy of Sciences, Dr. Geronimus received her undergraduate degree in political theory from Princeton University, her doctorate in behavioral sciences from the Harvard School of Public Health, and her postdoctoral training at Harvard Medical School.